CARDIOVASCULAR ENDOCRINOLOGY

CONTEMPORARY ENDOCRINOLOGY

P. Michael Conn, SERIES EDITOR

CARDIOVASCULAR ENDOCRINOLOGY

Shared Pathways and Clinical Crossroads

Edited by

VIVIAN A. FONSECA, MD

Tulane University Health Sciences Center, New Orleans, LO, USA

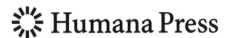 Humana Press

Editor
Vivian A. Fonseca
Tulane University Health
    Sciences Center
New Orleans, LO
USA
vfonseca@tulane.edu

ISBN: 978-1-58829-850-8   e-ISBN: 978-1-59745-141-3

Library of Congress Control Number: 2008933512

Printed on acid-free paper

9 8 7 6 5 4 3 2 1

springer.com

Preface

CARDIOVASCULAR ENDOCRINOLOGY

In the last two to three decades, cardiovascular disease and diabetes have emerged as a major public health problem. This is partly related to the epidemic of obesity, which plays a major role in the pathogenesis of both diabetes and cardiovascular disease. In addition, several other hormones and cytokines have been shown to play an important role in the regulation of the vascular system. This increase in the clinical problems of cardiovascular disease in a large segment of the population has brought together the two disciplines of vascular biology and endocrinology. This book highlights the many common pathophysiological processes involved in this epidemic and the common clinical manifestations that result from them.

The book has several important contributions from distinguished workers in the field. Derek Leroith begins with a novel view of the hormonal regulation of the vascular system, starting, not surprisingly, with pituitary and hypothalamic factors that may impact vascular disease.

The problems of diabetes and cardiovascular disease are extensively covered in a number of chapters, including a review of the epidemiology of the problem by James Meigs, and the important disruption of the nitric oxide signaling system, as well as the role of fatty acids and cytokines in the development of this problem, which are discussed by Bobby Nossaman and Gunther Boden, respectively.

Management of the problem of cardiovascular disease and diabetes in relation to screening of patients using modern cardiovascular techniques is discussed by Paolo Raggi, followed by discussions of the role of insulin (Dandona) and insulin sensitizers (Thethi), and their potential for impacting cardiovascular health.

Endocrine hypertension has long been recognized as an important contributed to cardiovascular morbidity, and the renin-angiotensin system plays a key role in not only endocrine-mediated hypertension, but hypertension in general. This system and its impact on cardiovascular events is discussed by Jim Sowers and followed by a discussion on microalbuminuria and chronic kidney disease by George Bakris.

Adiponectin has emerged as a natural endogenous vascular protective and anti-inflammatory substance of considerable importance in the context of cardiovascular endocrinology, and is reviewed by Mandeep Bajaj. Another important peptide hormone that affects vascular function is the group of natriuretic peptides, reviewed by Kailash Pandey.

Finally, the interaction of sexual dysfunction and cardiovascular disease has attracted much attention, and the overlap of these conditions and therapeutic approaches to overcome them are reviewed by Glen Matfin. Closely related is the effect of testosterone, often neglected as a player in vascular function and reviewed by Alan Seftel.

This textbook of cardiovascular endocrinology comes back full circle to the role of insulin-like growth factors and cardiovascular disease with the final contribution by Patrice Delafontaine.

Finally, I would like to dedicate this book to our many patients who have participated in clinical research to improve our understanding of their disease process. More importantly I wish to dedicate it to the people of New Orleans and wish that city a speedy recovery.

CONTENTS

Part IV Sex Hormones and Vascular Disease

Part V Of Interest

CONTRIBUTORS

MANDEEP BAJAJ, MD • *Division of Diabetes, Endocrinology and Metabolism and Molecular and Cellular Biology, Baylor College of Medicine, Houston, TX*

GEORGE BAKRIS, MD • *Department of Medicine, Hypertension Center, Endocrine Division, The University of Chicago, Chicago, IL*

GUENTHER BODEN, MD • *Divisions of Endocrinology/Diabetes/Metabolism, Temple University School of Medicine, Philadelphia, PA*

ISLAM BOLAD MBBS, MD, MRCP, FESC • *Section of Cardiology, Tulane University School of Medicine, New Orleans, LA*

AJAY CHAUDHURI, MD • *Division of Endocrinology, SUNY at Buffalo and Kaleida Health, Buffalo, NY*

PARESH DANDONA, MD, PhD • *Division of Endocrinology, SUNY at Buffalo and Kaleida Health, Buffalo, NY*

PATRICE DELAFONTAINE, MD • *Tulane University School of Medicine, New Orleans, LA*

DAVID S. FRANKEL, MD • *Department of Medicine, Massachusetts General Hospital, Boston, MA*

VIVIAN FONSECA, MD • *Tullis-Tulane Professor of Medicine, Department of Medicine and Pharmacology, Tulane University Health Sciences Center, New Orleans, LA*

HUSAM GHANIM, PhD • *Division of Endocrinology, SUNY at Buffalo and Kaleida Health, Buffalo, NY*

MEDHAVI JOGI, MD • *Department of Medicine, Baylor College of Medicine Houston, TX*

PHILIP J. KADOWITZ, PhD • *Department of Pharmacology, Tulane University Medical Center, New Orleans, LA*

L. ROMAYNE KURUKULASURIYA MD, FACE • *Diabetes Center, University of Missouri – Columbia, Columbia, MO*

DR. LAND, MD • *Case Western Reserve University, School of Medicine, Cleveland, OH*

DEREK LEROITH, MD, PhD • *Division of Endocrinology, Diabetes and Bone Diseases, Mount Sinai School of Medicine, New York, NY*

GLENN MATFIN, BSC (HONS), M.B. Ch.B., DGM, FFPM, FACE, FACP, FRCP • *Division of Endocrinology, Department of Medicine, New York University School of Medicine, New York, New York 10016, USA*

JAMES B. MEIGS, MD • *General Medicine Division, Clinical Epidemiology Unit and Diabetes Research Unit, Massachusetts General Hospital, Harvard Medical School, Boston, MA*

PRIYA MOHANTY, MD • *Division of Endocrinology, SUNY at Buffalo and Kaleida Health, Buffalo, NY*

SUBRAMANYAM N. MURTHY, PhD • *Department of Pharmacology and Department of Medicine, Tulane University Medical Center, New Orleans, LA*

BOBBY D. NOSSAMAN, MD • *Critical Care Medicine, Department of Anesthesiology Ochsner Health System, Department of Pharmacology, Tulane University Medical Center, New Orleans, LA*

KAILASH N. PANDEY, PhD • *Department of Physiology, Tulane University Health Sciences Center and School of Medicine, New Orleans, LA*

PAOLO RAGGI, MD • *Division of Cardiology, Emory University School of Medicine, Atlanta, GA*

PANTELIS A. SARAFIDIS, MD, PhD • *Department of Medicine, Hypertension Center, Endocrine Division, The University of Chicago, Chicago, IL*

ALLEN D. SEFTEL, MD • *Case Western Reserve University, School of Medicine, Cleveland, OH*

LESLEE J. SHAW, PhD • *Division of Cardiology, Emory University School of Medicine, Atlanta, GA*

SHIPRA SINGH • *Department of Medicine and Pharmacology, Tulane University Health Sciences Center, New Orleans, LA*

JAMES R. SOWERS, MD • *Diabetes Center, University of Missouri – Columbia, Columbia, MO*

TINA K. THETHI, MD • *Department of Medicine and Pharmacology, Tulane University Health Sciences Center, New Orleans, LA*

COLOR PLATES

Color Plate 1   Kaplan-Meier estimates of the probability (with 95% confidence intervals) of death from coronary heart disease in 1059 subjects with type 2 diabetes and 1378 nondiabetic subjects with and without prior myocardial infarction (MI) in a Finnish population-based study (Chapter 2, Fig. 1; *see* discussion on p. 21).

Color Plate 2   Example of myocardial perfusion performed by echocardiography after intravascular injection of echocontrast (microbubbles). The arrows point at an area of decreased perfusion of the inferior wall of the myocardium during dobutamine stress (panels B and C) (courtesy of Dr. Sanjiv Kaul, Oregon Health and Science University, Portland, OR) (Chapter 7, Fig. 3; *see* discussion on p. 101).

Color Plate 3   Examples of nuclear myocardial perfusion imaging of the left ventricular myocardium. Patient A shows a homogeneous distribution of the radioactive tracer both at rest and during stress. Patient B shows a moderate size defect in the anterior wall of the left ventricle (yellow arrows) during stress (top row images). The defect has disappeared (i.e., is reversible) during rest (bottom row images). Patient C demonstrates a large and fixed perfusion defect of the inferolateral wall (white arrow heads) and a partially reversible defect of the apex of the left ventricle (green arrows) (Chapter 7, Fig. 4; *see* discussion on p. 102).

Color Plate 4   An example of assessment of left ventricular function on PET imaging. The calculated left ventricular ejection fraction is 74%. The top row shows diastolic images of the left ventricle (the chamber is larger and the walls are thinner) while the bottom row shows systolic frames (the chamber is almost virtual and the walls are thick) (Chapter 7, Fig. 5; *see* discussion on p. 102).

Color Plate 5   Guidelines proposed by the American Diabetic Association on performance of exercise stress testing, with or without an imaging modality associated with it, in diabetic patients (modified from reference *(54)*) (Chapter 7, Fig. 10; *see* discussion on p. 112).

Color Plate 6   New standard of care from the American Diabetic Association on performance of exercise stress testing, with or without an imaging modality associated with it, in asymptomatic diabetic patients (modified from reference *(102)*) (Chapter 7, Fig. 11; *see* discussion on p. 112).

1 Hormonal Regulation of the Vascular System: An Overview

Ronald Tamler, MD, PhD,
and Derek LeRoith, MD, PhD

CONTENTS

SUMMARY

This chapter discusses hormonal influence on the vasculature. Catecholamines are the best-known and classic stimulators of vascular tone. The rennin–angiotensin–aldosterone system (RAAS) induces vasoconstriction and may damage the vasculature. Sex steroids have gender-dependent disparate genomic and rapid, nongenomic effects on the vasculature. Insulin may have beneficial properties, whereas growth hormone and IGF-1 imbalances are tied to coronary heart disease (CHD). Adipokines are produced in the fat tissue and also affect the vasculature in many ways. While this overview can only briefly touch on all the systems mentioned, later chapters provide greater depth to the reader.

Key Words: Insulin resistance, Hypertension, Coronary heart disease, Angiotensin, Estrogen, Testosterone

INTRODUCTION

When Thomas Addison discovered that the adrenal glands were essential for life *(1)* and later George Oliver and Edward Sharpey-Schafer purified adrenaline in the nineteenth century *(2)*, they were the first to discover the importance of hormonal control of the vasculature. In the

From: *Contemporary Endocrinology: Cardiovascular Endocrinology: Shared Pathways and Clinical Crossroads*
Edited by: V. A. Fonseca © Humana Press, New York, NY

twenty-first century, we are aware of a greater number of hormonal and nonhormonal vascular stimuli with highly complex interactions. Still, there is a sense that many pathways need to be better understood and many discoveries yet to be made.

Arterial blood pressure is influenced by vascular tone and cardiac output, both of which are subject to hormonal control. In addition to an inner coating with endothelium, arteries – particularly the resistance vessels, called arterioles – sport a surrounding muscular layer in the tunica media. This layer, directly and indirectly regulated by parasympathetic and hormonal influences, is responsible for arterial tone, a significant contributor to diastolic blood pressure. Meanwhile, the endothelium is influenced by a powerful vasorelaxant, endothelial-derived relaxing factor (EDRF), now identified as nitric oxide (NO) *(3)*, which in turn counteracts the vasoconstrictive effects of catecholamines and angiotensin II (ATII) *(4)*. Beyond acute vasoconstriction, chronic alterations of the vasculature, such as atherosclerosis are also hormonally influenced and can increase systemic blood pressure. Finally, cardiac output, the product of stroke volume and heart rate, affects systolic blood pressure and is regulated by parasympathetic and hormonal activity.

Hormones therefore influence the vasculature in multiple ways: by regulating volume status, modifying smooth muscle contractility directly and through the NO pathway, and, finally, by altering cardiac output.

In this chapter, we can only attempt to give a brief overview on what is known about how hormones control the cardiovascular system. We will address only a limited number of hormonal pathways as examples of the interaction between the endocrine and cardiovascular systems. The following chapters will provide a deeper and more thorough understanding of individual pathways.

1. Catecholamines

Catecholamines are a family of hormonally active amines derived from the amino acid tyrosine. Adrenaline (also called epinephrine) and dopamine can act centrally as neurotransmitters, whereas norepinephrine fulfills that role in the periphery. When found in the bloodstream, these compounds are typically spillover from neuronal ganglia *(5)* or synthesized in the adrenal medulla in response to sympathetic activation, the "fight or flight" reaction. General effects include increased heart rate, blood pressure, and stroke volume, but vascular catecholamine effects can vary and depend entirely on G-protein-coupled membrane receptors:

α1-Adrenoreceptors are divided into three subtypes (α1A, α1B, and α1D) with different efficiencies of activating phospholipase C via G-protein. Subsequently, the second messengers inositol triphosphate and diacylglycerol are increased and ultimately lead to calcium influx into the cell. The result is contraction of smooth muscle, leading to higher resistance and higher arterial blood pressure. α1-Adrenoreceptors are mainly stimulated by norepinephrine, but can also be activated by adrenaline.

α2-Receptors are also classified into three subtypes. They are coupled with a GTP-binding protein that inhibits adenylyl cyclase, eventually preventing the opening of Ca and K channels. α2 receptors are observed in noradrenergic neurons. While α1 receptors are typically found near sympathetic nerve terminals, α2 receptors are found extrajunctionally and are probably activated mainly by circulating catecholamines.

β-Adrenoreceptors are coupled to a stimulatory G-protein, leading to increased cAMP levels and calcium influx. They are also divided into three subtypes:

Cardiac β1 receptors counter vagal effects and they mediate positive inotropic, chronotropic, and dromotropic effects of catecholamines, mainly noradrenaline derived from sympathetic nerve activity. Over longer periods of time, these receptors, together with aldosterone from the renin-angiotensin-aldosterone system (RAAS), mediate cardiotoxicity. Selective inhibition of β1 receptors has proven an effective treatment *(6)*, but even greater survival benefit is seen with additional blockade of the RAAS *(7)*.

β2-Receptors mediate vasorelaxation and are stimulated by circulating epinephrine, but not by norepinephrine. Due to the selective response, a counterintuitive drop in blood pressure can sometimes be observed when adrenaline is administered and norepinephrine-sensitive α1 receptors are blocked. Depending on distribution and concentration of adrenoreceptors in the vasculature, vasodilation may outweigh vasoconstrictive effects. β2 receptors are found on the endothelium and are thought to mediate their vasodilatory effects through the NO pathway: removal of endothelium and pretreatment with L-NAME may both curb vasorelaxation *(8)*. β2-adrenoreceptor stimulation activates via increased cAMP levels cleaving of L-arginine and NO production, which in turn leads to cGMP formation and vasodilation.

β3 receptors also mediate vasodilation and are not blocked by propranolol or other β-blockers routinely used in practice *(9)*. However, a more fascinating function may lie in their mediation of lipolysis in visceral fat *(9)*, which in turn plays a role in obesity and the metabolic syndrome. Metabolically active adipose tissue enhances atherogenesis via inflammatory cytokines such as interleukin-6 (IL-6) or tumor necrosis factor-alpha (TNF-a) and directly regulates vasoconstriction via angiotensinogen *(10)*.

Dopamine can occupy alpha- and beta-adrenergic receptors when given in higher, pharmacologic concentrations, but mainly acts through five subclasses of D receptors. In the kidney, dopamine acts as an ATII antagonist by enhancing natriuresis via tubular D1-receptors and directly decreasing ATII production. The net effect is lower systemic blood pressure *(11)*.

2. Renin-angiotensin-aldosterone system (RAAS)

The glycoprotein renin is produced in the juxtaglomerular apparatus of the afferent renal arterioles in response to hyponatremia and hypotension. Renin cleaves angiotensinogen, which is mainly produced in the liver and is elevated in patients with visceral adiposity and the metabolic syndrome in general. The resulting biologically inactive ATI is converted to the vasoconstrictive ATII by angiotensin-converting enzyme (ACE) in the pulmonary vasculature. ACE-mediated vasoconstriction is potentiated by degradation of bradykinin, a vasodilatory agent. Cardiovascular effects of ATII throughout the body are mediated by the transmembranous AT1 receptor, which is coupled to a G-protein. Activation results in decreased cAMP levels with subsequent Ca influx and vasoconstriction and increased protein kinase C levels. The latter is a pathway shared with other hormonal regulators, such as insulin. In addition to systemic effects, there are several organ systems in which mRNA for all components of the RAAS can be found and thus operate independently: renal autocrine and paracrine activity of the RAAS in general and ATII in particular has been described for vasoconstriction of the afferent arterioles with subsequent reduction in renal blood flow *(12)*. It is also held responsible for enhanced tubular Na/H exchange and Na/K ATPase activity *(13)*, leading to sodium reabsorption, and modified tubuloglomerular feedback sensitivity *(14)*.

Similar to the kidney, the myocardium features receptors for renin, angiotensinogen, and ATII *(15)* in fibroblasts and myocytes, as do the endothelium and smooth muscle of the coronaries. In fact, most ATII acting on cardiac tissue is not derived from the circulation, but is rather the product of the local cardiac RAAS *(16)* and conversion by chymase *(17)*. Renin, glucocorticoids, estradiol, thyroid hormone, and atrial natriuretic peptide all increase local production of angiotensinogen *(18,19)*, and mechanical stretch of the myocardium leads to increased local ATII levels *(20)*. ATII can stimulate local production of angiotensinogen in the kidney and the heart, thus inducing positive feedback *(21)*.

ATII induces vasoconstriction via increased free radical production *(22)*, by modulating the endothelial NO pathway *(23)* and directly through its own AT1 receptor. However, its best-known endocrine effect is stimulation of aldosterone production in the adrenal gland. Interestingly, while aldosterone production is activated by systemic ATII, local RAAS effects from the zona glomerulosa *(24)* have also been described.

Aldosterone has long-known effects on sodium retention and hypertension *(25)*. Other effects are cardiac hypertrophy and vascular fibrosis *(26)*. It probably exhibits a contradictory effect in that it facilitates endothelial-dependent vasodilation and vascular smooth muscle cell (VSMC)-mediated vasoconstriction *(27)*. Nongenomic, rapid effects of aldosterone include dose-dependent myosin light-chain phosphorylation, which can be inhibited by spironolactone, and phosphatidylinositol 3-kinase (PI3k) inhibition in VSMCs. The result is a contraction, which apparently can also be generated by estradiol and hydrocortisone *(28)*. Aldosterone antagonists, such as eplerenone or spironolactone, have been shown to improve clinical outcomes in patients with heart disease *(29)* and exert protective effects on the endothelium *(30)*.

3. Glucocorticoids

Glucocorticoids may exert vascular effects by cross-stimulation of pathways used by other steroid hormones, such as aldosterone *(31)*. Produced in the adrenal cortex or administered as drugs, they exert nuclear effects by binding to a ubiquitous ligand-activated transcription factor *(32)*. Anti-inflammatory properties *(33)* and increased insulin resistance are well described. In animal models, highly dosed glucocorticoids nongenomically activate endothelial nitric oxide (eNOS) and thus improve endothelial function *(34)*. However, the opposite effect has been described as well, and generation of reactive oxidant species has been invoked as the provoking mechanism responsible for decreased endothelial reactivity *(35)*. While the exact mechanism of action on the vasculature demands further attention, it should be noted that patients with Cushing's disease, a state of chronic glucocorticoid excess, have increased carotid intima-media thickness *(36)* and a higher risk of cardiovascular disease *(37)* that may persist even beyond cure *(38)*.

4. Insulin

Insulin resistance is commonly seen in both obesity and type 2 diabetes, a condition associated with increased cardiovascular risk *(39)*. While many other factors such as hyperglycemia, hypertriglyceridemia, and inflammatory cytokines affect the vasculature, insulin itself has direct effects. Acting via the insulin receptor signaling pathways, particularly the PI3kinase/Akt pathways, insulin induces eNOS activity in endothelial cells, leading to increased NO production *(40)*. This in turn affects the vascular smooth cells and leads to vasodilation. On the other hand, insulin stimulates production of endothelin-1, PAI-1, as well as the adhesion molecules VCAM-1 and E-selectin in endothelial cells via the ERK pathway. Insulin is thus capable of inducing vasodilation in a NO-dependent manner, increasing blood flow to skeletal muscle, for example, which in turn increases glucose uptake in skeletal muscle *(41)*.

Insulin, in addition, can attenuate the contractility of VSMCs by opposing increases in cytosolic calcium through the voltage-dependent sensitive calcium channels. These effects are apparently also mediated by NO.

Under certain circumstances of insulin resistance, endothelial dysfunction can be explained by the altered state of the insulin-stimulated PI3k/Akt pathway. As in the case of skeletal muscle, hyperglycemia, hyperlipidemia, increased oxidative stress, and increased inflammatory cytokines inhibit the PI3k/Akt pathway. In contrast, the mitogen-activated protein

MAPK, and PI3 also leads to a higher availability of response elements for swifter vasodilatory mechanisms *(75)*.

Estrogens lead to rapid vasodilation by nongenomic pathways in men and women alike: membrane ERs, which are a product of the same transcript as the classic nuclear receptors, indirectly activate the MAPK and PI3k/Akt pathways within minutes *(77)*. Results of this nongenomic estrogen action are increased NO derived from eNOS and inducible NOS (iNOS) as well as endothelial rounding, a factor that makes it more difficult for leukocytes to adhere and promote atherogenesis.

Indirect vascular effects generated by estrogen include a favorable lipoprotein profile with decreased LDL and lipoprotein(a) levels as well as increased HDL levels, and modulation of hemostasis/fibrinolysis with decreased expression of PAI-1, tPA, and prothrombotic proteins *(76)*.

PROGESTERONE

The female gonadal steroid progesterone (Pg) mainly acts on classic reproductive tissues such as the placenta. A multitude of synthetic progesterones with varying degrees of androgenetic activity is in clinical use, mainly for contraceptive purposes. Although the Pg receptor is widely distributed throughout the vasculature *(78)*, little is known about its physiologic role. Vasorelaxant properties have been proposed after animal and in vitro data showed increased endothelial NOS activity *(77)*. In addition, enhancement of cyclooxygenase production and inhibited platelet aggregation have been demonstrated *(79)*. Similar to E2, Pg probably has rapid nongenomic effects, which by way of PI3k and protein kinase C generate a fast response in NO generation and on platelet function *(80)*.

Large clinical trials using HRT in postmenopausal women with E2 and Pg however found increased cardiovascular and cerebrovascular events *(64)*. Further investigation is required to reconcile the gap between the favorable physiologic data and poor outcomes in clinic trials. A prospective cohort study from the Framingham Heart Study that examined circulating estradiol in men found that those men with the highest estradiol levels had lower risk for cardiovascular events *(81)*. Men with defective mutations of estrogen synthesis or ERs have premature atherosclerosis which may be consistent with the view that estrogens yield some cardioprotective effect in men *(82,83)*. Indeed, the most recent prospective cohort study suggests higher endogenous estrogen levels are a better predictor of lower cardiovascular disease incidence than testosterone (T) or dehydroepiandrosterone sulfate (DHEAS) *(81)*.

ANDROGENS

DHEA and its sulfate (DHEAS) are produced in the adrenals and have mildly androgenic properties. Higher levels of DHEA and DHEAS correlate with lower incidence of cardiovascular disease. DHEA and DHEAS may serve as prohormones for downstream estrogenic hormones in men *(84–86)*. Of the many cohort studies investigating the correlation with cardiovascular disease *(81,87–91)*, one *(87)* suggested lower DHEAS levels in CHD survivors and two *(89,91)* delineated a trend toward benefit with higher DHEAS levels. However, a fairly recent prominently published study showed no benefit of DHEA supplementation in deficient men or women *(92)*.

The main androgen in humans is T, which is produced in the testicles and, to a lesser degree, in the ovaries and adrenals. T or the more potent dihydrotestosterone (DHT) interacts with the nuclear androgen receptor (AR) to cause changes in transcription. However, in vitro and in vivo studies have found T to be a rapid coronary vasodilator *(93–95)* with intravenous administration of T improving endothelial function in men with CHD *(96)*. These rapid changes are not blocked by pretreatment with the AR blocker Flutamide and therefore must follow a rapid, nongenomic pathway. In addition, T may act as a calcium channel blocker in the VSMC *(97)*.

T levels decrease in men as they age, and hypogonadism is estimated to affect more than 20% of men over the age of 60; however, men with CHD are known to have lower T levels than age-matched controls with normal coronary angiograms *(98–100)*. So far, the numerous prospective studies examining the relationship between endogenous T and cardiovascular disease incidence in men *(81,101–107)* have not shown a clear association. Androgens at supraphysiologic doses have been associated with the development of left ventricular hypertrophy *(108)*, heart failure *(109)*, and dilated cardiomyopathy *(110)*. However, salutary effects have been reported with physiologic doses of transdermal T in men with heart failure *(111)*. Low T is associated with greater atherosclerotic burden, and replacement with T improves aortic atherosclerosis in animal studies. This observation is only partly explained by a lipid effect *(112–115)*. Although the burden of atherosclerosis may be reduced with elevated T, it may paradoxically result in increased cardiovascular events from decreased plaque stability. In vitro data show that, in macrophages derived from men, androgen treatment upregulates pro-atherogenic genes associated with lipoprotein processing, cell-surface adhesion, extracellular signaling, coagulation, and fibrinolysis *(116)*.

Higher T levels in polycystic ovary syndrome (PCOS) are correlated with the development of the metabolic syndrome and diabetes in premenopausal women, and the decrease in E:T ratio has often been faulted for the increase in postmenopausal CHD. However, endothelial function in postmenopausal women correlates positively with T levels, while T is felt to protect against carotid plaque burden *(117,118)*.

7. Other hormonal systems

Parathyroid hormone (PTH) is known to impact the cardiovascular system in a negative way. Patients with hyperparathyroidism exhibit higher mortality *(119,120)* due to higher incidence of hypertension *(121)* and cardiovascular disease *(122)* as well as other components of the metabolic syndrome, such as insulin resistance *(123,124)*. The common denominator is impaired endothelial function *(125)*, proliferation of VSMCs *(126)*, and calcium influx into the VSMC mediated by the PTH/PTH-rp-receptor. The result is increased vascular tone *(127)*. It should be noted that, while this factor has not yet found its way into the societal and NIH guidelines for parathyroidectomy *(128)*, many authors have been advocating for long-term cardiovascular risk to be included in the decision-making process for surgery *(129)*.

A recently published randomized controlled study in patients with subclinical hypothyroidism showed that L-T4 supplementation improved endothelial function *(130)*. The authors mainly invoked improved lipid profile for the beneficial cardiovascular profile. Meanwhile, the more active T3 was found to reduce peripheral vascular resistance by NO-dependent endothelial mechanisms as well as increased SMVC susceptibility to noradrenaline *(131)*.

Adipokines are bioactive mediators secreted by the adipose tissue that often go beyond the traditional role of cytokines. Proinflammatory markers such as TNF-a, IL-6, and IL-1 act as disruptors of the insulin signaling cascade and endothelial function. Leptin, a medium-sized peptide of 167 amino acids abundantly secreted by adipocytes, has a multitude of receptors throughout the body and is implicated in effects beyond its traditionally invoked role in the control of appetite. So far, we know that leptin inhibits growth of VSMC *(132)*. High leptin levels are associated with decreased arterial distensibility *(133)* and increased cardiovascular mortality, particularly in patients with diabetes mellitus *(134,135)*. Resistin, which is 114 aminoacids long, is expressed by the bone marrow and peripheral mononuclear cells in humans, and controversy exists whether this peptide should be grouped with traditional adipokines *(136)*. It has been shown to promote inflammation *(137)* and proliferation of VSMC and endothelial cells *(138)*. Clinically, resistin appears to be linked to higher rates of cardiovascular disease in patients with diabetes *(139)*.

Adiponectin, which structurally belongs to the collagen family, is often described as the "good" adipokine: produced in the subcutaneous fat rather than visceral fat tissue, it is abundantly found in the bloodstream and is reduced in men, states of insulin resistance and cardiovascular disease *(140)*. Two receptors have so far been described, and although expression is ubiquitous, muscle and the liver are the main targets of adiponectin. They mediate activation of AMP kinase, PPARα, and, as a consequence, glucose uptake and fatty acid oxidation *(141)*. Thiazolidinediones (TZDs), which act as Peroxisome Proliferator-Activated Receptor (PPAR-γ) agonists, may unfold their beneficial effects on metabolism and endothelium alike by modulating expression of adiponectin and its receptors *(142)*.

CONCLUSION

As demonstrated in this brief overview, hormones influence the vasculature directly and indirectly. Catecholamines are the best-known and classic stimulators of vascular tone. The RAAS is an additional source of stimuli that may damage the vasculature. Sex steroids may show gender-dependent disparate genomic and rapid, nongenomic effects on the vasculature, and much research is needed to clarify the role of hormone supplementation. Insulin may have beneficial properties, whereas GH and IGF-1 are tied to CHD in both states of deficiency and excess. Finally, adipokines are a relatively novel group of agents that may directly, and through a variety of effects on hormonal axes and inflammatory pathways, regulate the vasculature. While this overview can only briefly touch on all the systems mentioned, later chapters provide greater depth to the reader.

REFERENCES

1. Addison T. On the Constitutional and Local Effects of Disease of the Suprarenal Capsules. London: S. Highley, 1855.
2. Oliver G, Schafer EA. On the physiological action of extract of the suprarenal capsules. *J Physiol (Lond)*. 1894; 16.
3. Marin E, Sessa WC. Role of endothelial-derived nitric oxide in hypertension and renal disease. *Curr Opin Nephrol Hypertens*. Mar 2007;16(2):105–110.
4. Toda N, Ayajiki K, Okamura T. Interaction of endothelial nitric oxide and angiotensin in the circulation. *Pharmacol Rev*. Mar 2007;59(1):54–87.
5. Teschemacher AG. Real-time measurements of noradrenaline release in periphery and central nervous system. *Auton Neurosci*. Jan 15 2005;117(1):1–8.
6. Guimaraes S, Moura D. Vascular adrenoceptors: an update. *Pharmacol Rev*. Jun 2001;53(2):319–356.
7. Shah NC, Pringle S, Struthers A. Aldosterone blockade over and above ACE-inhibitors in patients with coronary artery disease but without heart failure. *J Renin Angiotensin Aldosterone Syst*. Mar 2006;7(1): 20–30.
8. Ferro A, Queen LR, Priest RM, et al. Activation of nitric oxide synthase by beta 2-adrenoceptors in human umbilical vein endothelium in vitro. *Br J Pharmacol*. Apr 1999;126(8):1872–1880.
9. Fisher MH, Amend AM, Bach TJ, et al. A selective human beta3 adrenergic receptor agonist increases metabolic rate in rhesus monkeys. *J Clin Invest*. Jun 1 1998;101(11):2387–2393.
10. Rader DJ. Effect of insulin resistance, dyslipidemia, and intra-abdominal adiposity on the development of cardiovascular disease and diabetes mellitus. *Am J Med*. Mar 2007;120(3 Suppl 1):S12–S18.
11. Jose PA, Eisner GM, Felder RA. Dopamine and the kidney: a role in hypertension? *Curr Opin Nephrol Hypertens*. Mar 2003;12(2):189–194.

12. Miyata N, Park F, Li XF, Cowley AW, Jr. Distribution of angiotensin AT1 and AT2 receptor subtypes in the rat kidney. *Am J Physiol.* Sep 1999;277(3 Pt 2):F437–F446.

13. Garvin JL. Angiotensin stimulates bicarbonate transport and Na$^+$/K$^+$ ATPase in rat proximal straight tubules. *J Am Soc Nephrol.* Apr 1991;1(10):1146–1152.

14. Carey RM, Siragy HM. Newly recognized components of the renin-angiotensin system: potential roles in cardiovascular and renal regulation. *Endocr Rev.* Jun 2003;24(3):261–271.

15. Dostal DE, Baker KM. The cardiac renin-angiotensin system: conceptual, or a regulator of cardiac function? *Circ Res.* Oct 1 1999;85(7):643–650.

16. Danser AH, van Kesteren CA, Bax WA, et al. Prorenin, renin, angiotensinogen, and angiotensin-converting enzyme in normal and failing human hearts. Evidence for renin binding. *Circulation.* Jul 1 1997;96(1): 220–226.

17. Balcells E, Meng QC, Johnson WH, Jr., Oparil S, Dell'Italia LJ. Angiotensin II formation from ACE and chymase in human and animal hearts: methods and species considerations. *Am J Physiol.* Oct 1997;273(4 Pt 2):H1769–H1774.

18. Lindpaintner K, Jin M, Wilhelm MJ, et al. Intracardiac generation of angiotensin and its physiologic role. *Circulation.* Jun 1988;77(6 Pt 2):I18–I23.

19. Lindpaintner K, Jin MW, Niedermaier N, Wilhelm MJ, Ganten D. Cardiac angiotensinogen and its local activation in the isolated perfused beating heart. *Circ Res.* Sep 1990;67(3):564–573.

20. Sadoshima J, Xu Y, Slayter HS, Izumo S. Autocrine release of angiotensin II mediates stretch-induced hypertrophy of cardiac myocytes in vitro. *Cell.* Dec 3 1993;75(5):977–984.

21. Navar LG, Harrison-Bernard LM, Nishiyama A, Kobori H. Regulation of Intrarenal Angiotensin II in Hypertension: Am Heart Assoc; 2002.

22. Just A, Olson AJ, Whitten CL, Arendshorst WJ. Superoxide mediates acute renal vasoconstriction produced by angiotensin II and catecholamines by a mechanism independent of nitric oxide. *Am J Physiol Heart Circ Physiol.* Jan 2007;292(1):H83–H92.

23. Imanishi T, Kobayashi K, Kuroi A, et al. Effects of angiotensin II on NO bioavailability evaluated using a catheter-type NO sensor. *Hypertension.* Dec 2006;48(6):1058–1065.

24. Mulrow PJ, Franco-Saenz R. The adrenal renin-angiotensin system: a local hormonal regulator of aldosterone production. *J Hypertens.* 1996;14:173–176.

25. Brown NJ. Aldosterone and end-organ damage. *Curr Opin Nephrol Hypertens.* May 2005;14(3):235–241.

26. Duprez DA, Bauwens FR, De Buyzere ML, et al. Influence of arterial blood pressure and aldosterone on left ventricular hypertrophy in moderate essential hypertension. *Am J Cardiol.* Jan 21 1993;71(3):17A–20A.

27. Romagni P, Rossi F, Guerrini L, Quirini C, Santiemma V. Aldosterone induces contraction of the resistance arteries in man. *Atherosclerosis.* Feb 2003;166(2):345–349.

28. Gros R, Ding Q, Armstrong S, O'Neil C, Pickering JG, Feldman RD. Rapid effects of aldosterone on clonal human vascular smooth muscle cells. *Am J Physiol Cell Physiol.* Feb 2007;292(2):C788–C794.

29. Marcy TR, Ripley TL. Aldosterone antagonists in the treatment of heart failure. *Am J Health Syst Pharm.* Jan 1 2006;63(1):49–58.

30. Williams TA, Verhovez A, Milan A, Veglio F, Mulatero P. Protective effect of spironolactone on endothelial cell apoptosis. *Endocrinology.* May 2006;147(5):2496–2505.

31. Frey FJ, Odermatt A, Frey BM. Glucocorticoid-mediated mineralocorticoid receptor activation and hypertension. *Curr Opin Nephrol Hypertens.* Jul 2004;13(4):451–458.

32. Dittmar KD, Pratt WB. Folding of the glucocorticoid receptor by the reconstituted Hsp90-based chaperone machinery. The initial hsp90.p60.hsp70-dependent step is sufficient for creating the steroid binding conformation. *J Biol Chem.* May 16 1997;272(20):13047–13054.

33. Barnes PJ. Anti-inflammatory actions of glucocorticoids: molecular mechanisms. *Clin Sci (Lond).* Jun 1998;94(6):557–572.

34. Hafezi-Moghadam A, Simoncini T, Yang Z, et al. Acute cardiovascular protective effects of corticosteroids are mediated by non-transcriptional activation of endothelial nitric oxide synthase. *Nat Med.* May 2002;8(5): 473–479.

35. Brotman DJ, Girod JP, Garcia MJ, et al. Effects of short-term glucocorticoids on cardiovascular biomarkers. *J Clin Endocrinol Metab.* Jun 2005;90(6):3202–3208.

36. Albiger N, Testa RM, Almoto B, et al. Patients with Cushing's syndrome have increased intimal media thickness at different vascular levels: comparison with a population matched for similar cardiovascular risk factors. *Horm Metab Res.* Jun 2006;38(6):405–410.

37. Tauchmanova L, Rossi R, Biondi B, et al. Patients with subclinical Cushing's syndrome due to adrenal adenoma have increased cardiovascular risk. *J Clin Endocrinol Metab.* Nov 2002;87(11):4872–4878.

38. Colao A, Pivonello R, Spiezia S, et al. Persistence of increased cardiovascular risk in patients with Cushing's disease after five years of successful cure. *J Clin Endocrinol Metab.* Aug 1999;84(8):2664–2672.
39. Bansilal S, Farkouh ME, Fuster V. Role of insulin resistance and hyperglycemia in the development of atherosclerosis. *Am J Cardiol.* Feb 19 2007;99(4A):6B–14B.
40. Kim JA, Montagnani M, Koh KK, Quon MJ. Reciprocal relationships between insulin resistance and endothelial dysfunction: molecular and pathophysiological mechanisms. *Circulation.* Apr 18 2006;113(15): 1888–1904.
41. Lteif A, Vaishnava P, Baron AD, Mather KJ. Endothelin limits insulin action in obese/insulin-resistant humans. *Diabetes.* Mar 2007;56(3):728–734.
42. Grassi G. Sympathetic overdrive and cardiovascular risk in the metabolic syndrome. *Hypertens Res.* Nov 2006;29(11):839–847.
43. Grassi G, Quarti-Trevano F, Seravalle G, Dell'Oro R. Cardiovascular risk and adrenergic overdrive in the metabolic syndrome. *Nutr Metab Cardiovasc Dis.* Jul 2007;17(6):473–481.
44. Delafontaine P. Insulin-like growth factor I and its binding proteins in the cardiovascular system. *Cardiovasc Res.* Dec 1995;30(6):825–834.
45. Bornfeldt KE, Raines EW, Nakano T, Graves LM, Krebs EG, Ross R. Insulin-like growth factor-I and platelet-derived growth factor-BB induce directed migration of human arterial smooth muscle cells via signaling pathways that are distinct from those of proliferation. *J Clin Invest.* Mar 1994;93(3):1266–1274.
46. Gockerman A, Prevette T, Jones JI, Clemmons DR. Insulin-like growth factor (IGF)-binding proteins inhibit the smooth muscle cell migration responses to IGF-I and IGF-II. *Endocrinology.* Oct 1995;136(10): 4168–4173.
47. Pricci F, Pugliese G, Romano G, et al. Insulin-like growth factors I and II stimulate extracellular matrix production in human glomerular mesangial cells. Comparison with transforming growth factor-beta. *Endocrinology.* Mar 1996;137(3):879–885.
48. Hochberg Z, Hertz P, Maor G, Oiknine J, Aviram M. Growth hormone and insulin-like growth factor-I increase macrophage uptake and degradation of low density lipoprotein. *Endocrinology.* Jul 1992;131(1): 430–435.
49. Renier G, Clement I, Desfaits AC, Lambert A. Direct stimulatory effect of insulin-like growth factor-I on monocyte and macrophage tumor necrosis factor-alpha production. *Endocrinology.* Nov 1996;137(11): 4611–4618.
50. Colao A, Di Somma C, Salerno M, Spinelli L, Orio F, Lombardi G. The cardiovascular risk of GH-deficient adolescents. *J Clin Endocrinol Metab.* Aug 2002;87(8):3650–3655.
51. Maison P, Griffin S, Nicoue-Beglah M, Haddad N, Balkau B, Chanson P. Impact of growth hormone (GH) treatment on cardiovascular risk factors in GH-deficient adults: a meta-analysis of blinded, randomized, placebo-controlled trials. *J Clin Endocrinol Metab.* May 2004;89(5):2192–2199.
52. Burger AG, Monson JP, Colao AM, Klibanski A. Cardiovascular risk in patients with growth hormone deficiency: effects of growth hormone substitution. *Endocr Pract.* Nov-Dec 2006;12(6):682–689.
53. Laustsen PG, Russell SJ, Cui L, et al. Essential role of insulin and insulin-like growth factor 1 receptor signaling in cardiac development and function. *Mol Cell Biol.* Mar 2007;27(5):1649–1664.
54. Clayton RN. Cardiovascular function in acromegaly. *Endocr Rev.* Jun 2003;24(3):272–277.
55. Rosen T, Bengtsson BA. Premature mortality due to cardiovascular disease in hypopituitarism. *Lancet.* Aug 4 1990;336(8710):285–288.
56. Juul A, Scheike T, Davidsen M, Gyllenborg J, Jorgensen T. Low serum insulin-like growth factor I is associated with increased risk of ischemic heart disease: a population-based case–control study. *Circulation.* Aug 20 2002;106(8):939–944.
57. Ruotolo G, Bavenholm P, Brismar K, et al. Serum insulin-like growth factor-I level is independently associated with coronary artery disease progression in young male survivors of myocardial infarction: beneficial effects of bezafibrate treatment. *J Am Coll Cardiol.* Mar 1 2000;35(3):647–654.
58. Frystyk J, Ledet T, Moller N, Flyvbjerg A, Orskov H. Cardiovascular disease and insulin-like growth factor I. *Circulation.* Aug 20 2002;106(8):893–895.
59. Fischer F, Schulte H, Mohan S, et al. Associations of insulin-like growth factors, insulin-like growth factor binding proteins and acid-labile subunit with coronary heart disease. *Clin Endocrinol (Oxf).* Nov 2004;61(5):595–602.
60. Zumoff B, Troxler RG, O'Connor J, et al. Abnormal hormone levels in men with coronary artery disease. *Arteriosclerosis.* Jan–Feb 1982;2(1):58–67.
61. Bush TL. Noncontraceptive estrogen use and risk of cardiovascular disease: an overview and critique of the literature. *The Menopause: Biological and Clinical Consequences of Ovarian Failure: Evolution and Management. Norwell, Mass: Serono Symposia.* 1990:211–223.

62. Hsia J, Langer RD, Manson JE, et al. Conjugated equine estrogens and coronary heart disease: the Women's Health Initiative. *Arch Intern Med.* Feb 13 2006;166(3):357–365.

63. Anderson GL, Limacher M, Assaf AR, et al. Effects of conjugated equine estrogen in postmenopausal women with hysterectomy: the Women's Health Initiative randomized controlled trial. *Jama.* Apr 14 2004;291(14):1701–1712.

64. Hsia J, Criqui MH, Rodabough RJ, et al. Estrogen plus progestin and the risk of peripheral arterial disease: the Women's Health Initiative. *Circulation.* Feb 10 2004;109(5):620–626.

65. Barrett-Connor E, Goodman-Gruen D. Prospective study of endogenous sex hormones and fatal cardiovascular disease in postmenopausal women. *BMJ.* Nov 4 1995;311(7014):1193–1196.

66. Rosano GM, Vitale C, Fini M. Hormone replacement therapy and cardioprotection: what is good and what is bad for the cardiovascular system? *Ann N Y Acad Sci.* Dec 2006;1092:341–348.

67. Kato S, Sato T, Watanabe T, et al. Function of nuclear sex hormone receptors in gene regulation. *Can Chemother Pharmacol.* Nov 2005;56 Suppl 1:4–9.

68. Christodoulakos GE, Lambrinoudaki IV, Botsis DC. The cardiovascular effects of selective estrogen receptor modulators. *Ann N Y Acad Sci.* Dec 2006;1092:374–384.

69. Mendelsohn ME, Karas RH. The protective effects of estrogen on the cardiovascular system. *N Engl J Med.* Jun 10 1999;340(23):1801–1811.

70. Turgeon JL, Carr MC, Maki PM, Mendelsohn ME, Wise PM. Complex actions of sex steroids in adipose tissue, the cardiovascular system, and brain: Insights from basic science and clinical studies. *Endocr Rev.* Oct 2006;27(6):575–605.

71. Kuiper GG, Enmark E, Pelto-Huikko M, Nilsson S, Gustafsson JA. Cloning of a novel receptor expressed in rat prostate and ovary. *Proc Natl Acad Sci USA.* Jun 11 1996;93(12):5925–5930.

72. Kuiper GG, Carlsson B, Grandien K, et al. Comparison of the ligand binding specificity and transcript tissue distribution of estrogen receptors alpha and beta. *Endocrinology.* Mar 1997;138(3):863–870.

73. Haas E, Meyer MR, Schurr U, et al. Differential Effects of 17{beta}-Estradiol on Function and Expression of Estrogen Receptor {alpha}, Estrogen Receptor {beta}, and GPR30 in Arteries and Veins of Patients With Atherosclerosis. *Hypertension.* Apr 23 2007.

74. Watanabe T, Akishita M, Nakaoka T, et al. Estrogen receptor beta mediates the inhibitory effect of estradiol on vascular smooth muscle cell proliferation. *Cardiovasc Res.* Sep 1 2003;59(3):734–744.

75. Mendelsohn ME. Genomic and nongenomic effects of estrogen in the vasculature. *Am J Cardiol.* Jul 3 2002;90(1A):3F–6F.

76. Klouche M. Estrogens in human vascular diseases. *Ann N Y Acad Sci.* Nov 2006;1089:431–443.

77. Iruela-Arispe ML, Rodriguez-Manzaneque JC, Abu-Jawdeh G. Endometrial endothelial cells express estrogen and progesterone receptors and exhibit a tissue specific response to angiogenic growth factors. *Microcirculation.* Jun 1999;6(2):127–140.

78. Bergqvist A, Bergqvist D, Ferno M. Estrogen and progesterone receptors in vessel walls. Biochemical and immunochemical assays. *Acta Obstet Gynecol Scand.* Jan 1993;72(1):10–16.

79. Hermenegildo C, Oviedo PJ, Garcia-Martinez MC, Garcia-Perez MA, Tarin JJ, Cano A. Progestogens stimulate prostacyclin production by human endothelial cells. *Hum Reprod.* Jun 2005;20(6):1554–1561.

80. Selles J, Polini N, Alvarez C, Massheimer V. Nongenomic action of progesterone in rat aorta: role of nitric oxide and prostaglandins. *Cell Signal.* May 2002;14(5):431–436.

81. Arnlov J, Pencina MJ, Amin S, et al. Endogenous sex hormones and cardiovascular disease incidence in men. *Ann Intern Med.* Aug 1 2006;145(3):176–184.

82. Sudhir K, Chou TM, Messina LM, et al. Endothelial dysfunction in a man with disruptive mutation in oestrogen-receptor gene. *Lancet.* Apr 19 1997;349(9059):1146–1147.

83. Maffei L, Murata Y, Rochira V, et al. Dysmetabolic syndrome in a man with a novel mutation of the aromatase gene: effects of testosterone, alendronate, and estradiol treatment. *J Clin Endocrinol Metab.* Jan 2004;89(1):61–70.

84. Ebeling P, Koivisto VA. Physiological importance of dehydroepiandrosterone. *Lancet.* Jun 11 1994;343(8911):1479–1481.

85. Wu FC, von Eckardstein A. Androgens and coronary artery disease. *Endocr Rev.* Apr 2003;24(2):183–217.

86. Hayashi T, Esaki T, Muto E, et al. Dehydroepiandrosterone retards atherosclerosis formation through its conversion to estrogen: the possible role of nitric oxide. *Arterioscler Thromb Vasc Biol.* Mar 2000;20(3):782–792.

87. Barrett-Connor E, Goodman-Gruen D. The epidemiology of DHEAS and cardiovascular disease. *Ann N Y Acad Sci.* Dec 29 1995;774:259–270.

88. Berr C, Lafont S, Debuire B, Dartigues JF, Baulieu EE. Relationships of dehydroepiandrosterone sulfate in the elderly with functional, psychological, and mental status, and short-term mortality: a French community-based study. *Proc Natl Acad Sci USA.* Nov 12 1996;93(23):13410–13415.

89. Kiechl S, Willeit J, Bonora E, Schwarz S, Xu Q. No association between dehydroepiandrosterone sulfate and development of atherosclerosis in a prospective population study (Bruneck Study). *Arterioscler Thromb Vasc Biol.* Apr 2000;20(4):1094–1100.

90. Tilvis RS, Kahonen M, Harkonen M. Dehydroepiandrosterone sulfate, diseases and mortality in a general aged population. *Aging (Milano).* Feb 1999;11(1):30–34.

91. Trivedi DP, Khaw KT. Dehydroepiandrosterone sulfate and mortality in elderly men and women. *J Clin Endocrinol Metab.* Sep 2001;86(9):4171–4177.

92. Nair KS, Rizza RA, O'Brien P, et al. DHEA in elderly women and DHEA or testosterone in elderly men. *N Engl J Med.* Oct 19 2006;355(16):1647–1659.

93. Yue P, Chatterjee K, Beale C, Poole-Wilson PA, Collins P. Testosterone relaxes rabbit coronary arteries and aorta. *Circulation.* Feb 15 1995;91(4):1154–1160.

94. Webb CM, McNeill JG, Hayward CS, de Zeigler D, Collins P. Effects of testosterone on coronary vasomotor regulation in men with coronary heart disease. *Circulation.* Oct 19 1999;100(16):1690–1696.

95. Jones RD, Pugh PJ, Jones TH, Channer KS. The vasodilatory action of testosterone: a potassium-channel opening or a calcium antagonistic action? *Br J Pharmacol.* Mar 2003;138(5):733–744.

96. Ong PJ, Patrizi G, Chong WC, Webb CM, Hayward CS, Collins P. Testosterone enhances flow-mediated brachial artery reactivity in men with coronary artery disease. *Am J Cardiol.* Jan 15 2000;85(2):269–272.

97. Hall J, Jones RD, Jones TH, Channer KS, Peers C. Selective inhibition of L-type Ca^{2+} channels in A^7r^5 cells by physiological levels of testosterone. *Endocrinology.* Jun 2006;147(6):2675–2680.

98. English KM, Mandour O, Steeds RP, Diver MJ, Jones TH, Channer KS. Men with coronary artery disease have lower levels of androgens than men with normal coronary angiograms. *Eur Heart J.* Jun 2000;21(11):890–894.

99. Sieminska L, Wojciechowska C, Swietochowska E, et al. Serum free testosterone in men with coronary artery atherosclerosis. *Med Sci Monit.* May 2003;9(5):CR162–CR166.

100. Dobrzycki S, Serwatka W, Nadlewski S, et al. An assessment of correlations between endogenous sex hormone levels and the extensiveness of coronary heart disease and the ejection fraction of the left ventricle in males. *J Med Invest.* Aug 2003;50(3–4):162–169.

101. Barrett-Connor E, Khaw KT. Endogenous sex hormones and cardiovascular disease in men. A prospective population-based study. *Circulation.* Sep 1988;78(3):539–545.

102. Cauley JA, Gutai JP, Kuller LH, Dai WS. Usefulness of sex steroid hormone levels in predicting coronary artery disease in men. *Am J Cardiol.* Oct 1 1987;60(10):771–777.

103. Contoreggi CS, Blackman MR, Andres R, et al. Plasma levels of estradiol, testosterone, and DHEAS do not predict risk of coronary artery disease in men. *J Androl.* Sep–Oct 1990;11(5):460–470.

104. Harman SM, Metter EJ, Tobin JD, Pearson J, Blackman MR. Longitudinal effects of aging on serum total and free testosterone levels in healthy men. Baltimore Longitudinal Study of Aging. *J Clin Endocrinol Metab.* Feb 2001;86(2):724–731.

105. Hautanen A, Manttari M, Manninen V, et al. Adrenal androgens and testosterone as coronary risk factors in the Helsinki Heart Study. *Atherosclerosis.* Feb 1994;105(2):191–200.

106. Phillips GB, Yano K, Stemmermann GN. Serum sex hormone levels and myocardial infarction in the Honolulu Heart Program. Pitfalls in prospective studies on sex hormones. *J Clin Epidemiol.* 1988;41(12):1151–1156.

107. Yarnell JW, Beswick AD, Sweetnam PM, Riad-Fahmy D. Endogenous sex hormones and ischemic heart disease in men. The Caerphilly prospective study. *Arterioscler Thromb.* Apr 1993;13(4):517–520.

108. Karila TA, Karjalainen JE, Mantysaari MJ, Viitasalo MT, Seppala TA. Anabolic androgenic steroids produce dose-dependent increase in left ventricular mass in power atheletes, and this effect is potentiated by concomitant use of growth hormone. *Int J Sports Med.* Jul 2003;24(5):337–343.

109. Nieminen MS, Ramo MP, Viitasalo M, et al. Serious cardiovascular side effects of large doses of anabolic steroids in weight lifters. *Eur Heart J.* Oct 1996;17(10):1576–1583.

110. Ferrera PC, Putnam DL, Verdile VP. Anabolic steroid use as the possible precipitant of dilated cardiomyopathy. *Cardiology.* Mar–Apr 1997;88(2):218–220.

111. Malkin CJ, Pugh PJ, West JN, van Beek EJ, Jones TH, Channer KS. Testosterone therapy in men with moderate severity heart failure: a double-blind randomized placebo controlled trial. *Eur Heart J.* Jan 2006;27(1):57–64.

112. Arad Y, Badimon JJ, Badimon L, Hembree WC, Ginsberg HN. Dehydroepiandrosterone feeding prevents aortic fatty streak formation and cholesterol accumulation in cholesterol-fed rabbit. *Arteriosclerosis.* Mar–Apr 1989;9(2):159–166.

113. Alexandersen P, Haarbo J, Byrjalsen I, Lawaetz H, Christiansen C. Natural androgens inhibit male atherosclerosis: a study in castrated, cholesterol-fed rabbits. *Circ Res.* Apr 16 1999;84(7):813–819.

114. Hak AE, Witteman JC, de Jong FH, Geerlings MI, Hofman A, Pols HA. Low levels of endogenous androgens increase the risk of atherosclerosis in elderly men: the Rotterdam study. *J Clin Endocrinol Metab.* Aug 2002;87(8):3632–3639.

115. van den Beld AW, Bots ML, Janssen JA, Pols HA, Lamberts SW, Grobbee DE. Endogenous hormones and carotid atherosclerosis in elderly men. *Am J Epidemiol.* Jan 1 2003;157(1):25–31.

116. Ng MK, Quinn CM, McCrohon JA, et al. Androgens up-regulate atherosclerosis-related genes in macrophages from males but not females: molecular insights into gender differences in atherosclerosis. *J Am Coll Cardiol.* Oct 1 2003;42(7):1306–1313.

117. Montalcini T, Gorgone G, Gazzaruso C, Sesti G, Perticone F, Pujia A. Role of endogenous androgens on carotid atherosclerosis in non-obese postmenopausal women. *Nutr Metab Cardiovasc Dis.* Dec 2007;17(10):705–711.

118. Montalcini T, Gorgone G, Gazzaruso C, Sesti G, Perticone F, Pujia A. Endogenous testosterone and endothelial function in postmenopausal women. *Coron Artery Dis.* Feb 2007;18(1):9–13.

119. Palmer M, Ljunghall S, Akerstrom G, et al. Patients with primary hyperparathyroidism operated on over a 24-year period: temporal trends of clinical and laboratory findings. *J Chronic Dis.* 1987;40(2):121–130.

120. Wermers RA, Khosla S, Atkinson EJ, et al. Survival after the diagnosis of hyperparathyroidism: a population-based study. *Am J Med.* Feb 1998;104(2):115–122.

121. Duprez D, Bauwens F, De Buyzere M, et al. Relationship between parathyroid hormone and left ventricular mass in moderate essential hypertension. *J Hypertens Suppl.* Dec 1991;9(6):S116–S117.

122. Dalberg K, Brodin LA, Juhlin-Dannfelt A, Farnebo LO. Cardiac function in primary hyperparathyroidism before and after operation. An echocardiographic study. *Eur J Surg.* Mar 1996;162(3):171–176.

123. Lundgren E, Ljunghall S, Akerstrom G, Hetta J, Mallmin H, Rastad J. Case–control study on symptoms and signs of "asymptomatic" primary hyperparathyroidism. *Surgery.* Dec 1998;124(6):980–985; discussion 985–986.

124. Nainby-Luxmoore JC, Langford HG, Nelson NC, Watson RL, Barnes TY. A case-comparison study of hypertension and hyperparathyroidism. *J Clin Endocrinol Metab.* Aug 1982;55(2):303–306.

125. Baykan M, Erem C, Gedikli O, et al. Impairment of flow-mediated vasodilatation of brachial artery in patients with Cushing's Syndrome. *Endocrine.* Jun 2007;31(3):300–304.

126. Lundgren E, Szabo E, Ljunghall S, Bergstrom R, Holmberg L, Rastad J. Population based case–control study of sick leave in postmenopausal women before diagnosis of hyperparathyroidism. *BMJ.* Sep 26 1998;317(7162):848–851.

127. Hanson AS, Linas SL. Parathyroid hormone/adenylate cyclase coupling in vascular smooth muscle cells. *Hypertension.* Apr 1994;23(4):468–475.

128. Bilezikian JP, Potts JT, Jr., Fuleihan Gel H, et al. Summary statement from a workshop on asymptomatic primary hyperparathyroidism: a perspective for the 21st century. *J Bone Miner Res.* Nov 2002;17 Suppl 2:N2–N11.

129. Eigelberger MS, Cheah WK, Ituarte PH, Streja L, Duh QY, Clark OH. The NIH criteria for parathyroidectomy in asymptomatic primary hyperparathyroidism: are they too limited? *Ann Surg.* Apr 2004;239(4):528–535.

130. Razvi S, Ingoe L, Keeka G, Oates C, McMillan C, Weaver JU. The beneficial effect of L-thyroxine on cardiovascular risk factors, endothelial function, and quality of life in subclinical hypothyroidism: randomized, crossover trial. *J Clin Endocrinol Metab.* May 2007;92(5):1715–1723.

131. Napoli R, Guardasole V, Angelini V, et al. Acute effects of triiodothyronine on endothelial function in human subjects. *J Clin Endocrinol Metab.* Jan 2007;92(1):250–254.

132. Bohlen F, Kratzsch J, Mueller M, et al. Leptin inhibits cell growth of human vascular smooth muscle cells. *Vascul Pharmacol.* Jan 2007;46(1):67–71.

133. Singhal A, Farooqi IS, Cole TJ, et al. Influence of leptin on arterial distensibility: a novel link between obesity and cardiovascular disease? *Circulation.* Oct 8 2002;106(15):1919–1924.

134. Wolk R, Berger P, Lennon RJ, Brilakis ES, Johnson BD, Somers VK. Plasma leptin and prognosis in patients with established coronary atherosclerosis. *J Am Coll Cardiol.* Nov 2 2004;44(9):1819–1824.

135. Reilly MP, Iqbal N, Schutta M, et al. Plasma leptin levels are associated with coronary atherosclerosis in type 2 diabetes. *J Clin Endocrinol Metab.* Aug 2004;89(8):3872–3878.

136. Koerner A, Kratzsch J, Kiess W. Adipocytokines: leptin – the classical, resistin – the controversial, adiponectin – the promising, and more to come. *Best Pract Res Clin Endocrinol Metab.* Dec 2005;19(4):525–546.

137. Bokarewa M, Nagaev I, Dahlberg L, Smith U, Tarkowski A. Resistin, an adipokine with potent proinflammatory properties. *J Immunol.* May 1 2005;174(9):5789–5795.

138. Calabro P, Samudio I, Willerson JT, Yeh ET. Resistin promotes smooth muscle cell proliferation through activation of extracellular signal-regulated kinase 1/2 and phosphatidylinositol 3-kinase pathways. *Circulation.* Nov 23 2004;110(21):3335–3340.

139. Reilly MP, Lehrke M, Wolfe ML, Rohatgi A, Lazar MA, Rader DJ. Resistin is an inflammatory marker of atherosclerosis in humans. *Circulation.* Feb 22 2005;111(7):932–939.
140. Matsuzawa Y, Funahashi T, Kihara S, Shimomura I. Adiponectin and metabolic syndrome. *Arterioscler Thromb Vasc Biol.* Jan 2004;24(1):29–33.
141. Gil-Campos M, Canete RR, Gil A. Adiponectin, the missing link in insulin resistance and obesity. *Clin Nutr.* Oct 2004;23(5):963–974.
142. Lihn AS, Pedersen SB, Richelsen B. Adiponectin: action, regulation and association to insulin sensitivity. *Obes Rev.* Feb 2005;6(1):13–21.

I DIABETES AND CARDIOVASCULAR DISEASE

2 Epidemiology and Prevention of Cardiovascular Disease in Diabetes

David S. Frankel, MD *and James B. Meigs,* MD

CONTENTS

SUMMARY

Diabetes is a common disease with a rapidly increasing prevalence. Diabetic patients are at markedly increased risk for development of coronary artery disease (CAD) and heart failure and, further, when they develop these diseases, they have worse outcomes including higher mortality. This mandates an aggressive approach to reducing cardiovascular risk in all diabetic patients. Good evidence has shown that tight blood pressure (BP), lipid and glycemic control, as well as smoking cessation, all substantially decrease the risk of cardiovascular disease and death.

Key Words: Diabetes, Cardiovascular disease, Epidemiology, Prevention, Risk factor modification, Blood pressure, Lipids, Glycemic control

From: *Contemporary Endocrinology: Cardiovascular Endocrinology: Shared Pathways and Clinical Crossroads*
Edited by: V. A. Fonseca © Humana Press, New York, NY

Abbreviations: ACE – angiotensin converting enzyme, ARB – angiotensin II receptor blocker, BP – blood pressure, CAD – coronary artery disease, CCB – calcium channel blocker, DCCT – Diabetes Control and Complications Trial, HbA1c – hemoglobin A1C, LDL – low density lipoprotein, MI – myocardial infarction, NCEP – National Cholesterol Education Program, SBP – systolic blood pressure, UKPDS – United Kingdom Prospective Diabetes Study

PREVALENCE OF DIABETES

The prevalence of diabetes is substantial throughout the world, with type 2 diabetes comprising 90–95% of cases. In the US, an estimated 20.8 million people, or 7.0% of the population, have diabetes, with 14.6 million cases diagnosed and 6.2 million undiagnosed. Even more concerning, 41 million Americans have pre-diabetes, defined as impaired fasting glucose or impaired glucose tolerance. The prevalence of diabetes is lowest among young people (0.22% of those under age 20) but increases with age, such that 9.6% of people over age 20 and 20.9% of people over age 60 have diabetes. While men have a slightly higher prevalence of diabetes in the US, both sexes are largely affected, with 10.5% of men and 8.8% of women over the age of 20 having diabetes. The prevalence of diabetes is increased among minority populations. Among adults over the age of 20, the prevalence of diabetes (diagnosed and undiagnosed) among non-Hispanic whites is 8.7%. After adjusting for population age differences, American Indian and Alaska Natives are 2.2 times as likely to have diabetes as non-Hispanic whites. Similarly, non-Hispanic blacks living in America are 1.8 times, Puerto Rican Americans 1.8 times, Mexican Americans 1.7 times, and Asian Americans living in California are 1.5 times are as likely to have diabetes as non-Hispanic whites *(1)*.

The prevalence of diabetes in the US is growing at an alarming rate, with a 38% increase among those aged 40–74 from 1980 to 1990 *(2)*, 1.5 million new cases of diabetes diagnosed in 2005, and 2 million adolescents, aged 12–19, with pre-diabetes *(1)*.

IMPACT OF DIABETES ON HEALTH AND HEALTHCARE COSTS

The impact of diabetes on health is staggering. According to US death certificates in 2002, diabetes was the sixth leading cause of death, contributing to 224,092 deaths. As diabetes is frequently underreported on death certificates, this likely represents an underestimation of its true impact. The risk of death among people with diabetes is twice that of nondiabetics *(1)*. While those with diabetes are at increased risk for microvascular complications, including retinopathy, nephropathy, and neuropathy, it is the macrovascular complications, including CAD, cerebrovascular disease, and peripheral arterial disease, which extract the greatest toll. In the United Kingdom Prospective Diabetes Study (UKPDS), macrovascular endpoints occurred more than three times as frequently as microvascular endpoints *(3)*. Further, heart disease accounts for more than 75% of deaths in diabetes and shortens life expectancy by about 10 years *(4)*.

The economic burden of diabetes in the US is equally impressive, with an estimated cost of $132 billion in 2002. Direct costs comprised $92 billion, including diabetes care, chronic diabetes-related complications, and excess prevalence of general medical conditions. Indirect costs comprised $40 billion, including 88 million lost or restricted workdays, as well as substantial mortality and permanent disability due to diabetes. Compared to a nondiabetic patient, whose healthcare costs averaged $2560 in 2002, caring for a diabetes patient cost $13,243 (an increase of more than 30% from 1997). In fact, one of out every 10 US healthcare dollars is now spent on diabetes and its complications. Again, heart disease is by far the most costly complication of diabetes, accounting for $17.6 billion dollars in annual expenditures *(5)*.

DIABETES AS A RISK FACTOR FOR CORONARY ARTERY DISEASE

People with diabetes are at a markedly increased risk for cardiovascular disease and mortality. Data from the Framingham Heart Study, published in the late 1970s, showed that men and women with diabetes had a respective twofold and threefold increased risk for development of CAD, peripheral arterial disease, and stroke, compared to nondiabetics *(6)*. While this association holds for all patients with diabetes, it is probably even stronger among those with type 1 diabetes *(7)*. A study of 292 young people with type 1 diabetes demonstrated a staggering 35% mortality rate due to CAD by age 55 *(8)*. A Finnish study of 2400 adult subjects showed that in 7 years of follow-up, patients with type 2 diabetes without a history of prior myocardial infarction (MI) actually had a higher rate of MI and stroke, and only slightly lower rate of death from cardiovascular causes than nondiabetics with a history of prior MI (20.2%, 10.3%, and 15.4% vs. 18.8%, 7.2%, and 15.9%, respectively) *(9)* (*see* Fig. 1 and Color Plate 1). It is based on such data that the National Cholesterol Education Program (NCEP) considers diabetes to be a CAD equivalent in determining cardiovascular risk and cholesterol treatment goals *(10)*.

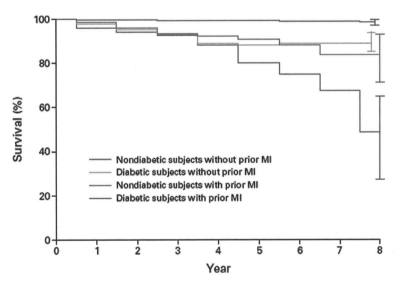

Fig. 1. Kaplan-Meier estimates of the probability (with 95% confidence intervals) of death from coronary heart disease in 1059 subjects with type 2 diabetes and 1378 nondiabetic subjects with and without prior myocardial infarction (MI) in a Finnish population-based study. (*see* Color Plate 1) Reprinted, by permission, from Haffner, SM et al. Mortality from coronary heart disease in subjects with type 2 diabetes and in nondiabetic subjects with and without prior myocardial infarction. New Engl J Med 1998; 339:229–34.

OUTCOME AMONG DIABETES PATIENTS WITH CORONARY ARTERY DISEASE

Patients with diabetes have worse outcomes following MI than do patients without diabetes. An approximately double mortality rate has been shown in studies with short-term (28 days) *(11)*, intermediate-term (2–4 years) *(12,13)*, and long-term (34 years) *(14)* follow-up. This increased risk is mediated through elevated rates of subsequent MI, stroke, and development of heart failure *(12)*. Further, the increased mortality following MI applies to all patients with diabetes: type 1 and type 2, young and old *(15)*, male and especially female *(13,14)*.

DIABETES AS A RISK FACTOR FOR HEART FAILURE

Heart failure is another cause of substantial morbidity and mortality in patients with diabetes. Among a large sample of Medicare diabetic patients aged 65 years or older, the prevalence of heart failure was found to be 22.3% in 1994 with a subsequent incidence rate of 12.6 per 100 person-years *(16)*. A cohort study of type 2 diabetes subjects found a 2.5-fold increased risk for development of heart failure compared to nondiabetics *(17)*. Risk factors for development of heart failure in diabetes include increasing age, poor glycemic control, increasing BMI, ischemic heart disease, peripheral vascular disease, and nephropathy *(16–19)*. In addition to increased rates of CAD and hypertension leading to more ischemic and hypertensive cardiomyopathies, there is also a distinct entity known as "diabetic cardiomyopathy"*(20)*.

The mechanism for the development of diabetic cardiomyopathy is only partially understood, leading to both systolic and diastolic dysfunction. People with diabetes have been shown to have decreased baseline ejection fraction and decreased augmentation in response to exercise (cardiac reserve) *(21–23)*. They have also been shown to have increased left ventricular mass and wall thickness, even when controlled for body mass index and BP *(24)*. This, in addition to autonomic dysfunction, both predispose to diastolic dysfunction *(23,25)*.

OUTCOMES AMONG DIABETES PATIENTS WITH HEART FAILURE

Diabetes patients with heart failure have dramatically higher mortality rates than diabetes patients without heart failure (32.7 vs. 3.7 deaths per 100 person-years) *(16)*. Further, among those with established heart failure, patients with diabetes, especially females, have modestly increased rates of heart failure hospitalization and all-cause mortality compared to nondiabetics *(26,27)*. While this increased risk applies to both systolic and diastolic heart failure *(27)*, in further analysis from the Studies of Left Ventricular Dysfunction (SOLVD) Prevention and Treatment trials, the effect appears to be confined to those with ischemic cardiomyopathy *(28)*.

SECONDARY PREVENTION OF CARDIOVASCULAR DISEASE IN DIABETES – BLOOD PRESSURE CONTROL

Diabetes patients have a high incidence of hypertension, which is likely mediated by multiple factors, including diabetic nephropathy, hyperinsulinemia, extracellular fluid volume expansion, and increased arterial stiffness. Numerous randomized controlled trials have shown that lowering BP leads to lower rates of both macrovascular and microvascular complications. The UKPDS randomized 1148 participants with type 2 diabetes to tight BP control (aiming for <150/85 mm Hg) using captopril or atenolol versus less tight BP control (aiming for <180/105 mm Hg). A difference of 10/5 mm Hg between the two groups was achieved and at 9 years of follow-up, the tight control group had a 24% relative risk reduction in diabetes-related endpoints, including 32% reduction in death related to diabetes, 44% reduction in strokes, and 37% reduction in microvascular endpoints, mainly diabetic retinopathy *(29)*.

The same group subsequently showed that the larger the decrease in BP, the larger the benefit. For each 10 mm Hg decrease in systolic BP (SBP), the risk of death related to diabetes was decreased by 17% and the risk of diabetes complications decreased by 12%. No threshold was identified below which further BP reduction was not beneficial; those with SBP <120 mm Hg had the lowest risk *(30)*. See Fig. 2.

A small number of studies have provided contradictory results, raising the possibility that extremely low BP can be harmful. For example, in a post-hoc analysis of data from the Irbesartan Diabetic Nephropathy Trial (IDNT), BP <120/85 mm Hg was associated with increased adverse cardiovascular events *(31)*. Particularly, excessively low diastolic BP in patients with CAD may be problematic, as the heart is perfused mostly during diastole. This was suggested in a post-hoc analysis of data from the International Verapamil-Trandolapril Study, in which 22,000 patients with CAD and hypertension had a higher rate of all-cause death and MI when the diastolic BP was lowered beneath 84 mm Hg *(32)*. Still, there are significant methodological flaws in these retrospective analyses. In the IDNT trial, those who ended up achieving SBP

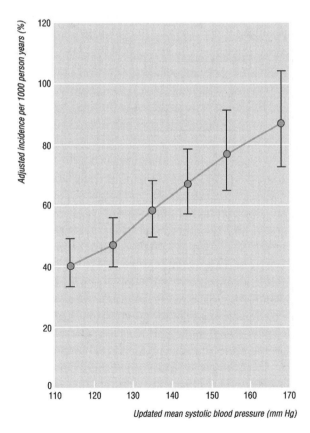

Fig. 2. Incidence rate (with 95% confidence interval) of any aggregate endpoint (death, macrovascular, and microvascular complications) as it relates to mean systolic blood pressure, adjusted for age, sex, and ethnic group, in UKPDS 36. Reproduced with permission from the BMJ Publishing Group, from Adler AI, et al. Association of systolic blood pressure with macrovascular and microvascular complications of type 2 diabetes (UKPDS 36): prospective observational study. Br Med J 2000; 321:412–9.

<120 mm Hg had more history of heart disease and heart failure at baseline. Thus, lower BP is more likely to be a marker of worse heart failure at baseline, than a cause of adverse cardiovascular events. Further, the number of subjects achieving SBP <120 mm Hg was small, limiting the power to draw meaningful conclusions.

Therefore, the weight of evidence overwhelmingly supports aggressive BP lowering. The American Diabetes Association recommends a goal of less than 130/80 mm Hg *(33)*. It remains uncertain whether there is benefit in BP reduction lower than these goals, but the epidemiological data, at least, support a "lower is better" approach.

While it is clear that aggressive BP lowering is essential, the choice of initial agent is more controversial. There are numerous well-designed, randomized controlled trials demonstrating the superiority of diuretics, angiotensin-converting enzyme (ACE) inhibitors, angiotensin II receptor blockers (ARB), and, to a lesser extent, beta-blockers over placebo. The Antihypertensive and Lipid-Lowering Treatment to Prevent Heart Attack Trial (ALLHAT) enrolled 33,000 patients with hypertension and at least one additional CAD risk factor. Participants were randomized to chlorthalidone (diuretic), amlodipine (dihydropyridine calcium channel blocker (CCB)), and lisinopril (ACE). Among participants with diabetes, outcomes were similar in 5 years of follow-up in all three groups, with the exception of fewer incident cases of heart failure in the diuretic group, compared to both the CCB and ACE inhibitor groups *(34)*. Further support for thiazide diuretic use is provided by the Systolic Hypertension in the Elderly Program Cooperative Research Group (SHEP) in which participants older than age 60 with diabetes and isolated systolic hypertension (SBP >160 mm Hg and diastolic BP <90 mm Hg) had lower rates of cardiovascular morbidity and mortality when treated with chlorthalidone compared to placebo *(35)*.

Support for ACE inhibitor as first-line treatment in diabetes patients was provided by the Heart Outcomes Prevention Evaluation (HOPE) Study in which 9000 patients with vascular disease or diabetes plus one other CAD risk factor, but no known heart failure or low ejection fraction, were randomized to treatment with ramipril or placebo. Patients randomized to ramipril had a lower incidence of death, MI, and stroke *(36)*.

The Losartan Intervention for Endpoint Reduction in Hypertension (LIFE) Study randomized participants with diabetes, hypertension, and signs of left ventricular hypertrophy on electrocardiogram to losartan (ARB) or atenolol (beta-blocker). Those assigned to losartan had a lower incidence of cardiovascular morbidity and mortality *(37)*, as well as greater regression of left ventricular hypertrophy, independent of BP response *(38)*.

ACE inhibitors and ARBs are especially effective at preventing and treating diabetic nephropathy. MICRO-HOPE, a substudy of the HOPE trial focusing on microvascular complications, found that diabetic participants without proteinuria treated with ramipril had a 24% relative risk reduction for the development of proteinuria over the following 4.5 years *(39)*. Further, the Effects of Losartan on Renal and Cardiovascular Outcomes (RENAAL) trial showed that losartan (ARB) as compared to placebo, reduced the combined endpoint of doubling of baseline serum creatinine, development of end-stage renal disease, or death, by 16% in those with type 2 diabetes and established nephropathy (proteinuria and elevated serum creatinine at baseline) *(40)*.

While there is little data demonstrating the superiority of beta-blockers to placebo for BP control in diabetes patients without CAD, data from the UKPDS 39 demonstrated equivalence of atenolol (beta-blocker) to captopril (ACE inhibitor) for BP reduction, as well as for prevention of macrovascular and microvascular endpoints. Of note, fewer patients assigned to the beta-blocker group complied with their medical regimen, and average weight gain was greater *(41)*. In contrast, for patients with established CAD, including those with diabetes, there is extensive data supporting beta-blockers as first-line antihypertensives. For example, an ad-hoc analysis of data from the Bezafibrate Infarction Prevention (BIP)] trial showed that diabetes participants with CAD treated with beta-blockers had a 44% reduction in all-cause mortality and a 42% reduction in cardiac mortality compared to patients not taking beta-blockers, over 3 years of follow-up *(42)*. However, concerns exist about worsened glycemic control, as well as masking symptoms of hypoglycemia and possibly exacerbating peripheral vascular disease. In the Glycemic Effects in Diabetes Mellitus (GEMINI) trial, carvedilol (combined alpha- and beta-blocker) was compared to metoprolol (beta-blocker only) in diabetes patients already taking ACE inhibitors or ARBs. Carvedilol did not increase hemoglobin A1C (HbA1c), while metoprolol did. Further, insulin sensitivity was improved by carvedilol and not metoprolol. Progression to microalbuminuria was less frequent in the carvedilol group *(43)*.

The Systolic Hypertension in Europe (Syst-Eur) group showed the superiority of dihydropyridine CCBs to placebo in a post-hoc analysis of 500 diabetic participants over the age of 60 with isolated systolic hypertension. Those randomized to treatment with nitrendipine (CCB) had a markedly decreased overall and cardiovascular mortality *(44)*. However, several head-to-head trials have demonstrated the inferiority of CCBs to ACE inhibitors. For example, the Appropriate Blood Pressure Control in Diabetes (ABCD) trial randomized patients to treatment with nislodipine (CCB) or enalapril (ACE). While BP control was equivalent, those randomized to the CCB group had a higher incidence of fatal and nonfatal MI *(45)*. Most recently, the Anglo-Scandinavian Cardiac Outcomes Trial (ASCOT) showed that a regimen of amlodipine (CCB) adding perindopril (ACE inhibitor) as needed to achieve BP goals was superior to a regimen of atenolol (beta-blocker) adding bendroflumethiazide (thiazide), with fewer cardiovascular events and procedures and lower all-cause mortality (both overall and among diabetic subjects). Of note, the primary endpoint (nonfatal MI and fatal CAD) was not significantly different between treatment groups *(46)*.

In summary, aggressive BP control is essential to preventing the macrovascular and microvascular complications of diabetes. BP should be lowered to at least 130/80 mm Hg and likely lower. Multiple antihypertensives will be required in most patients to achieve this goal. Evidence supports the use of thiazides, ACE inhibitors, or ARBs for first-line treatment of hypertension in diabetes. Thiazides are particularly effective in elderly patients with systolic hypertension. ACE inhibitors and ARBs have the additional, important benefit of protecting against nephropathy. ARBs have been shown to be beneficial in patients with left ventricular hypertrophy. Beta-blockers, especially carvedilol, can be used as first-line antihypertensives in diabetes patients with known CAD. CCBs can be added to first-line agents when further BP reduction is required.

SECONDARY PREVENTION OF CARDIOVASCULAR DISEASE IN DIABETES – LIPID CONTROL

As noted above, type 2 diabetes patients without a history of prior MI have been shown to have a higher risk of MI and stroke, and only slightly lower rate of cardiovascular death than nondiabetics with a history of prior MI *(9)*. This has led the NCEP to classify diabetes as a "coronary heart disease equivalent," emphasizing the importance of lowering lipids aggressively.

Benefit for lipid lowering among diabetic participants was first demonstrated in subgroup analyses of trials for secondary prevention of CAD (i.e., preventing recurrent events in patients with established CAD). The Scandinavian Simvastatin Survival Study (4S) randomized 4444 patients with previous MI or angina and elevated baseline low-density lipoprotein (LDL) cholesterol (median 186 mg/dl) to simvastatin (HMG CoA reductase inhibitor or statin) or placebo. Among the 202 diabetic participants, those randomized to simvastatin had a 43% relative risk reduction in total mortality, a 55% reduction in major coronary heart disease events, and a 37% reduction in all atherosclerotic events over 5 years of follow-up. Within the treatment group, the risk reduction among diabetic participants was greater both in relative and absolute terms than among nondiabetics *(47)*.

The Cholesterol and Recurrent Events (CARE) trial extended these findings to patients with established CAD and intermediate baseline LDL (median 136 mg/dl). Among the 586 participants with diabetes, those randomized to treatment with pravastatin had a relative risk reduction of 25% in coronary events and 32% in revascularization procedures over 5 years of follow-up, when compared to those randomized to placebo *(48)*.

The Pravastatin or Atorvastatin Evaluation and Infection Therapy (PROVE IT) trial conducted by the Thrombolysis in Myocardial Infarction (TIMI) group suggested than an even more aggressive approach is warranted among patients presenting with an acute coronary syndrome. A total number of 4000 patients, with median baseline LDL 106 mg/dl, were randomized to pravastatin 40 mg (standard therapy) or atorvastatin 80 mg (intensive therapy). The median LDL achieved by standard therapy was 95 mg/dl. The median LDL achieved by aggressive therapy was 68 mg/dl. Over 2 years of follow-up, those randomized to the aggressive treatment group had a 16% relative risk reduction in the composite endpoint of death or major cardiovascular events (most significantly unstable angina requiring hospitalization). The relative risk reduction was even greater among the 734 diabetic participants, although this group was not large enough to demonstrate statistical significance *(49)*.

Other randomized trials have demonstrated the effectiveness of statins for the primary prevention of CAD (i.e., prevention of first CAD event) among all participants and especially diabetic ones. For example, within the Heart Protection Study, 3000 diabetes patients without known cardiovascular disease were randomized to treatment with simvastatin 40 mg or placebo. Among the simvastatin-treated patients, there was a 31% relative risk reduction in the rate of first major vascular event (nonfatal MI, coronary death, stroke, or revascularization). This effect was apparent even for diabetic participants with baseline LDL <116 mg/dl *(50)*.

The Collaborative Atorvastatin Diabetes Study (CARDS) is unique in that it enrolled exclusively patients with diabetes. This primary prevention trial of nearly 3000 subjects, with median baseline LDL 117 mg/dl, randomized participants to treatment with atorvastatin 10 mg or placebo. The median LDL on treatment was 77 mg/dl, and 25% of patients achieved an LDL of <65 mg/dl. The trial was terminated early because of a 37% relative risk reduction in acute coronary heart disease events, coronary revascularization, and stroke. Death was reduced by 27%, of borderline statistical significance *(51)* (see Fig. 3) *(51)*.

Based on the above trials, as well as additional trials not reviewed here, the NCEP recommended the following in Adult Treatment Plan III, updated in 2004. All diabetes patients should be considered at high risk for development of cardiovascular disease and should therefore be treated aggressively, with an LDL goal <100 mg/dL. If LDL exceeds 100 mg/dL, therapeutic lifestyle changes should be initiated, including reductions in dietary total and saturated fat, weight loss in overweight patients, and aerobic exercise. Statin therapy can be considered for a baseline LDL 100–129 mg/dL and should be initiated for LDL 100–129 mg/dL despite therapeutic lifestyle changes or a baseline LDL ≥130 mg/dL. Additionally, based on data from HPS and PROVE IT, diabetes patients with known CAD can be considered to be at very high risk, with an optional LDL goal <70 mg/dl. Once treatment with a statin is initiated, doses should be titrated up to achieve at least a 30–40% reduction in LDL *(52)*.

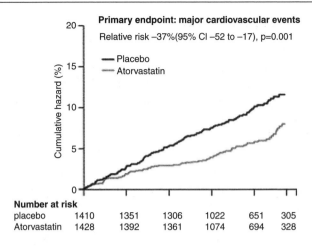

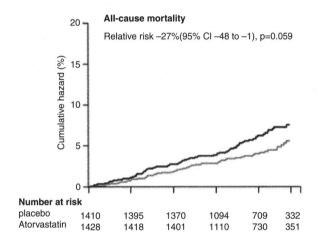

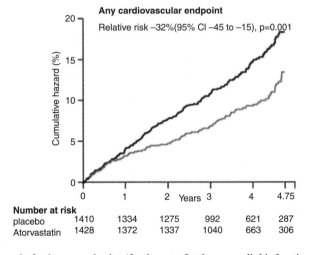

Fig. 3. Cumulative hazard of primary endpoint (fatal or nonfatal myocardial infarction, unstable angina, coronary revascularization, fatal or nonfatal stroke) by treatment with atorvastatin 10 mg vs. placebo, in CARDS. Reprinted with permission from Elsevier Science (From Colhoun et al. Primary prevention of cardiovascular disease with atorvastatin in type 2 diabetes in the Collaborative Atorvastatin Diabetes Study (CARDS): multicentre randomised placebo-controlled trial. The Lancet 2004; 364:685–96).

SECONDARY PREVENTION OF CARDIOVASCULAR DISEASE IN DIABETES – GLYCEMIC CONTROL

Tight glycemic control reduces the risk of both microvascular and macrovascular complications in people with diabetes. The Diabetes Control and Complications Trial (DCCT) first demonstrated that intensive insulin therapy decreased the risk of retinopathy, nephropathy, and neuropathy (microvascular complications) in patients with type 1 diabetes. Over 1400 participants, aged 13–39, were randomized to intensive or conventional insulin therapy. Intensive

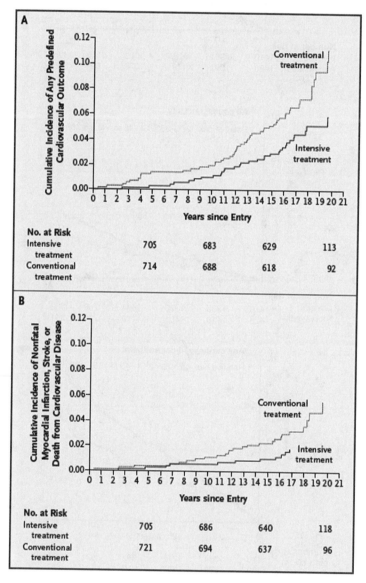

Fig. 4. Cumulative incidence of any of the predefined cardiovascular disease outcomes, including confirmed angina and need for coronary revascularization (panel A) and restricted to nonfatal myocardial infarction, stroke, or death from cardiovascular disease (panel B), by intensive glycemic control vs. conventional treatment in DCCT. Reprinted, by permission, from DM Nathan et al. Intensive diabetes treatment and cardiovascular disease in patients with type 1 diabetes. New Engl J Med 2005; 353:2643–53.

therapy involved three or more daily insulin injections or an insulin pump. Patients were followed for a mean of 6.5 years. At the end of the trial, the mean HbA1c was 7.4% in the intensive group and 9.1% in the conventional group. Greater than 50% reductions were achieved in development of retinopathy, proteinuria, and clinical neuropathy *(53)*.

The initial 6.5 years of follow-up demonstrated a trend toward decreased major cardiovascular events, but did not reach statistical significance, as patients were young with low absolute event rates *(54)*. However, the Epidemiology of Diabetes Interventions and Complications (EDIC) study extended follow-up an additional 11 years with excellent subject retention. During these 11 years, nearly all patients were treated with intensive insulin therapy, including 94% of those from the original conventional therapy group. Follow-up from the EDIC study demonstrated that intensive insulin treatment during the DCCT phase (first 6.5 years) decreased the risk of MI, stroke, and cardiovascular death by 57% over 16 years of follow-up *(55)*. See Fig. 4.

The UKPDS demonstrated that tight glycemic control also reduces the risk of microvascular complications in patients with type 2 diabetes. Nearly 4000 participants were randomized to intensive glycemic control, with a sulfonylurea or insulin, or to conventional treatment with diet alone. At the end of 10 years of follow-up, the mean HbA1c was 7.0% in the intensive group and 7.9% in the conventional group. The intensive group had 12% fewer diabetes-related events, mainly driven by 25% fewer microvascular endpoints, including the need for retinal photocoagulation *(56)*.

Decrease in macrovascular endpoints in type 2 diabetes has not yet been definitively demonstrated in randomized controlled trials of glycemic control. However, observational studies have documented a correlation of HbA1c to cardiovascular endpoints. A meta-analysis of 13 observational studies suggested an increase in relative risk of cardiovascular disease of 18% for every increase in HbA1c of 1% *(57)*. Similar observational studies have found an association between higher glucose levels and increased incidence of heart failure, even when adjusted for CAD *(18,19)*.

There is good evidence that intensive glycemic control reduces not only microvascular, but also macrovascular endpoints, in patients with type 1 and likely type 2 diabetes. The American Diabetes Association recommends lowering HbA1c to a goal of <7% for patients in general and as close to normal (<6%) as possible in individual patients, without causing significant hypoglycemia *(58)*.

SECONDARY PREVENTION OF CARDIOVASCULAR DISEASE IN DIABETES – SMOKING CESSATION

Smoking is common among people with diabetes. A 1989 survey of 2400 diabetes participants found that 27.3% were smokers, compared to 25.9% of the general population *(59)*. As has been well established in the general population, smokers with diabetes are at greater risk for death *(60)*. A dose–response relationship has been established between number of cigarettes smoked and risk for CAD *(61)*. Further, smoking leads to greater rates of microvascular complications, including nephropathy, neuropathy, and retinopathy *(62–64)*.

Mortality is related to duration of smoking, and risk returns toward normal years after quitting *(65)*. Smoking cessation programs have been shown to be successful in patients with diabetes and therefore need to be a high priority *(66)*.

SUMMARY

Diabetes is a common problem with a steadily increasing prevalence. People with diabetes develop cardiovascular disease at markedly increased rates, and have worse outcomes following cardiovascular events. Rates of cardiovascular disease can be controlled through aggressive risk factor modification. Blood pressure should be lowered to at least 130/80 mm Hg and likely lower, using thiazides, ACE inhibitors, or ARBs for first-line treatment, or beta-blockers in diabetes patients with known CAD. LDL cholesterol should be treated with a statin to a goal <100 mg/dl and in those with known CAD, can be treated to a goal <70 mg/dl. Once started, statins should be titrated to achieve at least a 30–40% LDL reduction. Blood sugar should be lowered as close to normal (HbA1c <6%) as possible, without causing significant hypoglycemia. All smokers should be encouraged to quit and offered smoking cessation interventions. Aspirin should be given as secondary prevention to diabetes patients who have had cardiovascular events, and as primary prevention to those over the age of 40 or with additional CAD risk factors *(58)*. Target-driven, intensified interventions aimed at multiple risk factors are likely the best strategy for preventing the epidemic in cardiovascular disease that is likely to result from the rising diabetes epidemic *(67)*.

ACKNOWLEDGMENTS

Dr Meigs is supported by an American Diabetes Association Career Development Award, has been the recipient of research grants from GlaxoSmithKline, Pfizer, and Wyeth, and has served on Advisory boards for GlaxoSmithKline, Merck, Pfizer, and Lilly.

REFERENCES

1. American-Diabetes-Association. National Diabetes Fact Sheet, 2005.
2. Harris MI, Flegal KM, Cowie CC, et al. Prevalence of diabetes, impaired fasting glucose, and impaired glucose tolerance in U.S. adults. The Third National Health and Nutrition Examination Survey, 1988–1994. Diabetes Care 1998; 21:518–24.
3. Turner RC, Holman RR. The UK Prospective Diabetes Study. UK Prospective Diabetes Study Group. Ann Med 1996; 28:439–44.
4. Wingard DL, Barrett-Connor E. Heart Disease and Diabetes. In: Harris MI, ed. Diabetes in America. Bethesda: National Institutes of Health, 1995:429–456.
5. Hogan P, Dall T, Nikolov P. Economic costs of diabetes in the US in 2002. Diabetes Care 2003; 26:917–32.
6. Kannel WB, McGee DL. Diabetes and cardiovascular disease. The Framingham study. JAMA 1979; 241: 2035–8.
7. Barrett-Connor E, Orchard TJ. Insulin-dependent diabetes mellitus and ischemic heart disease. Diabetes Care 1985; 8 Suppl 1:65–70.
8. Krolewski AS, Kosinski EJ, Warram JH, et al. Magnitude and determinants of coronary artery disease in juvenile-onset, insulin-dependent diabetes mellitus. Am J Cardiol 1987; 59:750–5.
9. Haffner SM, Lehto S, Ronnemaa T, Pyorala K, Laakso M. Mortality from coronary heart disease in subjects with type 2 diabetes and in nondiabetic subjects with and without prior myocardial infarction. N Engl J Med 1998; 339:229–34.
10. Third Report of the National Cholesterol Education Program (NCEP) Expert Panel on Detection, Evaluation, and Treatment of High Blood Cholesterol in Adults (Adult Treatment Panel III) final report. Circulation 2002; 106:3143–421.
11. Miettinen H, Lehto S, Salomaa V, et al. Impact of diabetes on mortality after the first myocardial infarction. The FINMONICA Myocardial Infarction Register Study Group. Diabetes Care 1998; 21:69–75.
12. Malmberg K, Yusuf S, Gerstein HC, et al. Impact of diabetes on long-term prognosis in patients with unstable angina and non-Q-wave myocardial infarction: results of the OASIS (Organization to Assess Strategies for Ischemic Syndromes) Registry. Circulation 2000; 102:1014–9.
13. Mukamal KJ, Nesto RW, Cohen MC, et al. Impact of diabetes on long-term survival after acute myocardial infarction: comparability of risk with prior myocardial infarction. Diabetes Care 2001; 24:1422–7.

14. Abbott RD, Donahue RP, Kannel WB, Wilson PW. The impact of diabetes on survival following myocardial infarction in men vs women. The Framingham Study. JAMA 1988; 260:3456–60.
15. Chyun D, Vaccarino V, Murillo J, Young LH, Krumholz HM. Cardiac outcomes after myocardial infarction in elderly patients with diabetes mellitus. Am J Crit Care 2002; 11:504–19.
16. Bertoni AG, Hundley WG, Massing MW, Bonds DE, Burke GL, Goff DC, Jr. Heart failure prevalence, incidence, and mortality in the elderly with diabetes. Diabetes Care 2004; 27:699–703.
17. Nichols GA, Gullion CM, Koro CE, Ephross SA, Brown JB. The incidence of congestive heart failure in type 2 diabetes: an update. Diabetes Care 2004; 27:1879–84.
18. Barzilay JI, Kronmal RA, Gottdiener JS, et al. The association of fasting glucose levels with congestive heart failure in diabetic adults > or =65 years: the Cardiovascular Health Study. J Am Coll Cardiol 2004; 43:2236–41.
19. Iribarren C, Karter AJ, Go AS, et al. Glycemic control and heart failure among adult patients with diabetes. Circulation 2001; 103:2668–73.
20. Bertoni AG, Tsai A, Kasper EK, Brancati FL. Diabetes and idiopathic cardiomyopathy: a nationwide case–control study. Diabetes Care 2003; 26:2791–5.
21. Mustonen JN, Uusitupa MI, Laakso M, et al. Left ventricular systolic function in middle-aged patients with diabetes mellitus. Am J Cardiol 1994; 73:1202–8.
22. Mildenberger RR, Bar-Shlomo B, Druck MN, et al. Clinically unrecognized ventricular dysfunction in young diabetic patients. J Am Coll Cardiol 1984; 4:234–8.
23. Zarich SW, Nesto RW. Diabetic cardiomyopathy. Am Heart J 1989; 118:1000–12.
24. Devereux RB, Roman MJ, Paranicas M, et al. Impact of diabetes on cardiac structure and function: the strong heart study. Circulation 2000; 101:2271–6.
25. Scognamiglio R, Avogaro A, Casara D, et al. Myocardial dysfunction and adrenergic cardiac innervation in patients with insulin-dependent diabetes mellitus. J Am Coll Cardiol 1998; 31:404–12.
26. Shindler DM, Kostis JB, Yusuf S, et al. Diabetes mellitus, a predictor of morbidity and mortality in the Studies of Left Ventricular Dysfunction (SOLVD) Trials and Registry. Am J Cardiol 1996; 77:1017–20.
27. Gustafsson I, Brendorp B, Seibaek M, et al. Influence of diabetes and diabetes–gender interaction on the risk of death in patients hospitalized with congestive heart failure. J Am Coll Cardiol 2004; 43:771–7.
28. Dries DL, Sweitzer NK, Drazner MH, Stevenson LW, Gersh BJ. Prognostic impact of diabetes mellitus in patients with heart failure according to the etiology of left ventricular systolic dysfunction. J Am Coll Cardiol 2001; 38:421–8.
29. Tight blood pressure control and risk of macrovascular and microvascular complications in type 2 diabetes: UKPDS 38. UK Prospective Diabetes Study Group. BMJ 1998; 317:703–13.
30. Adler AI, Stratton IM, Neil HA, et al. Association of systolic blood pressure with macrovascular and microvascular complications of type 2 diabetes (UKPDS 36): prospective observational study. BMJ 2000; 321:412–9.
31. Berl T, Hunsicker LG, Lewis JB, et al. Impact of achieved blood pressure on cardiovascular outcomes in the Irbesartan Diabetic Nephropathy Trial. J Am Soc Nephrol 2005; 16:2170–9.
32. Messerli FH, Mancia G, Conti CR, et al. Dogma disputed: can aggressively lowering blood pressure in hypertensive patients with coronary artery disease be dangerous? Ann Intern Med 2006; 144:884–93.
33. Arauz-Pacheco C. Hypertension Management in Adults with Diabetes: American Diabetes Association: Clinical Practice Recommendations 2004: Position Statement. Diabetes Care 2004; 27:S65–S67.
34. Major outcomes in high-risk hypertensive patients randomized to angiotensin-converting enzyme inhibitor or calcium channel blocker vs diuretic: The Antihypertensive and Lipid-Lowering Treatment to Prevent Heart Attack Trial (ALLHAT). JAMA 2002; 288:2981–97.
35. Curb JD, Pressel SL, Cutler JA, et al. Effect of diuretic-based antihypertensive treatment on cardiovascular disease risk in older diabetic patients with isolated systolic hypertension. Systolic Hypertension in the Elderly Program Cooperative Research Group. JAMA 1996; 276:1886–92.
36. Yusuf S, Sleight P, Pogue J, Bosch J, Davies R, Dagenais G. Effects of an angiotensin-converting-enzyme inhibitor, ramipril, on cardiovascular events in high-risk patients. The Heart Outcomes Prevention Evaluation Study Investigators. N Engl J Med 2000; 342:145–53.
37. Lindholm LH, Ibsen H, Dahlof B, et al. Cardiovascular morbidity and mortality in patients with diabetes in the Losartan Intervention for Endpoint reduction in hypertension study (LIFE): a randomised trial against atenolol. Lancet 2002; 359:1004–10.
38. Okin PM, Devereux RB, Liu JE, et al. Regression of electrocardiographic left ventricular hypertrophy predicts regression of echocardiographic left ventricular mass: the LIFE study. J Hum Hypertens 2004; 18:403–9.
39. Effects of ramipril on cardiovascular and microvascular outcomes in people with diabetes mellitus: results of the HOPE study and MICRO-HOPE substudy. Heart Outcomes Prevention Evaluation Study Investigators. Lancet 2000; 355:253–9.

40. Brenner BM, Cooper ME, de Zeeuw D, et al. Effects of losartan on renal and cardiovascular outcomes in patients with type 2 diabetes and nephropathy. N Engl J Med 2001; 345:861–9.

41. Efficacy of atenolol and captopril in reducing risk of macrovascular and microvascular complications in type 2 diabetes: UKPDS 39. UK Prospective Diabetes Study Group. BMJ 1998; 317:713–20.

42. Jonas M, Reicher-Reiss H, Boyko V, et al. Usefulness of beta-blocker therapy in patients with non-insulin-dependent diabetes mellitus and coronary artery disease. Bezafibrate Infarction Prevention (BIP) Study Group. Am J Cardiol 1996; 77:1273–7.

43. Bakris GL, Fonseca V, Katholi RE, et al. Metabolic effects of carvedilol vs metoprolol in patients with type 2 diabetes mellitus and hypertension: a randomized controlled trial. JAMA 2004; 292:2227–36.

44. Tuomilehto J, Rastenyte D, Birkenhager WH, et al. Effects of calcium-channel blockade in older patients with diabetes and systolic hypertension. Systolic Hypertension in Europe Trial Investigators. N Engl J Med 1999; 340:677–84.

45. Estacio RO, Jeffers BW, Hiatt WR, Biggerstaff SL, Gifford N, Schrier RW. The effect of nisoldipine as compared with enalapril on cardiovascular outcomes in patients with non-insulin-dependent diabetes and hypertension. N Engl J Med 1998; 338:645–52.

46. Dahlof B, Sever PS, Poulter NR, et al. Prevention of cardiovascular events with an antihypertensive regimen of amlodipine adding perindopril as required versus atenolol adding bendroflumethiazide as required, in the Anglo-Scandinavian Cardiac Outcomes Trial-Blood Pressure Lowering Arm (ASCOT-BPLA): a multicentre randomised controlled trial. Lancet 2005; 366:895–906.

47. Pyorala K, Pedersen TR, Kjekshus J, Faergeman O, Olsson AG, Thorgeirsson G. Cholesterol lowering with simvastatin improves prognosis of diabetic patients with coronary heart disease. A subgroup analysis of the Scandinavian Simvastatin Survival Study (4S). Diabetes Care 1997; 20:614–20.

48. Goldberg RB, Mellies MJ, Sacks FM, et al. Cardiovascular events and their reduction with pravastatin in diabetic and glucose-intolerant myocardial infarction survivors with average cholesterol levels: subgroup analyses in the cholesterol and recurrent events (CARE) trial. The Care Investigators. Circulation 1998; 98: 2513–9.

49. Cannon CP, Braunwald E, McCabe CH, et al. Intensive versus moderate lipid lowering with statins after acute coronary syndromes. N Engl J Med 2004; 350:1495–504.

50. Collins R, Armitage J, Parish S, Sleigh P, Peto R. MRC/BHF Heart Protection Study of cholesterol-lowering with simvastatin in 5963 people with diabetes: a randomised placebo-controlled trial. Lancet 2003; 361: 2005–16.

51. Colhoun HM, Betteridge DJ, Durrington PN, et al. Primary prevention of cardiovascular disease with atorvastatin in type 2 diabetes in the Collaborative Atorvastatin Diabetes Study (CARDS): multicentre randomised placebo-controlled trial. Lancet 2004; 364:685–96.

52. Grundy SM, Cleeman JI, Merz CN, et al. Implications of recent clinical trials for the National Cholesterol Education Program Adult Treatment Panel III guidelines. Circulation 2004; 110:227–39.

53. The effect of intensive treatment of diabetes on the development and progression of long-term complications in insulin-dependent diabetes mellitus. The Diabetes Control and Complications Trial Research Group. N Engl J Med 1993; 329:977–86.

54. Effect of intensive diabetes management on macrovascular events and risk factors in the Diabetes Control and Complications Trial. Am J Cardiol 1995; 75:894–903.

55. Nathan DM, Cleary PA, Backlund JY, et al. Intensive diabetes treatment and cardiovascular disease in patients with type 1 diabetes. N Engl J Med 2005; 353:2643–53.

56. Intensive blood-glucose control with sulphonylureas or insulin compared with conventional treatment and risk of complications in patients with type 2 diabetes (UKPDS 33). UK Prospective Diabetes Study (UKPDS) Group. Lancet 1998; 352:837–53.

57. Selvin E, Marinopoulos S, Berkenblit G, et al. Meta-analysis: glycosylated hemoglobin and cardiovascular disease in diabetes mellitus. Ann Intern Med 2004; 141:421–31.

58. American-Diabetes-Association. Standards of medical care in diabetes – 2006. Diabetes Care 2006; 29 Suppl 1:S4–S42.

59. Ford ES, Malarcher AM, Herman WH, Aubert RE. Diabetes mellitus and cigarette smoking. Findings from the 1989 National Health Interview Survey. Diabetes Care 1994; 17:688–92.

60. Moy CS, LaPorte RE, Dorman JS, et al. Insulin-dependent diabetes mellitus mortality. The risk of cigarette smoking. Circulation 1990; 82:37–43.

61. Al-Delaimy WK, Manson JE, Solomon CG, et al. Smoking and risk of coronary heart disease among women with type 2 diabetes mellitus. Arch Intern Med 2002; 162:273–9.

62. Chaturvedi N, Stephenson JM, Fuller JH. The relationship between smoking and microvascular complications in the EURODIAB IDDM Complications Study. Diabetes Care 1995; 18:785–92.

63. Chase HP, Garg SK, Marshall G, et al. Cigarette smoking increases the risk of albuminuria among subjects with type I diabetes. JAMA 1991; 265:614–7.

64. Mitchell BD, Hawthorne VM, Vinik AI. Cigarette smoking and neuropathy in diabetic patients. Diabetes Care 1990; 13:434–7.

65. Chaturvedi N, Stevens L, Fuller JH. Which features of smoking determine mortality risk in former cigarette smokers with diabetes? The World Health Organization Multinational Study Group. Diabetes Care 1997; 20:1266–72.

66. Canga N, De Irala J, Vara E, Duaso MJ, Ferrer A, Martinez-Gonzalez MA. Intervention study for smoking cessation in diabetic patients: a randomized controlled trial in both clinical and primary care settings. Diabetes Care 2000; 23:1455–60.

67. Gaede P, Vedel P, Larsen N, Jensen GV, Parving HH, Pedersen O. Multifactorial intervention and cardiovascular disease in patients with type 2 diabetes. N Engl J Med 2003; 348:383–93.

3 Disruption of the Nitric Oxide Signaling System in Diabetes

Bobby D. Nossaman, MD, Subramanyam N. Murthy, PhD, and Philip J. Kadowitz, PhD

CONTENTS

SUMMARY

Diabetes has become a national and international epidemic with the incidence of diabetes expecting to double by the year 2030. The metabolic and structural abnormalities observed in diabetic patients, in patients with the metabolic syndrome, and now being observed in the post-surgical intensive care unit, have all been associated with the development of endothelial dysfunction. Recent studies suggest that this finding of endothelial dysfunction may be due to decreased bioavailability of a key signaling molecule, nitric oxide (NO), which is due to disruption of the endothelial nitric oxide synthase (eNOS)/soluble guanylate cyclase/cyclic guanosine monophosphate (cGMP)-dependent pathway. Disruption of this pathway results in an oxidative and nitrosative stress state that accelerates the progression and the complications of cardiovascular disease found in diabetes. The purpose of this chapter is to review current information about the disruption of this important signaling system especially in the context of diabetes.

Research Support: NIH Grant HL62000, HL77421, ES10018, and RR16456.

From: *Contemporary Endocrinology: Cardiovascular Endocrinology: Shared Pathways and Clinical Crossroads*
Edited by: V. A. Fonseca © Humana Press, New York, NY

Key Words: Nitric oxide, Diabetes, Endothelial dysfunction, Endothelial nitric oxide synthase, Cyclic GMP pathway, Oxidative stress, Nitrosative stress, Insulin resistance

INTRODUCTION

Types of Diabetes

Diabetes is a costly and a major national and international health problem, with an estimated global prevalence of 170 million. This finding is expected to double by 2030 due to increases in population growth, aging, urbanization, and the increasing prevalence of obesity and physical inactivity *(1–4)*.

"Type 2 diabetes" accounts for 90% of diabetes and occurs mainly in adults, but is now being reported in adolescents and children *(5,6)*. It is characterized by the development of insulin resistance and is often associated with obesity, hypertension, and dyslipidemia *(7–9)*. The main etiology for mortality in these patients is the accelerated development of atherosclerosis and subsequent end-organ damage *(1,10–13)*. Moreover, the insulin resistance found in type 2 diabetes is associated with vascular dysfunction/damage, impaired fibrinolysis, and low-grade inflammation that is independent of obesity and poor glycemic control *(4,9,14)*. Patients with the metabolic syndrome or patients with pre-diabetes are also associated with increased cardiovascular mortality, suggesting that the findings of atherogenic vascular changes begin prior to the onset of overt diabetes. Endothelial dysfunction appears to be the initial lesion seen in patients with cardiovascular risk factors *(10,15,16)*.

"Type 1 diabetes" occurs predominantly in children and in young adults, and accounts for 5%–10% of diagnosed cases. It is characterized by the development of an insulin deficiency due to the destruction of pancreatic beta cells *(1,17–20)*.

"Gestational diabetes" accounts for a small percentage and usually resolves following delivery. However, these patients are more likely to develop overt diabetes within 10 years of this obstetrical complication and therefore should have long-term follow-up to ameliorate this increased risk *(21–24)*. Maternal vascular endothelial dysfunction contributes to the increased incidence of cardiovascular disorders in women with gestational diabetes, and than treatment of gestational diabetes reduces serious perinatal morbidity *(24,25)*.

"Diabetes of injury" develops in critically ill patients and is associated with an increase in adverse outcome in patients with prolonged critical illness *(26,28)*. The use of intensive insulin therapy to maintain control of postoperative hyperglycemia improves mortality and morbidity in critically ill surgical patients, whereas the benefit for other patient populations, such as patients in medical intensive care units or in hospitalized patients who do not require intensive care but who do present with stress-induced hyperglycemia, remains to be proved *(26)*. Moreover, if intensive insulin therapy is implemented during surgery, it may improve or worsen mortality, neurologic outcome, or the incidence of critical illness polyneuropathy/myopathy *(27–37)*.

Assessment for Diabetes

Hyperglycemia was the most prominent routine laboratory measurement seen in both types of diabetes; however, the recent discovery of elevated seromarkers of oxidative and nitrosative stress can be found in patients who have pre-diabetes, insulin resistance, metabolic syndrome, following surgical stress, and can be even observed in diabetic patients with well-controlled glycemia *(2,21,38–50)*.

Although biomarkers such as total cholesterol, low-density lipoprotein (LDL) cholesterol, and hemoglobin A1c (HbA1c) are routinely used in the detection and management of cardiovascular disease including diabetes, the development of specific biomarkers could be used to study endothelial function as surrogate markers of cardiovascular risk, like those seen in patients with pre-diabetes, metabolic syndrome, or insulin resistance. Serial assessments of these biomarkers could indirectly assess the clinical efficacy of current or potential treatments, or these biomarkers could be directly targeted as a means of therapy, although initial results are discouraging *(37,39,51–55)*. However, the administration of insulin/glucose-insulin-potassium regimen has been shown to suppress production of tumor necrosis factor-alpha, interleukin-6, macrophage migration inhibitory factor, free radicals, and enhance the synthesis of endothelial NO, but these findings are not supported in other studies *(37,56)*.

Risks in Diabetes

All diabetic patients, whether type 1 or 2, have a twofold to eightfold increase in the risk of developing cardiovascular disease, peripheral arterial disease, and congestive heart failure *(6,14,57,58)*. Moreover, 80% of individuals with diabetes die from cardiovascular disease and have a worse prognosis for survival, as mortality from cardiovascular disease is almost three times higher in patients with diabetes than which is found in the general population *(6,57,58)*.

VASCULAR ENDOTHELIUM

The vascular endothelium consists of a continuous cellular monolayer lining the blood vessels, and has important homeostatic functions. It participates in highly active metabolic and regulatory functions, including control of coagulation and fibrinolysis, platelet and leukocyte interactions within the vessel lumen, interactions with lipoproteins, regulation of smooth muscle cell growth, and control of vascular tone. The normal endothelium maintains a relaxed vascular tone, with low levels of oxidative and nitrosative stress. This lining also maintains an antiproliferative, anti-inflammatory, and anti-apoptotic environment within the vessel wall through the functions of vasodilation, platelet inhibition, and anti-inflammation through the secretion of NO, prostacyclin, and endothelium-derived hyperpolarization factor, and in the suppression of formation of endothelin-1 and of angiotensin II *(48,59–63)*. However, the endothelium is extremely vulnerable and this lining may be disturbed by a number of endogenous and exogenous factors. These factors include psychological and physical stress, and disease states including atherosclerosis, hypertension, aging, inflammation, and diabetes that transform the lining from a quiescent state to an activated state marked by vasospasm, inflammation, leukocyte and platelet adhesion and aggregation, thrombosis, abnormal vascular proliferation, atherosclerosis, and hypertension *(64–75)*.

NO SYNTHASE/SOLUBLE GUANYLATE CYCLASE/CYCLIC GMP-DEPENDENT PATHWAY

It now appears that the production of NO from the endothelium is the most important event not only for regulation of vasomotor tone in the arterial bed, but also for maintaining the anti-inflammatory and antithrombotic properties in the vascular bed *(76–78)*. In the endothelium, NO is generated by the conversion of L-arginine to L-citrulline by the constitutive enzyme, eNOS, and this isoform is responsible for most of the vascular NO produced *(78–80)*. Although both the L- and D-enantiomers of arginine are present within the human circulation, only L-arginine is recognized by eNOS *(81,82)*. Biochemical factors, such as acetylcholine or bradykinin, or shear stress, activate membrane receptors on the endothelial cells, cause an influx of calcium, and activation of eNOS generating NO *(76,78,79,83,84)*. The NO generated within vascular endothelial cells, diffuses into vascular smooth muscle, stimulates guanylate cyclase to generate cGMP that eventually induces vasodilation. This process is termed endothelium-dependent vasodilation. However, clinically used nitrosodonors, such as nitroglycerin and sodium nitroprusside, can directly release NO or release NO following cleavage from an enzymatic reaction. The NO that is released from these donors acts via the same signaling pathway as endogenously produced NO to produce relaxation of vascular smooth muscle and vasodilation. This process is termed endothelium-independent vasodilation *(76,78,81)*.

ENDOTHELIAL DYSFUNCTION

Endothelial dysfunction is defined as an imbalance in the formation of relaxing and contracting factors, procoagulant and anticoagulant mediators, and growth-inhibiting and -promoting substances, with a resultant shift of endothelial function toward a reduced vasodilator, proinflammatory, prothrombotic state as shown in Fig. 1 *(85–87)*. Furthermore, ongoing injury to the endothelium results in cellular dysfunction with impaired release of endogenous NO *(88,89)*. Endothelial dysfunction is hypothesized to be an early stage of the atherosclerotic process and results from chronic exposure to cardiovascular risk factors. Indeed, endothelial dysfunction is integral to the pathogenesis of atherosclerosis and diabetes as the development of insulin resistance, metabolic syndrome, and atherosclerosis follow similar pathways *(15,40,78,90–93)*.

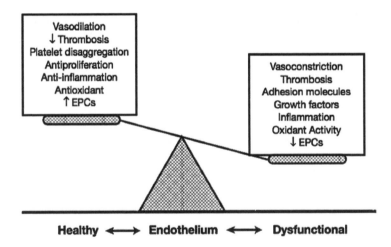

Fig. 1. Endothelial dysfunction is defined as an imbalance in the formation of relaxing and contracting factors, procoagulant and anticoagulant mediators, growth-inhibiting and -promoting substances, with a shift of endothelial function towards reduced vasodilator, proinflammatory, and prothrombotic state *(87)*.

INFLUENCES OF DIABETES ON THE VASCULAR WALL

The detection of hyperglycemia and elevated glycosylated hemoglobin (HbA1c) was, until recently, considered to be the only early laboratory methods of detection for the presence of type 2 diabetes. However, recent studies suggest that the use of biomarkers of oxidative and nitrosative stress may be the earliest manifestation for the presence of endothelial dysfunction in the development of diabetes. Moreover, some of these studies suggest that this dysfunction may be due to reduced bioavailability of endothelial-derived NO (Fig. 2) *(39,40,51–55,94–97)*.

Dysfunction of the eNOS/soluble guanylate cyclase/cGMP system is a common mechanism by which cardiovascular risk factors such as diabetes, hypertension, smoking, dyslipidemia, vascular inflammation, menopause, hyperhomocysteinemia, and sedentary lifestyle mediate their deleterious effects on the vascular wall *(2,9,98–104)*.

The Role of the Endothelium in Diabetes

Although the pathogenesis and progression of cardiovascular disease in diabetes is multi-factorial and can be affected by metabolic or other factors, the presence of atherosclerosis is a major factor *(10,105)*. The hypothesis that the initial lesion of atherosclerosis is endothelial dysfunction has been documented in patients with diabetes, in individuals with insulin resistance, or those at high risk for developing type 2 diabetes *(10,106–110)*. Clinically, endothelial dysfunction can be measured with changes in the seromarkers produced by the vasculature *(39,51–55)*, or by measuring the degree of blunting of the NO-dependent vasodilatory endothelial response to acetylcholine or the degree of reactive hyperemia following short-term arterial obstruction *(111–122)*.

The Effect of Diabetes on eNOS Substrate and Cofactors

The decrease in the bioavailability of endogenous NO that is seen in diabetes can be due to a deficiency of the NOS substrate, L-arginine, or due to decreased availability of one or more cofactors essential for optimal functioning of NOS (Fig. 2). Other factors that contribute include post-translational control mechanisms, and uncoupling of receptor-mediated signal transduction *(40,50,80,123–128)*.

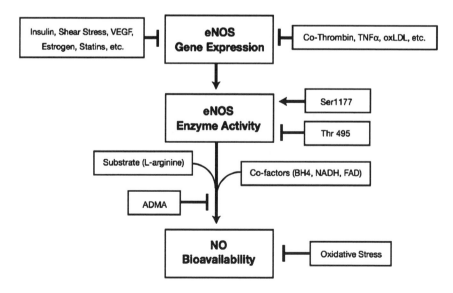

Fig. 2. Diagram demonstrating the factors and co-factors that lead to decreased NO bioavailability *(128)*.
Source: Redrawn from Yang & Ming *(128)*.

L-Arginine Deficiency

"Conditionally essential nutrients" (CENs) are organic compounds that are ordinarily produced by the body in amounts sufficient to meet its physiological requirements. However, in stressful conditions, such as cardiovascular disease, biosynthesis may be inadequate. Under these circumstances, these CENs become essential nutrients, comparable to vitamins. The CENs of primary importance in cardiovascular disease are coenzyme Q10, L-carnitine, propionyl-L-carnitine, and L-arginine (129,130). L-arginine is usually not rate-limiting except during high demand states, such as observed in atheroscleropathy associated with type 2 diabetes (131). Reductions in L-arginine may decrease eNOS activity in the diabetic vascular bed (132,133). Dietary supplementation of L-arginine may help protect arteries against atherosclerosis since chronic L-arginine supplementation is known to improve insulin sensitivity and endothelial function as observed in nonobese type 2 diabetic patients and in experimental models of diabetes (134–137). L-Arginine supplementation improves endothelial function in smokers as well as in patients with hypercholesterolemia, and hypertension (99). Dietary supplementations with fish oils or flavanol-rich cocoa, caseinate, or soy protein have also been shown to augment endothelium-dependent relaxation (138–140).

The modern Western diet, with its excess of refined products such as sugar and fats, often contains a deficiency of nutrients such as zinc, selenium, and vitamins A, B, C, and E. However, adequate intake of these nutrients can help minimize diabetic complications (141–146). For example, the antioxidant, vitamin C, has been shown to improve endothelium-dependent vasodilation in patients with either insulin-dependent or non-insulin-dependent diabetes mellitus. These studies support the hypothesis that in diabetes oxygen-derived free radicals inactivate NO and contribute to abnormal vascular reactivity (147,148).

Post-Translational Control Mechanisms

Historically eNOS has been thought to be a constitutively expressed enzyme regulated by calcium and calmodulin. However, it is becoming clear that eNOS activity and subsequent release of NO can be regulated by post-translational control mechanisms, such as eNOS phosphorylation and activation of RhoA/Rho-kinase. In addition, protein–protein interactions as seen with heat shock protein 90 (Hsp90) and with caveolin-1 may modulate the duration and magnitude of NO release (124,149).

eNOS Phosphorylation

Regulation of endothelial NO synthesis by multisite eNOS phosphorylation occurs in response to a wide variety of humoral, mechanical, and pharmacological stimuli. This regulation involves numerous kinases and phosphatases (150). Production of reactive-oxygen species (ROS) is increased in patients with diabetes, especially in diabetics with poor glycemic control. The increase in ROS is associated with a perturbation of signaling pathways (151–153).

Multiple protein kinases including Ser/Thr kinase Akt/PKB (protein kinase B), cAMP-dependent protein kinase, and the AMP-activated protein kinase, activate eNOS by phosphorylation of Ser-1177 in response to various stimuli (Fig. 2). For example, in endothelial cells there is a transient increase in Ser-1177 phosphorylation associated with a concomitant decrease in Thr-495 phosphorylation during vascular endothelial growth factor (VEGF) signaling (154), whereas in endothelial cells during protein kinase C signaling, inhibition of eNOS activity occurs via phosphorylation of Thr-495 and dephosphorylation of Ser-1177. Protein kinase A signaling, on the contrary, involves phosphorylation of Ser-1177 and dephosphorylation of Thr-495 to activate eNOS *(154,155)*.

The Ser/Thr kinase Akt/PKB pathway is involved in the metabolic effects of insulin and this pathway is remarkably well conserved across a broad range of species *(156)*. Recent studies in human endothelial cells suggest that insulin activates eNOS by PKB-mediated phosphorylation at Ser-1177 *(157–159)*. However in hyperglycemia, eNOS activity decreases due to an impairment of eNOS phosphorylation at Ser-1177 *(149,159,160)*, but this finding has not been found in all studies *(161)*.

In addition to phosphorylation of Ser-1177 as being a critical requirement for eNOS activation, phosphorylation of eNOS at Ser-633 also increases eNOS activity. Regulated phosphorylation of eNOS also occurs at Ser-114 and Ser-615; however, the functions of these phosphorylation sites remain controversial *(150)*. Finally, recent studies in endothelial cells suggest that the phosphorylation/dephosphorylation cycle of Thr-497 (the Thr-495 equivalent in bovine endothelial cells) may be an important mechanism that determines whether eNOS generates NO or generates superoxide anion *(155)*.

RhoA/Rho-Kinase Pathway

Rho signaling pathways serve homeostatic functions under normal physiological conditions, but appear to be highly activated under conditions of inflammation. Moreover with sustained activation, pathological consequences are observed in occlusive diseases ranging from atherosclerosis to restenosis injury *(162)*. When Rho-kinase is activated, eNOS expression is inhibited, whereas inhibition of Rho kinase results in an increase in eNOS expression (see Fig. 3) *(163)*.

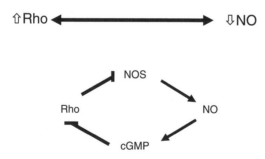

Fig. 3. Diagram demonstrating the balance of Rho activation leading to inhibition of nitric oxide synthase in inflammatory states *(170)*.

Smooth muscle contraction is mediated by phosphorylation of myosin light chain (MLC) via the Ca^{2+}/calmodulin-dependent activation of MLC kinase and actin/myosin cross-bridge formation *(164,165)*. Smooth muscle relaxation is mediated by dephosphorylation of MLC via MLC phosphatase *(166)*. A principle regulator of MLC phosphatase is Rho-kinase, which belongs to the serine/threonine kinase family. RhoA, a GTP-binding protein, mediates agonist-induced activation of Rho-kinase *(167–169)*. It was previously found that the Rho-kinase protein expression was increased in diabetic rabbit corporal tissue, suggesting that RhoA/Rho-kinase signaling pathway contributes to diabetes-related ED *(165)*. In studies using an animal model, we observed downregulation of eNOS expression by RhoA/Rho-kinase that contributed to diabetes-related vascular dysfunction *(170).*

Hsp90 and Caveolin-1

Recent studies have shown that eNOS activity and NO release can also be regulated by post-translational control mechanisms (phosphorylation) and by protein–protein interactions (with caveolin-1 and Hsp90) *(124).* Hsp90 and caveolin-1 act as major activators of eNOS. High glucose levels can impair eNOS activity via alterations in Hsp90 interactions affecting eNOS function and thereby reducing NO production *(149,171).* It appears that translocation of Hsp90 by high glucose levels is the mechanism by which diabetes impairs eNOS activity and hence reduces NO production *(171).* However, metformin, a drug commonly used in combination therapy for the treatment of type 1 and type 2 diabetes, increases NO release by increasing eNOS association with Hsp90 *(172).*

Unlike the effect of Hsp90 interacting with eNOS, the binding of caveolin-1 to eNOS (in the caveolae) partially inhibits eNOS activity by occupying a calmodulin-binding site *(172,173).* Caveolae are vesicular invaginations in the plasma membrane that mediate the intracellular transport of lipids such as cholesterol *(174).* Receptor activation or humoral and mechanical stimuli, such as estrogen and shear stress, induce redistribution of eNOS away from plasma membrane caveolae to internal membrane structures. This removes tonic inhibition and results in eNOS activation *(172).*

eNOS Uncoupling and the Oxidative Stress State

Uncoupling of constitutive NOS can result in overproduction of superoxide and peroxynitrite. These two potent cellular oxidants switch eNOS from a NO-producing enzyme to a superoxide-producing enzyme, a phenomenon termed eNOS uncoupling. In this uncoupled state, electrons are diverted to molecular oxygen rather than to L-arginine. This results in the production of superoxide instead of NO, which decreases the functional activity of eNOS. The mechanism underlying eNOS uncoupling appears to be through oxidation of the zinc thiolate cluster of eNOS and the cofactor tetrahydro-L-biopterin (BH4), and the decreased availability of the NOS substrate, L-arginine, have been proposed to lead to monomerization of eNOS, increased production of ROS, and reduced NO production by the enzyme *(175).* The major oxidant of leukocyte-derived myeloperoxidase, hypochlorous acid, has been reported to oxidize the zinc-thiolate center of eNOS and uncouples the enzyme *(142).*

Methylated L-Arginines

In several human diseases, such as hyperhomocysteinemia, hypertension, and diabetes, there are increases in serum levels of methylated L-arginines, such as asymmetrical dimethylarginine (ADMA) and monomethylarginine (L-NMMA). These endogenously produced amino acids inhibit all three isoforms of NOS, and are synthesized during the methylation of protein arginine residues. ADMA cannot be used as a substrate by eNOS for the formation of NO. Furthermore, ADMA inhibits NOS that decreases NO bioavailability (Fig. 2) *(176–178).* Recently, it has been demonstrated that plasma levels of ADMA are elevated in patients with diabetes, nonfatal stroke, myocardial infarction, and renal dysfunction, *(132,179).* In patients with type 2 diabetes, intensive correction of hyperglycemia was associated with a reduction in the levels of ADMA (Fig. 2) *(111,180).*

Oxidized LDL

The oxidation of LDL is an early event found in atherosclerosis and that oxidized LDL (oxLDL) contributes to atherosclerosis *(181)*. Studies suggest that oxLDL is able to decrease local endothelial uptake of L-arginine. This effect leads to local depletion of L-arginine, eNOS uncoupling, and overproduction of superoxide anions from oxygen *(182,183)*. Moreover, endothelial cells from diabetic patients are more likely to undergo endothelial apoptosis due to the action of glycated LDL *(184)*.

In animal studies and in small-scale human trials, administration of the antioxidants, vitamins E or C, was found to attenuate diabetes-associated vascular dysfunction, such as lowering oxLDL, and decreasing oxidiative stress *(185–189)*. However, larger clinical trials failed to demonstrate any beneficial therapeutic effect of vitamins C and E in diabetic patients with cardiovascular disease *(190–194)*.

Tetrahydrobiopterin (BH4)

eNOS is responsible for most of the vascular NO produced. Normal function of eNOS requires dimerization of the enzyme, the availability of the substrate, L-arginine, and the essential cofactor, BH4 *(80)*. BH4 stabilizes the active dimeric form of eNOS to facilitate electron transfer from the reductase domain to the oxygenase domain of NOS that increases L-arginine binding (Fig. 4) *(195)*.

Exposure of endothelial cells to high concentrations of glucose leads to disruption of the zinc-thiolate cluster on eNOS (where the BH4-binding site is located), which reduces intracellular BH4 bioavailability *(175)* (Fig. 4). This action results in decreased production and increased consumption of NO, and increased generation of free radicals, such as superoxide and peroxynitrite *(196)*. Furthermore, BH4 is highly sensitive to oxidation by peroxynitrite. BH4 levels also regulate proliferation of normal endothelial cells and a BH4 deficiency impairs NO-dependent proliferation of these cells *(197)*. This transformation of eNOS from a protective enzyme to a contributor to oxidative stress has been observed in patients with cardiovascular risk factors *(80,198)*. Dietary supplementation with BH4 improves endothelial function in diabetic patients *(199)*. In addition, administration of folic acid and infusions of vitamin C are able to restore eNOS functionality, most probably by enhancing BH4 levels *(80)*. As BH4 plays an

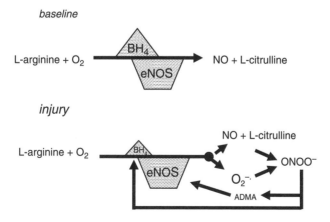

Fig. 4. Diagram depicting eNOS uncoupling *(175)*.

important role in regulating eNOS and structure activity, increasing levels of endothelial BH4 and/or protecting it from oxidation may be a viable therapeutic option to restore NO-mediated endothelial function in diabetes and in other vascular disease states *(200,201)*.

NITROSATIVE STRESS STATE

Inducible NOS Activation

In contrast to beneficial effects of NO produced from eNOS, the generation of NO from inducible NOS (iNOS), can be stimulated in vascular tissues in response to inflammatory mediators. This level of NO expression is not normally found in healthy cells, but is observed when the endothelium is activated in response to proinflammatory signals *(202)*. The elevated production of NO is more deleterious if it is associated with increased formation of ROS, particularly superoxide *(48,203)*. Diabetes is associated with oxidative stress and increased expression of iNOS, and may produce peroxynitrite. Peroxynitrite assaults the vascular endothelium, vascular smooth muscle, and the myocardium, leading to cardiovascular dysfunction. Increased production of peroxynitrite not only causes nitrosative stress, which is cytotoxic to tissues, but also reduces the bioavailability of functional NO and contributes to impaired endothelium-mediated relaxation *(48,204)*. The presence of increased oxidative and nitrosative stress play important roles in the development and progression of cardiovascular disease found in diabetes *(2,10,21,40,42,48,58,203,205–207)*.

Peroxynitrite

Endothelial cells produce NO and the combination of NO with superoxide in hyperglycemic studies results in the production of peroxynitrite. Peroxynitrite reacts with protein and nonprotein thiol groups resulting in injury in most cell types *(208–213)*. Studies support a pathologic role for endogenous peroxynitrite formation in diabetes, as increased levels of nitrotyrosine, a biomarker of peroxynitrite, is reported in plasma and in the platelets of diabetic patients *(214,215)*. Nitrotyrosine is harmful to endothelial cells as it may contribute to vascular endothelial dysfunction through promotion of DNA damage and/or apoptosis *(216)*. Moreover, high-glucose conditions can alter prostacyclin synthase, which further suppresses the vasodilatory, growth-inhibiting, antithrombotic, and antiadhesive effects of the endothelium and promotes the release of potent vasoconstrictor, prothrombotic, growth- and adhesion-promoting agents, such as thromboxane A2 *(50,217,218)*.

Peroxynitrite has been reported to attack various biomolecules, leading to compromised cardiovascular function in diabetes via numerous mechanisms *(219–221)*. Studies in our laboratory have shown that the cytotoxic effects of peroxynitrite may have been overemphasized. Although the toxic effects of peroxynitrite on vascular smooth muscle, endothelial cells, and platelets have been described in many studies, it has also been reported that peroxynitrite has protective effects in ischemia reperfusion injury models *(222–228)*. Peroxynitrite has been shown to have vasorelaxant properties and to induce vasodilation in the anesthetized rat *(229)*. In addition to having vasodilator activity, it has been reported that tachyphylaxis develops to the response, and peroxynitrite impairs vasodilator and vasoconstrictor responses *(230–234)*. The mechanism by which peroxynitrite relaxes vascular smooth muscle has been reported to involve the release of NO, the activation of soluble guanylate cyclase, and the accumulation of cGMP in vascular smooth muscle cells *(235–237)*. It has been postulated that the rapid reaction of NO and superoxide may provide a mechanism for disposal of excess superoxide and to prolong the vasodilator actions of NO *(238–240)*. We found that repeated injections of peroxynitrite did not alter responses to vasoconstrictor or vasodilator agents, including acetylcholine, indicating that vasoconstrictor and vasodilator mechanisms, including endothelium-dependent responses, were not altered by short-term exposure to peroxynitrite. Our findings are consistent with the hypothesis that peroxynitrite is rapidly converted in the circulation to a compound that has the properties of an NO donor and it is possible that NO formation may mediate the vasodilator response to peroxynitrite *(241,242)*.

Poly(ADP-ribose) Polymerase

Peroxynitrite can attack certain biomolecules through a number of pathways that can lead to the compromised cardiovascular function seen in diabetes *(219–221)*. Although nitrosative stress results in many damaging cellular effects, it is the effect on cellular DNA, which is the most damaging to cellular function. Nitrosative stress induces DNA single-strand breaks and leads to overactivation of a DNA repair enzyme, poly(ADP-ribose) polymerase (PARP) *(48,243–247)*.

PARP comprise a family of enzymes that catalyzes poly(ADP-ribosyl)ation of DNA-binding proteins. PARP is one of the most abundant nuclear proteins, and functions as a DNA nick sensor enzyme. However, in response to excessive oxidative- or nitrosative-mediated DNA single-strand breaks, activation of PARP initiates an energy-consuming, inefficient cellular metabolic cycle that leads to functional impairment of affected cells, such as seen in beta-cells of the pancreas or in vascular endothelial cells, which eventually promotes cellular dysfunction and necrotic cell death *(48,246,248,249)*.

PARP also appears to modulate the course of inflammation by regulating the activation of nuclear factor kappa B that regulates the expression of genes involved in inflammation and in diabetic vascular dysfunction *(48,243,249,250)*.

MITOCHONDRIA

Abnormal endothelial function plays a pivotal role in the pathogenesis of diabetic complications due to vascular damage which develop as a consequence of chronic diabetes. One pathophysiological sequence revolves around the metabolic abnormalities triggered as a result of overproduction of superoxide by the mitochondrial electron transport chain. NO can influence mitochondrial respiratory activity, through direct effects on the respiratory chain or indirectly via modulation of mitochondrial calcium accumulation. At pathological concentrations, NO can cause irreversible changes in respiratory function and can also interact with ROS to form reactive-nitrogen species (RNS), which may further impair mitochondrial respiration and can even lead to opening of mitochondrial permeability transition pores and cellular death. Diabetes, as well as aging, and heart failure are associated with increased generation of ROS that alters the regulatory balance of NO in the mitochondria *(251,252)*. Overproduction of mitochondrial superoxide increases DNA strand breaks that activate PARP, an enzyme involved in DNA repair. However, PARP activation results in inhibition of glyceraldehyde-3-phosphate dehydrogenase (GAPDH) by poly-ADP-ribosylation. Inhibition of GAPDH activity decreases the amount of ATP available to cells. Additionally, activation of PARP results in depletion of NAD and ATP, with both processes leading to acute endothelial dysfunction in diabetic blood vessels and contributes to the development of diabetic complications *(253)*.

Redox Signaling

Free radicals and related ROS such as O$_2$-, HO-, ONOO-, and ROO- are associated with endothelial dysfunction. These ROS are constantly produced in small amounts; however, hyperglycemia from uncontrolled glucose regulation, causes autoxidation of glucose, glycation of proteins, and increased flux through the polyol pathway that leads to decreased NO bioavailability. These processes play important roles in diabetic complications that accelerate tissue damage via generation of ROS *(254)*.

Autoxidation

In diabetes, sustained hyperglycemia produces increased intracellular concentrations of glucose metabolites in endothelial cells. Increased intracellular metabolism of glucose leads to overproduction of nicotinamide adenine dinucleotide (NADH) (Fig. 5).

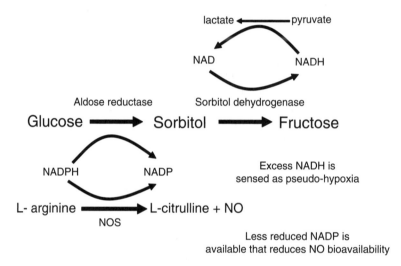

Fig. 5. Excess glucose (hyperglycemia) results in metabolism to fructose and generates nicotinamide adenine dinucleotide (NADH) in the process. Overproduction of NADH leads to the body's perception of hypoxia. Moreover, hyperglycemia also results in the consumption of nicotinamide adenine dinucleotide phosphate (NADPH), which leads to less protection against ROS toxicity. Once formed, ROS deplete antioxidant defenses, rendering the affected cells and tissues more susceptible to oxidative damage.

Excess NADH produces excess mitochondrial protons with electrons now transferring to oxygen and producing ROS *(152,255)*. ROS reduce NO bioavailability and also inhibit the synthesis of prostacyclin *(256)* (Fig. 5).

Advanced Glycation End-Products

Nonenzymatic glycation is implicated in the development of various diseases such as Alzheimer's and diabetes that have been shown to accelerate the physiologic process of aging. An increase in the generation of ROS can occur by glucose autoxidation and by nonenzymatic glycation. Both of these processes lead to the formation of advanced glycation end-products (AGEs) *(255,257)*. AGEs are proteins or lipids that become glycated after exposure to sugars, referred to as the Maillard, or Browning, reaction. Scientists have been interested in the Maillard reaction as it is associated with food spoilage. AGEs, especially glyceraldehyde-derived AGEs, play an important role in the pathogenesis of angiopathy in diabetic patients *(258)*.

AGEs contribute to a variety of vascular complications through the formation of cross-links between molecules in the basement membrane of the extracellular matrix *(21,259)*. AGEs also block NO activity in the endothelium and cause the production of ROS *(259,260)*.

Polyol Pathway

Two enzymes, aldose reductase (AR) and sorbitol dehydrogenase (SDH), contribute to ROS generation. There is strong evidence that AR, the first and rate-limiting enzyme of the polyol pathway that converts glucose to fructose, plays a key role in the pathogenesis of microvascular complications. AR uses NADPH for reduction of glucose to sorbitol. Under normal conditions sorbitol production by AR is a minor reaction, whereas under conditions of hyperglycemia, up to 35% of glucose is metabolized by this pathway *(261,262)*. Recent work demonstrated that exposure to NO donors or L-arginine significantly decreased AR activity and sorbitol accumulation in diabetic tissues *(263)*. However, clinical trials of the AR inhibitors were disappointing and several pharmaceutical companies abandoned further development of this line of drugs, although the development of new AR inhibitors is warranted.

SDH oxidizes sorbitol to fructose with a concurrent increase in NADH levels. Increased NADH can be used by NADPH oxidases to produce superoxide production *(21)*.

There are three potential mechanisms for the polyol pathway to contribute to oxidative stress. AR activity depletes its cofactor NADPH, which is also required for glutathione reductase to regenerate GSH. Under hyperglycemic conditions, glucose is channeled into the polyol pathway resulting in a substantial depletion of NADPH and decreases in GSH levels. AR activity diminishes the cellular antioxidant capacity during hyperglycemia. Oxidation of sorbitol to fructose by SDH induces oxidative stress as its cofactor NAD^+ is converted to NADH, with increased levels of NADH as the substrate for NADH oxidase to generate ROS. The polyol pathway converts glucose to fructose. Because fructose and its metabolites, fructose-3-phosphate and 3-deoxyglucosone, are more potent nonenzymatic glycation agents than glucose, the flux of glucose through the polyol pathway increases formation of AGEs. AGEs are known to increase oxidative stress *(264)*.

Insulin Resistance

Insulin resistance in most cases is believed to manifest at the cellular level via post-receptor defects in insulin signaling. Insulin resistance has been described in several diseases that increase cardiovascular risk and mortality, including diabetes, obesity, hypertension, metabolic syndrome, and heart failure *(265)*. Insulin resistance syndrome consists of the presence of glucose intolerance, hyperinsulinemia, dyslipidemia, hypertension, and is a component of the metabolic syndrome that also includes central obesity and hypercoagulability *(266–269)*. The evolving epidemic of obesity will generate a large increase in type 2 diabetes with a significant increase in cardiovascular morbidity and mortality *(1–4)*. It is now being recognized that the major antecedent of this type of diabetes, insulin resistance, is the major pathologic mechanism for the development of premature cardiovascular disease as these patients have increased secretion of proinflammatory cytokines and increased circulating levels of free fatty acids that decrease the release of endothelium-derived NO *(4,40,266)*. Increased plasma levels of fatty acids inhibit glucose transport by inhibiting the insulin receptor *(266)*. Proinflammatory cytokines and cellular adhesion molecules, such as tumor necrosis factor-alpha, interleukin-6, -8, and -10, von Willebrand factor, high-sensitivity C-reactive protein, tissue plasminogen activator, and plasminogen activator inhibitor-1, are expressed by vascular and blood cells during stimulation by growth factors, such as VEGF, that contribute to a low-grade, chronic systemic inflammation *(9,10,40,266)*.

In contrast, the novel polypeptide, adiponectin has a decreased expression in patients with insulin resistance. It has been suggested that several agents, such as tumor necrosis factor-alpha, could mediate their effects on insulin metabolism through modulating adiponectin secretion from adipocytes *(40,270–274)*. Adiponectin has been shown to modulate endothelial function and has an inhibitory effect on vascular smooth muscle cell proliferation and is involved in the modulation of inflammation *(40,134,270,275,276)*. Thiazolidinediones are currently used in patients with type 2 diabetes to improve insulin sensitivity and improve endothelial dysfunction. Thiazolidinediones have a direct effect on adiponectin, as this class of drugs have been shown to interfere with expression and release of mediators of insulin resistance and with subsequent improvement of insulin sensitivity *(277,278)*. Adiponectin has anti-inflammatory and antiatherogeneic effects as well as multiple beneficial effects on metabolism *(270,273,278–281)*.

CONCLUSION

Endothelial dysfunction, characterized by impaired NO availability, constitutes an early step in the pathogenesis of atherosclerotic disease and diabetes. Studies have shown that impaired endothelium-dependent vasodilation predicts cardiovascular events *(282)*. Dysfunction of the eNOS/soluble guanylate cyclase/cGMP system is a common mechanism by which several cardiovascular risk factors mediate deleterious effects on the vascular wall. Among them are vascular inflammation, sedentary lifestyle, menopause, hypercholesterolemia, hypertension, smoking, hyperhomocysteinemia, and diabetes *(2,9,98–104)*. Atherosclerosis in patients with diabetes surfaces earlier and is more aggressive, with cardiovascular complications contributing to the majority of diabetes-related deaths *(6,21)*.

Deficiency of endothelial-derived NO is believed to be the primary defect that links insulin resistance and endothelial dysfunction. NO deficiency results from decreased synthesis, in combination with exaggerated breakdown in tissues by high levels of ROS and RNS species. Endothelial dysfunction contributes to impaired insulin action, by altering transcapillary passage of insulin to target tissues, impaired expansion of the capillary network, with attenuation of blood flow to metabolically active tissues. This establishes a positive feedback cycle in which progressive endothelial dysfunction and disturbances in glucose and lipid metabolism occur secondary to insulin resistance. Vascular damage from lipid deposition and oxidative stress triggers an inflammatory reaction and the release of chemoattractants and cytokines that worsens insulin resistance and endothelial dysfunction. From the clinical standpoint, much experimental evidence supports the concept that therapies that improve insulin resistance and endothelial function reduce cardiovascular morbidity and mortality *(16)*. The main goals in the restoration of endothelial function are optimal glycemic control, lipid lowering, cessation of smoking, normalization of blood pressure, improvement in the release of endothelial NO, antioxidants to scavenge free oxygen radicals, normalization of homocysteine levels, and decreasing hyperinsulinemia *(105)*.

Identification of the earliest sign of vascular dysfunction may offer the best opportunity to interfere with pathogenic mechanisms and to avoid progression of diabetic vasculopathy. It appears that endothelial dysfunction meets this criterion, and therefore intervention at the earliest stages of endothelial dysfunction offers opportunity to prevent the fatal consequences of diabetes. As the human and economic costs of this epidemic are enormous, a concerted, global effort will be required to address this diabetes epidemic *(1)*.

Recent clinical data have raised new questions about the pharmacological approach to intensive management of diabetes to reduce cardiovascular events. Firstly, a meta-analysis suggested that rosiglitazone may increase the risk of cardiovascular events *(283)*, in contrast with the PROACTIVE trial with pioglitazone, discussed above. The methodology and the conclusions of the meta-analysis remain controversial, but it still raises questions about differences between drugs within a class and also questions the utility of some of the surrogate and mechanistic data we have presented in this review. On the other hand, other clinical trials do not support the meta-analysis and we will have to wait for the completion of long term trials to address this question *(284,285)*.

REFERENCES

1. Wild S, Roglic G, Green A, Sicree R, King H. Global Prevalence of Diabetes: Estimates for the year 2000 and projections for 2030. Diabetes Care 2004;27(5):1047–53.
2. Winer N, Sowers JR. Diabetes and arterial stiffening. Adv Cardiol 2007;44:245–51.
3. Ogden CLP, Carroll MD, Curtin LR, McDowell MA, Tabak CJ, Flegal KM. Prevalence of overweight and obesity in the United States, 1999–2004. JAMA 2006;295(13):1549–55.
4. Nigro J, Osman N, Dart AM, Little PJ. Insulin resistance and atherosclerosis. Endocr Rev 2006;27(3):242–59.
5. Triggle CR, Howarth A, Cheng ZJ, Ding H. Twenty-five years since the discovery of endothelium-derived relaxing factor (EDRF): does a dysfunctional endothelium contribute to the development of type 2 diabetes? Can J Physiol Pharmacol 2005;83(8–9):681–700.
6. Howard BV, Rodriguez BL, Bennett PH, et al. Prevention Conference VI: Diabetes and Cardiovascular Disease: Writing Group I: Epidemiology. Circulation 2002;105(18):e132–7.
7. Caballero AE. Endothelial dysfunction, inflammation, and insulin resistance: a focus on subjects at risk for type 2 diabetes. Curr Diab Rep 2004;4(4):237–46.
8. Groop PH, Forsblom C, Thomas MC. Mechanisms of disease: Pathway-selective insulin resistance and microvascular complications of diabetes. Nat Clin Prac Endocrinol Metab 2005;1(2):100–10.
9. Natali A, Toschi E, Baldeweg S, et al. Clustering of insulin resistance with vascular dysfunction and low-grade inflammation in type 2 diabetes. Diabetes 2006;55(4):1133–40.
10. Shahab A. Why does diabetes mellitus increase the risk of cardiovascular disease? Acta Med Indones 2006;38(1):33–41.
11. Sarafidis PA, Ruilope LM. Insulin resistance, hyperinsulinemia, and renal injury: mechanisms and implications. Am J Nephrol 2006;26(3):232–44.
12. Hartge MM, Kintscher U, Unger T. Endothelial dysfunction and its role in diabetic vascular disease. Endocrinol Metab Clin North Am 2006;35(3):551–60, viii–ix.
13. Candido R, Zanetti M. Current perspective. Diabetic vascular disease: from endothelial dysfunction to atherosclerosis. Italian Heart Journal: Official Journal of the Italian Federation of Cardiology 2005;6(9): 703–20.
14. Beckman JA, Creager MA, Libby P. Diabetes and atherosclerosis: epidemiology, pathophysiology, and management. JAMA 2002;287(19):2570–81.
15. Quiñones MJ, Nicholas SB, Lyon CJ. Insulin resistance and the endothelium. Curr Diab Rep 2005;5(4):246–53.
16. Cersosimo E, DeFronzo RA. Insulin resistance and endothelial dysfunction: the road map to cardiovascular diseases. Diabetes Metab Res Rev 2006;22(6):423–36.
17. Lee M-S, Chang I, Kim S. Death effectors of beta-cell apoptosis in type 1 diabetes. Mol Genet Metab 2004;83(1–2):82–92.
18. Araki E, Oyadomari S, Mori M. Endoplasmic reticulum stress and diabetes mellitus. Intern Med 2003;42(1): 7–14.
19. Delaney CA, Tyrberg B, Bouwens L, Vaghef H, Hellman B, Eizirik DL. Sensitivity of human pancreatic islets to peroxynitrite-induced cell dysfunction and death. FEBS Lett 1996;394(3):300–6.
20. Mauricio D, Mandrup-Poulsen T. Apoptosis and the pathogenesis of IDDM: a question of life and death. Diabetes 1998;47(10):1537–43.
21. Jay D, Hitomi H, Griendling KK. Oxidative stress and diabetic cardiovascular complications. Free Radical Biology and Medicine 2006;40(2):183–92.
22. Lee AJ, Hiscock RJ, Wein P, Walker SP, Permezel M. Gestational diabetes mellitus: clinical predictors and long-term risk of developing type 2 diabetes: A retrospective cohort study using survival analysis. Diabetes Care 2007;30(4):878–83.

23. Hung TW, Yang XL, Chan JCN, et al. Progression to impaired glucose regulation, diabetes and metabolic syndrome in Chinese women with a past history of gestational diabetes. Diabetes/Metabolism Research and Reviews 2007;9999(9999):n/a.

24. Knock GA, McCarthy AL, Lowy C, Poston L. Association of gestational diabetes with abnormal maternal vascular endothelial function. Br J Obstet Gynaecol 1997;104(2):229–34.

25. Crowther CA, Hiller JE, Moss JR, et al. Effect of treatment of gestational diabetes mellitus on pregnancy outcomes. N Engl J Med 2005;352(24):2477–86.

26. Van den Berghe G, Wilmer A, Hermans G, et al. Intensive insulin therapy in the medical ICU (see comment). N Engl J Med 2006;354(5):449–61.

27. Nisoli E, Clementi E, Carruba MO, Moncada S. Defective mitochondrial biogenesis: a hallmark of the high cardiovascular risk in the metabolic syndrome? Circ Res 2007;100(6):795–806.

28. Van den Berghe G, Wilmer A, Milants I, et al. Intensive insulin therapy in mixed medical/surgical intensive care units: benefit versus harm. Diabetes 2006;55(11):3151–9.

29. Vanhorebeek I, Van den Berghe G. Diabetes of injury: novel insights. Endocrinology & Metabolism Clinics of North America 2006;35(4):859–72.

30. Van den Berghe G. Does tight blood glucose control during cardiac surgery improve patient outcome? Ann Intern Med 2007;146(4):307–8.

31. Gandhi GY, Nuttall GA, Abel MD, et al. Intensive intraoperative insulin therapy versus conventional glucose management during cardiac surgery: a randomized trial. Ann Intern Med 2007;146(4):233–43.

32. Mesotten D, Van den Berghe G. Clinical potential of insulin therapy in critically ill patients. Drugs 2003;63(7):625–36.

33. Egi M, Bellomo R, Stachowski E, et al. Intensive insulin therapy in postoperative intensive care unit patients: a decision analysis (see comment). Am J Respiratory & Critical Care Med 2006;173(4):407–13.

34. Gandhi GY, Nuttall GA, Abel MD, et al. Intensive intraoperative insulin therapy versus conventional glucose management during cardiac surgery: a randomized trial (see comment). Annals of Internal Medicine 2007;146(4):233–43.

35. Hermans G, Wilmer A, Meersseman W, et al. Impact of intensive insulin therapy on neuromuscular complications and ventilator dependency in the medical intensive care unit (see comment). Am J Respiratory & Critical Care Med 2007;175(5):480–9.

36. Mitchell I, Knight E, Gissane J, et al. A phase II randomised controlled trial of intensive insulin therapy in general intensive care patients. Critical Care & Resuscitation 2006;8(4):289–93.

37. Hoedemaekers CW, Pickkers P, Netea MG, van Deuren M, Van der Hoeven JG. Intensive insulin therapy does not alter the inflammatory response in patients undergoing coronary artery bypass grafting: a randomized controlled trial (ISRCTN95608630). Critical care (London, England) 2005;9(6):R790–7.

38. Hayden MR, Tyagi SC. Myocardial redox stress and remodeling in metabolic syndrome, type 2 diabetes mellitus, and congestive heart failure. Med Sci Monit 2003;9(7):SR35–52.

39. Tsukahara H. Biomarkers for oxidative stress: clinical application in pediatric medicine. Curr Med Chem 2007;14(3):339–51.

40. Rask-Madsen C, King GL. Mechanisms of disease: endothelial dysfunction in insulin resistance and diabetes. Nat Clin Pract Endocrinol Metab 2007;3(1):46–56.

41. Valko M, Leibfritz D, Moncol J, Cronin MTD, Mazur M, Telser J. Free radicals and antioxidants in normal physiological functions and human disease. Int J Biochem Cell Biol 2007;39(1):44–84.

42. Yung LM, Leung FP, Yao X, Chen Z-Y, Huang Y. Reactive oxygen species in vascular wall. Cardiovasc Hematol Disord Drug Targets 2006;6(1):1–19.

43. Seckin D, Ilhan N, Ertugrul S. Glycaemic control, markers of endothelial cell activation and oxidative stress in children with type 1 diabetes mellitus. Diabetes Res Clin Pract 2006;73(2):191–7.

44. Lo H-C, Lin S-C, Wang Y-M. The relationship among serum cytokines, chemokine, nitric oxide, and leptin in children with type 1 diabetes mellitus. Clin Biochem 2004;37(8):666–72.

45. Allen DA, Yaqoob MM, Harwood SM. Mechanisms of high glucose-induced apoptosis and its relationship to diabetic complications. J Nutr Biochem 2005;16(12):705–13.

46. Hoeldtke RD. Nitrosative stress in early Type 1 diabetes. David H. P. Streeten Memorial Lecture. Clin Auton Res 2003;13(6):406–21.

47. Llorens S, Nava E. Cardiovascular diseases and the nitric oxide pathway. Curr Vasc Pharmacol 2003;1(3):335–46.

48. Pacher P, Obrosova IG, Mabley JG, Szabó C. Role of nitrosative stress and peroxynitrite in the pathogenesis of diabetic complications. Emerging new therapeutical strategies. Curr Med Chem 2005;12(3):267–75.

49. Soriano FG, Nogueira AC, Caldini EG, et al. Potential role of poly(adenosine 5'-diphosphate-ribose) polymerase activation in the pathogenesis of myocardial contractile dysfunction associated with human septic shock. Critical Care Med 2006;34(4):1073–9.

50. Zou M-H, Cohen R, Ullrich V. Peroxynitrite and vascular endothelial dysfunction in diabetes mellitus. Endothelium 2004;11(2):89–97.

51. Nambi V, Ballantyne C. Role of biomarkers in developing new therapies for vascular disease. World Journal of Surgery 2007;31(4):676–81.

52. Zoppini G, Targher G, Zamboni C, et al. Effects of moderate-intensity exercise training on plasma biomarkers of inflammation and endothelial dysfunction in older patients with type 2 diabetes. Nutr Metab Cardiovasc Dis 2006;16(8):543–9.

53. Matteucci E, Passerai S, Mariotti M, et al. Dietary habits and nutritional biomarkers in Italian type 1 diabetes families: evidence of unhealthy diet and combined-vitamin-deficient intakes. Eur J Clin Nutr 2005;59(1): 114–22.

54. Ding H, Triggle CR. Endothelial cell dysfunction and the vascular complications associated with type 2 diabetes: assessing the health of the endothelium. Vasc Health Risk Manag 2005;1(1):55–71.

55. Miyata T, Kurokawa K. A detective story for biomedical footprints towards new therapeutic interventions in diabetic nephropathy. Intern Med 2003;42(12):1165–71.

56. Das UN. Insulin: an endogenous cardioprotector. Curr Opin Crit Care 2003;9(5):375–83.

57. Grundy SM, Howard B, Smith S, Jr, Eckel R, Redberg R, Bonow RO. Prevention Conference VI: Diabetes and Cardiovascular Disease: Executive Summary: Conference Proceeding for Healthcare Professionals From a Special Writing Group of the American Heart Association. Circulation 2002;105(18):2231–9.

58. Haidara MA, Yassin HZ, Rateb M, Ammar H, Zorkani MA. Role of oxidative stress in development of cardiovascular complications in diabetes mellitus. Curr Vasc Pharmacol 2006;4(3):215–27.

59. Fitzgerald SM, Kemp-Harper BK, Tare M, Parkington HC. Role of endothelium-derived hyperpolarizing factor in endothelial dysfunction during diabetes. Clin Exp Pharmacol Physiol 2005;32(5–6):482–7.

60. Dandona P, Aljada A. Advances in diabetes for the millennium: diabetes and the endothelium. MedGenMed 2004;6(3 Suppl):6.

61. Quon MJ. Reciprocal relationships between insulin resistance and endothelial dysfunction: insights from therapeutic interventions. Zhong Nan Da Xue Xue Bao Yi Xue Ban 2006;31(3):305–12.

62. Cheng ZJ, Vapaatalo H, Mervaala E. Angiotensin II and vascular inflammation. Medical Science Monitor 2005;11(6):RA194–205.

63. Toda N, Ayajiki K, Okamura T. Interaction of endothelial nitric oxide and angiotensin in the circulation. Pharmacol Rev 2007;59(1):54–87.

64. Vapaatalo H, Mervaala E. Clinically important factors influencing endothelial function. Med Sci Monit 2001;7(5):1075–85.

65. Fernández N, Jancar S, Sánchez CM. Blood and endothelium in immune complex-mediated tissue injury. Trends Pharmacol Sci 2004;25(10):512–7.

66. Szekanecz Z, Koch AE. Vascular endothelium and immune responses: implications for inflammation and angiogenesis. Rheum Dis Clin North Am 2004;30(1):97–114.

67. Tan KT, Lip GYH. Platelets, atherosclerosis and the endothelium: new therapeutic targets? Expert Opin Investig Drugs 2003;12(11):1765–76.

68. Tarkka T, Sipola A, Jamsa T, et al. Adenoviral VEGF-A gene transfer induces angiogenesis and promotes bone formation in healing osseous tissues. J Gene Med 2003;5(7):560–6.

69. Aird WC. The role of the endothelium in severe sepsis and multiple organ dysfunction syndrome. Blood 2003;101(10):3765–77.

70. Hippenstiel S, Suttorp N. Interaction of pathogens with the endothelium. Thromb Haemost 2003;89(1): 18–24.

71. d'Alessio P. Endothelium as a pharmacological target. Curr Opin Investig Drugs 2001;2(12):1720–4.

72. Levi M, ten Cate H, van der Poll T. Endothelium: interface between coagulation and inflammation. Crit Care Med 2002;30(5 Suppl):S220–4.

73. Meroni PL, Raschi E, Testoni C, Tincani A, Balestrieri G. Antiphospholipid antibodies and the endothelium. Rheum Dis Clin North Am 2001;27(3):587–602.

74. Hack CE, Zeerleder S. The endothelium in sepsis: source of and a target for inflammation. Crit Care Med 2001;29(7 Suppl):S21–7.

75. Willerson JT, Kereiakes DJ. Endothelial dysfunction. Circulation 2003;108(17):2060–1.

76. Moncada S, Palmer RMJ, Higgs EA. Nitric oxide: Physiology, pathophysiology, and pharmacology. Pharmacol Rev 1991;43(2):109–42.

77. Dandona P. Endothelium, inflammation, and diabetes. Curr Diab Rep 2002;2(4):311–5.

78. Gornik HL, Creager MA. Arginine and endothelial and vascular health. J Nutr 2004;134(10):2880S–7.

79. Palmer RMJ, Ashton DS, Moncada S. Vascular endothelial cells synthesize nitric oxide from L-arginine. Nature 1988;333(6174):664–6.

80. Förstermann U, Münzel T. Endothelial nitric oxide synthase in vascular disease: from marvel to menace. Circulation 2006;113(13):1708–14.

81. Moncada S, Higgs A. The L-arginine-nitric oxide pathway. N Engl J Med 1993;329(27):2002–12.

82. Ouviña SM, La GRD, Zanaro NL, Palmer L, Sassetti B. Endothelial dysfunction, nitric oxide and platelet activation in hypertensive and diabetic type II patients. Thromb Res 2001;102(2):107–14.

83. Wotherspoon F, Browne DL, Meeking DR, et al. The contribution of nitric oxide and vasodilatory prostanoids to bradykinin-mediated vasodilation in Type 1 diabetes. Diabet Med 2005;22(6):697–702.

84. Tran D, Lowy A, Howes JB, Howes LG. Effects of cerivastatin on forearm vascular responses, blood pressure responsiveness and ambulatory blood pressure in type 2 diabetic men. Diabetes Obes Metab 2005;7(3):273–81.

85. De Meyer GRY, Herman AG. Vascular endothelial dysfunction. Prog Cardiovasc Dis 1997;39(4):325–42.

86. Endemann DH, Schiffrin EL. Endothelial dysfunction. J Am Soc Nephrol 2004;15(8):1983–92.

87. Nossaman BD, Gur S, Kadowitz PJ. Gene and stem cell therapy in the treatment of erectile dysfunction and pulmonary hypertension; potential treatments for the common problem of endothelial dysfunction. Curr Gene Ther 2007;7(2):131–53.

88. Dandona P, Aljada A. Advances in diabetes for the millennium: diabetes and the endothelium. Medgenmed [Computer File]: Medscape General Medicine 2004;6(3 Suppl):6.

89. Fitzgerald SM, Kemp-Harper BK, Tare M, Parkington HC. Role of endothelium-derived hyperpolarizing factor in endothelial dysfunction during diabetes. Clinical & Experimental Pharmacology & Physiology 2005;32(5–6):482–7.

90. Hsueh WA, Quiñones MJ. Role of endothelial dysfunction in insulin resistance. Am J Cardiol 2003;92(4A):10J–7J.

91. Leclercq B, Jaimes EA, Raij L. Nitric oxide synthase and hypertension. Curr Opin Nephrol Hypertens 2002;11(2):185–9.

92. Tooke J. The association between insulin resistance and endotheliopathy. Diabetes Obes Metab 1999;(1 Suppl 1):S17–22.

93. Conger JD. Endothelial regulation of vascular tone. Hosp Pract (Off Ed) 1994;29(10):117–22, 25–6.

94. Hink U, Li H, Mollnau H, et al. Mechanisms underlying endothelial dysfunction in diabetes mellitus. Circ Res 2001;88(2):E14–22.

95. Brunner H, Cockcroft JR, Deanfield J, et al. Endothelial function and dysfunction. Part II: Association with cardiovascular risk factors and diseases. A statement by the Working Group on Endothelins and Endothelial Factors of the European Society of Hypertension. J Hypertens 2005;23(2):233–46.

96. Mather KJ, Lteif A, Steinberg HO, Baron AD. Interactions between endothelin and nitric oxide in the regulation of vascular tone in obesity and diabetes. Diabetes 2004;53(8):2060–6.

97. Steinberg HO, Baron AD. Vascular function, insulin resistance and fatty acids. Diabetologia 2002;45(5):623–34.

98. Boger RH. Asymmetric dimethylarginine, an endogenous inhibitor of nitric oxide synthase, explains the "L-arginine paradox" and acts as a novel cardiovascular risk factor. J Nutr 2004;134(10):2842S–7.

99. Siasos G, Tousoulis D, Antoniades C, Stefanadi E, Stefanadis C. L-Arginine, the substrate for NO synthesis: an alternative treatment for premature atherosclerosis? Int J Cardiol 2007;116(3):300–8.

100. Shimasaki Y, Saito Y, Yoshimura M, et al. The effects of long-term smoking on endothelial nitric oxide synthase mRNA expression in human platelets as detected with real-time quantitative RT-PCR. Clin Appl Thromb Hemost 2007;13(1):43–51.

101. Forgione MA, Loscalzo J. Oxidant stress as a critical determinant of endothelial function. Drug News Perspect 2000;13(9):523–9.

102. Cooke JP. Therapeutic interventions in endothelial dysfunction: endothelium as a target organ. Clin Cardiol 1997;20(11 Suppl 2):II-45–51.

103. Signorello, Viviani, Armani, et al. Homocysteine, reactive oxygen species and nitric oxide in type 2 diabetes mellitus. Thromb Res 2006.

104. Tawakol A, Omland T, Gerhard M, Wu JT, Creager MA. Hyperhomocyst(e)inemia is associated with impaired endothelium-dependent vasodilation in humans. Circulation 1997;95(5):1119–21.

105. Najemnik C, Sinzinger H, Kritz H. Endothelial dysfunction, atherosclerosis and diabetes. Acta Med Austriaca 1999;26(5):148–53.

106. Calles-Escandon J, Cipolla M. Diabetes and endothelial dysfunction: a clinical perspective. Endocr Rev 2001;22(1):36–52.

107. Liu Y, Freedman BI. Genetics of progressive renal failure in diabetic kidney disease. Kidney Int Suppl 2005(99):S94–7.

108. Kao WHL, Hsueh W-C, Rainwater DL, et al. Family history of type 2 diabetes is associated with increased carotid artery intimal-medial thickness in Mexican Americans. Diabetes Care 2005;28(8):1882–9.

109. Slyper AH. Clinical review 168: What vascular ultrasound testing has revealed about pediatric atherogenesis, and a potential clinical role for ultrasound in pediatric risk assessment. J Clin Endocrinol Metab 2004;89(7):3089–95.

110. McAllister AS, Atkinson AB, Johnston GD, McCance DR. Endothelial function in offspring of Type 1 diabetic patients with and without diabetic nephropathy. Diabet Med 1999;16(4):298–303.

111. Yasuda S, Miyazaki S, Kanda M, et al. Intensive treatment of risk factors in patients with type-2 diabetes mellitus is associated with improvement of endothelial function coupled with a reduction in the levels of plasma asymmetric dimethylarginine and endogenous inhibitor of nitric oxide synthase. Eur Heart J 2006;27(10):1159–65.

112. Title LM, Ur E, Giddens K, McQueen MJ, Nassar BA. Folic acid improves endothelial dysfunction in type 2 diabetes – an effect independent of homocysteine-lowering. Vasc Med 2006;11(2):101–9.

113. Pena AS, Wiltshire E, MacKenzie K, et al. Vascular endothelial and smooth muscle function relates to body mass index and glucose in obese and nonobese children. J Clin Endocrinol Metab 2006;91(11):4467–71.

114. Madsen PL, Scheuermann FM, Neubauer S, Channon K, Clarke K. Haemoglobin and flow-mediated vasodilation. Clin Sci (Lond) 2006;110(4):467–73.

115. Dogra GK, Watts GF, Chan DC, Stanton K. Statin therapy improves brachial artery vasodilator function in patients with Type 1 diabetes and microalbuminuria. Diabet Med 2005;22(3):239–42.

116. Yugar-Toledo JC, Tanus-Santos JE, Sabha M, et al. Uncontrolled hypertension, uncompensated type II diabetes, and smoking have different patterns of vascular dysfunction. Chest 2004;125(3):823–30.

117. Henry RMA, Ferreira I, Kostense PJ, et al. Type 2 diabetes is associated with impaired endothelium-dependent, flow-mediated dilation, but impaired glucose metabolism is not; The Hoorn Study. In: Atherosclerosis. 1 ed; 2004:49–56.

118. Hashimoto M, Miyamoto Y, Matsuda Y, Akita H. New methods to evaluate endothelial function: Non-invasive method of evaluating endothelial function in humans. J Pharmacol Sci 2003;93(4):405–8.

119. Desouza C, Parulkar A, Lumpkin D, Akers D, Fonseca VA. Acute and prolonged effects of sildenafil on brachial artery flow-mediated dilatation in type 2 diabetes. Diabetes Care 2002;25(8):1336–9.

120. McFarlane R, McCredie RJ, Bonney MA, et al. Angiotensin converting enzyme inhibition and arterial endothelial function in adults with Type 1 diabetes mellitus. Diabet Med 1999;16(1):62–6.

121. Ifrim S, Vasilescu R. Early detection of atherosclerosis in type 2 diabetic patients by endothelial dysfunction and intima-media thickness. Rom J Intern Med 2004;42(2):343–54.

122. Beishuizen ED, Tamsma JT, Jukema JW, et al. The effect of statin therapy on endothelial function in type 2 diabetes without manifest cardiovascular disease. Diabetes Care 2005;28(7):1668–74.

123. Honing ML, Morrison PJ, Banga JD, Stroes ES, Rabelink TJ. Nitric oxide availability in diabetes mellitus. Diabetes Metab Rev 1998;14(3):241–9.

124. Sessa WC. Regulation of endothelial derived nitric oxide in health and disease. Mem Inst Oswaldo Cruz 2005;100(Suppl 1):15–8.

125. Santilli F, Cipollone F, Mezzetti A, Chiarelli F. The role of nitric oxide in the development of diabetic angiopathy. Horm Metab Res 2004;36(5):319–35.

126. Förstermann U. Janus-faced role of endothelial NO synthase in vascular disease: uncoupling of oxygen reduction from NO synthesis and its pharmacological reversal. Biol Chem 2006;387(12):1521–33.

127. Münzel T, Daiber A, Ullrich V, Mülsch A. Vascular consequences of endothelial nitric oxide synthase uncoupling for the activity and expression of the soluble guanylyl cyclase and the cGMP-dependent protein kinase. Arterioscler Thromb Vasc Biol 2005;25(8):1551–7.

128. Yang Z, Ming X-F. Recent advances in understanding endothelial dysfunction in atherosclerosis. Clin Med Res 2006;4(1):53–65.

129. Kendler BSP, FACN. Supplemental conditionally essential nutrients in cardiovascular disease therapy. J Cardiovas Nurs 2006;21(1):916.

130. Galli F, Rossi R, Di SP, Floridi A, Canestrari F. Protein thiols and glutathione influence the nitric oxide-dependent regulation of the red blood cell metabolism. Nitric Oxide 2002;6(2):186–99.

131. Hayden MR, Tyagi SC. Is type 2 diabetes mellitus a vascular disease (atheroscleropathy) with hyperglycemia a late manifestation? The role of NOS, NO, and redox stress. Cardiovasc Diabetol 2003;2:2.

132. Yamagishi, Ueda, Okuda. A possible involvement of crosstalk between advanced glycation end products (AGEs) and asymmetric dimethylarginine (ADMA), an endogenous nitric oxide synthase inhibitor in accelerated atherosclerosis in diabetes. Med Hypotheses 2007.

133. Avogaro A, Toffolo G, Kiwanuka E, de KSV, Tessari P, Cobelli C. L-arginine-nitric oxide kinetics in normal and type 2 diabetic subjects: a stable-labelled 15N arginine approach. Diabetes 2003;52(3):795–802.

134. Lucotti P, Setola E, Monti LD, et al. Beneficial effects of a long-term oral L-arginine treatment added to a hypocaloric diet and exercise training program in obese, insulin-resistant type 2 diabetic patients. Am J Physiol Endocrinol Metab 2006;291(5):E906–12.

135. Kohli R, Meininger CJ, Haynes TE, Yan W, Self JT, Wu G. Dietary L-arginine supplementation enhances endothelial nitric oxide synthesis in streptozotocin-induced diabetic rats. J Nutr 2004;134(3):600–8.

136. Pieper GM, Siebeneich W, Dondlinger LA. Short-term oral administration of L-arginine reverses defective endothelium-dependent relaxation and cGMP generation in diabetes. Eur J Pharmacol 1996;317(2–3):317–20.

137. Fu WJ, Haynes TE, Kohli R, et al. Dietary L-arginine supplementation reduces fat mass in Zucker diabetic fatty rats. J Nutr 2005;135(4):714–21.

138. McVeigh GE, Brennan GM, Johnston GD, et al. Dietary fish oil augments nitric oxide production or release in patients with type 2 (non-insulin-dependent) diabetes mellitus. Diabetologia 1993;36(1):33–8.

139. Hollenberg NK. Vascular action of cocoa flavanols in humans: the roots of the story. J Cardiovasc Pharmacol 2006;47(Suppl 2):S99–102; discussion S19–21.

140. Westphal, Taneva, Kastner, et al. Endothelial dysfunction induced by postprandial lipemia is neutralized by addition of proteins to the fatty meal. Atherosclerosis 2006;185(2):313–9.

141. Sprietsma JE. Modern diets and diseases: NO–zinc balance. Under Th1, zinc and nitrogen monoxide (NO) collectively protect against viruses, AIDS, autoimmunity, diabetes, allergies, asthma, infectious diseases, atherosclerosis and cancer. Med Hypotheses 1999;53(1):6–16.

142. Xu J, Xie Z, Reece R, Pimental D, Zou M-H. Uncoupling of endothelial nitric oxidase synthase by hypochlorous acid: role of NAD(P)H oxidase-derived superoxide and peroxynitrite. Arterioscler Thromb Vasc Biol 2006;26(12):2688–95.

143. Ayaz M, Turan B. Selenium prevents diabetes-induced alterations in $[Zn^{2+}]i$ and metallothionein level of rat heart via restoration of cell redox cycle. Am J Physiol Heart Circ Physiol 2006;290(3):H1071–80.

144. Song Y, Wang J, Li X-k, Cai L. Zinc and the diabetic heart. Biometals 2005;18(4):325–32.

145. Zou MH, Shi C, Cohen RA. Oxidation of the zinc-thiolate complex and uncoupling of endothelial nitric oxide synthase by peroxynitrite. J Clin Invest 2002;109(6):817–26.

146. Kowluru RA, Koppolu P, Chakrabarti S, Chen S. Diabetes-induced activation of nuclear transcriptional factor in the retina, and its inhibition by antioxidants. Free Radic Res 2003;37(11):1169–80.

147. Timimi FK, Ting HH, Haley EA, Roddy MA, Ganz P, Creager MA. Vitamin C improves endothelium-dependent vasodilation in patients with insulin-dependent diabetes mellitus. J Am Coll Cardiol 1998;31(3):552–7.

148. Ting HH, Timimi FK, Boles KS, Creager SJ, Ganz P, Creager MA. Vitamin C improves endothelium-dependent vasodilation in patients with non-insulin-dependent diabetes mellitus. J Clin Invest 1996;97(1):22–8.

149. Lin L-Y, Lin C-Y, Ho F-M, Liau CS. Up-regulation of the association between heat shock protein 90 and endothelial nitric oxide synthase prevents high glucose-induced apoptosis in human endothelial cells. J Cell Biochem 2005;94(1):194–201.

150. Mount PF, Kemp BE, Power DA. Regulation of endothelial and myocardial NO synthesis by multi-site eNOS phosphorylation (see comment). [Review] [71 refs]. J Mol Cell Cardiol 2007;42(2):271–9.

151. Okon EB, Chung AWY, Rauniyar P, et al. Compromised arterial function in human type 2 diabetic patients. Diabetes 2005;54(8):2415–23.

152. Niedowicz DM, Daleke DL. The role of oxidative stress in diabetic complications. Cell Biochem Biophys 2005;43(2):289–330.

153. Son SM, Whalin MK, Harrison DG, Taylor WR, Griendling KK. Oxidative stress and diabetic vascular complications. Curr Diab Rep 2004;4(4):247–52.

154. Michell BJ, Chen Z, Tiganis T, et al. Coordinated control of endothelial nitric-oxide synthase phosphorylation by protein kinase C and the cAMP-dependent protein kinase. J Biol Chem 2001;276(21):17625–8.

155. Lin MI, Fulton D, Babbitt R, et al. Phosphorylation of threonine 497 in endothelial nitric-oxide synthase coordinates the coupling of L-arginine metabolism to efficient nitric oxide production. J Biol Chem 2003;278(45):44719–26.

156. Whiteman EL, Cho H, Birnbaum MJ. Role of Akt/protein kinase B in metabolism. Trends Endocrinol Metab 2002;13(10):444–51.

157. Dimmeler S, Fleming I, Fisslthaler B, Hermann C, Busse R, Zeiher AM. Activation of nitric oxide synthase in endothelial cells by Akt-dependent phosphorylation. Nature 1999;399(6736):601–5.

158. Fulton D, Gratton J-P, McCabe TJ, et al. Regulation of endothelium-derived nitric oxide production by the protein kinase Akt. Nature 1999;399(6736):597–601.

159. Federici M, Menghini R, Mauriello A, et al. Insulin-dependent activation of endothelial nitric oxide synthase is impaired by O-linked glycosylation modification of signaling proteins in human coronary endothelial cells. Circulation 2002;106(4):466–72.

160. Du XL, Edelstein D, Dimmeler S, Ju Q, Sui C, Brownlee M. Hyperglycemia inhibits endothelial nitric oxide synthase activity by posttranslational modification at the Akt site. J Clin Invest 2001;108(9):1341–8.
161. Salt IP, Morrow VA, Brandie FM, Connell JMC, Petrie JR. High glucose inhibits insulin-stimulated nitric oxide production without reducing endothelial nitric-oxide synthase Ser1177 phosphorylation in human aortic endothelial cells. J Biol Chem 2003;278(21):18791–7.
162. Seasholtz TM, Brown JH. Rho signaling in vascular diseases. Mol Interv 2004;4(6):348–57.
163. Laufs U, Liao JK. Post-transcriptional regulation of endothelial nitric oxide synthase mRNA stability by Rho GTPase. J Biol Chem 1998;273(37):24266–71.
164. Mills TM, Lewis RW, Wingard CJ, Linder AE, Jin L, Webb RC. Vasoconstriction, RhoA/Rho-kinase and the erectile response. Int J Impot Res 2003;15 (Suppl 5):S20–4.
165. Chang S, Hypolite JA, Changolkar A, Wein AJ, Chacko S, DiSanto ME. Increased contractility of diabetic rabbit corpora smooth muscle in response to endothelin is mediated via Rho-kinase beta. Int J Impot Res 2003;15(1):53–62.
166. Feng J, Ito M, Ichikawa K, et al. Inhibitory phosphorylation site for Rho-associated kinase on smooth muscle myosin phosphatase. J Biol Chem 1999;274(52):37385–90.
167. Gong MC, Gorenne I, Read P, et al. Regulation by GDI of RhoA/Rho-kinase-induced Ca^{2+} sensitization of smooth muscle myosin II. Am J Physiol Cell Physiol 2001;281(1):C257–69.
168. Chitaley K, Wingard CJ, Clinton WR, et al. Antagonism of Rho-kinase stimulates rat penile erection via a nitric oxide-independent pathway. Nat Med 2001;7(1):119–22.
169. Rees RW, Foxwell NA, Ralph DJ, Kell PD, Moncada S, Cellek S. Y-27632, a Rho-kinase inhibitor, inhibits proliferation and adrenergic contraction of prostatic smooth muscle cells. J Urol 2003;170(6 Pt 1):2517–22.
170. Bivalacqua, Liu, Musicki, Champion, Burnett. Endothelial nitric oxide synthase keeps erection regulatory function balance in the penis. Eur Urol 2006.
171. Lei H, Venkatakrishnan A, Yu S, Kazlauskas A. Protein kinase A-dependent translocation of Hsp90{alpha} impairs endothelial nitric-oxide synthase activity in high glucose and diabetes. J Biol Chem 2007;282(13):9364–71.
172. Davis BJ, Xie Z, Viollet B, Zou M-H. Activation of the AMP-activated kinase by antidiabetes drug metformin stimulates nitric oxide synthesis in vivo by promoting the association of heat shock protein 90 and endothelial nitric oxide synthase. Diabetes 2006;55(2):496–505.
173. Garcia-Cardena G, Fan R, Shah V, et al. Dynamic activation of endothelial nitric oxide synthase by Hsp90. Nature 1998;392(6678):821–4.
174. Hayashi T, Juliet PAR, Miyazaki A, Ignarro LJ, Iguchi A. High glucose downregulates the number of caveolae in monocytes through oxidative stress from NADPH oxidase: implications for atherosclerosis. Biochim Biophys Acta 2007;1772(3):364–72.
175. Zou M-H, Shi C, Cohen RA. Oxidation of the zinc-thiolate complex and uncoupling of endothelial nitric oxide synthase by peroxynitrite. J Clin Invest 2002;109(6):817–26.
176. Lin KY, Ito A, Asagami T, et al. Impaired nitric oxide synthase pathway in diabetes mellitus: role of asymmetric dimethylarginine and dimethylarginine dimethylaminohydrolase. Circulation 2002;106(8):987–92.
177. Toth J, Racz A, Kaminski PM, Wolin MS, Bagi Z, Koller A. Asymmetrical dimethylarginine inhibits shear stress-induced nitric oxide release and dilation and elicits superoxide-mediated increase in arteriolar tone. Hypertension 2007;49(3):563–8.
178. Beltowski J, Kedra A. Asymmetric dimethylarginine (ADMA) as a target for pharmacotherapy. Pharmacol Rep 2006;58(2):159–78.
179. Krzyzanowska K, Mittermayer F, Shnawa N, et al. Asymmetrical dimethylarginine is related to renal function, chronic inflammation and macroangiopathy in patients with Type 2 diabetes and albuminuria. Diabet Med 2007;24(1):81–6.
180. Worthley MI, Holmes AS, Willoughby SR, et al. The deleterious effects of hyperglycemia on platelet function in diabetic patients with acute coronary syndromes mediation by superoxide production, resolution with intensive insulin administration. J Am Coll Cardiol 2007;49(3):304–10.
181. Stocker R, Keaney JF, Jr. Role of oxidative modifications in atherosclerosis. Physiological Reviews 2004;84(4):1381–478.
182. Posch K, Simecek S, Wascher TC, et al. Glycated low-density lipoprotein attenuates shear stress-induced nitric oxide synthesis by inhibition of shear stress-activated L-arginine uptake in endothelial cells. Diabetes 1999;48(6):1331–7.
183. Vergnani L, Hatrik S, Ricci F, et al. Effect of native and oxidized low-density lipoprotein on endothelial nitric oxide and superoxide production: key role of L-arginine availability. Circulation 2000;101(11):1261–6.
184. Artwohl M, Graier WF, Roden M, et al. Diabetic LDL triggers apoptosis in vascular endothelial cells. Diabetes 2003;52(5):1240–7.

185. Hirooka Y, Eshima K, Setoguchi S, Kishi T, Egashira K, Takeshita A. Vitamin C improves attenuated angiotensin II-induced endothelium-dependent vasodilation in human forearm vessels. Hypertens Res 2003;26(12):953–9.

186. Wigg SJ, Tare M, Forbes J, et al. Early vitamin E supplementation attenuates diabetes-associated vascular dysfunction and the rise in protein kinase C-beta in mesenteric artery and ameliorates wall stiffness in femoral artery of Wistar rats. Diabetologia 2004;47(6):1038–46.

187. Carr A, Frei B. The role of natural antioxidants in preserving the biological activity of endothelium-derived nitric oxide. Free Radic Biol Med 2000;28(12):1806–14.

188. Delles C, Schneider MP, Oehmer S, Fleischmann I, Fleischmann EF, Schmieder RE. Increased response of renal perfusion to the antioxidant vitamin C in type 2 diabetes. Nephrol Dial Transplant 2004;19(10): 2513–8.

189. De YL, Yu D, Bateman RM, Brock GB. Oxidative stress and antioxidant therapy: their impact in diabetes-associated erectile dysfunction. In: J Androl. 5 ed; 2004:830–6.

190. Chen H, Karne RJ, Hall G, et al. High-dose oral vitamin C partially replenishes vitamin C levels in patients with Type 2 diabetes and low vitamin C levels but does not improve endothelial dysfunction or insulin resistance. Am J Physiol Heart Circ Physiol 2006;290(1):H137–45.

191. McSorley PT, Bell PM, Young IS, et al. Endothelial function, insulin action and cardiovascular risk factors in young healthy adult offspring of parents with Type 2 diabetes: effect of vitamin E in a randomized double-blind, controlled clinical trial. Diabet Med 2005;22(6):703–10.

192. McQueen MJ, Lonn E, Gerstein HC, Bosch J, Yusuf S. The HOPE (Heart Outcomes Prevention Evaluation) Study and its consequences. Scand J Clin Lab Invest Suppl 2005;240:143–56.

193. Miller ER, 3rd, Pastor-Barriuso R, Dalal D, Riemersma RA, Appel LJ, Guallar E. Meta-analysis: high-dosage vitamin E supplementation may increase all-cause mortality (see comment) (summary for patients in Ann Intern Med. 2005 Jan 4;142(1):I40; PMID: 15537683). Annal Int Med 2005;142(1):37–46.

194. Heart Protection Study Collaborative G. MRC/BHF Heart Protection Study of antioxidant vitamin supplementation in 20,536 high-risk individuals: a randomised placebo-controlled trial (see comment) (summary for patients in J Fam Pract. 2002 Oct;51(10):810; PMID: 12401142). Lancet 2002;360(9326):23–33.

195. Vasquez-Vivar J, Kalyanaraman B, Martasek P, et al. Superoxide generation by endothelial nitric oxide synthase: The influence of cofactors. PNAS 1998;95(16):9220–5.

196. Chew GT, Watts GF. Coenzyme Q10 and diabetic endotheliopathy: oxidative stress and the "recoupling hypothesis". QJM 2004;97(8):537–48.

197. Marinos RS, Zhang W, Wu G, Kelly KA, Meininger CJ. Tetrahydrobiopterin levels regulate endothelial cell proliferation. Am J Physiol Heart Circ Physiol 2001;281(2):H482–9.

198. Alp NJ, Channon KM. Regulation of endothelial nitric oxide synthase by tetrahydrobiopterin in vascular disease. Arterioscler Thromb Vasc Biol 2004;24(3):413–20.

199. Heitzer T, Krohn K, Albers S, Meinertz T. Tetrahydrobiopterin improves endothelium-dependent vasodilation by increasing nitric oxide activity in patients with Type II diabetes mellitus. Diabetologia 2000;43(11): 1435–8.

200. Cai S, Khoo J, Mussa S, Alp NJ, Channon KM. Endothelial nitric oxide synthase dysfunction in diabetic mice: importance of tetrahydrobiopterin in eNOS dimerisation. Diabetologia 2005;48(9):1933–40.

201. Alp NJ, Mussa S, Khoo J, et al. Tetrahydrobiopterin-dependent preservation of nitric oxide-mediated endothelial function in diabetes by targeted transgenic GTP-cyclohydrolase I overexpression. J Clin Invest 2003;112(5):725–35.

202. Herman AG, Moncada S. Therapeutic potential of nitric oxide donors in the prevention and treatment of atherosclerosis. Eur Heart J 2005;26(19):1945–55.

203. Ceriello A. Oxidative stress and diabetes-associated complications. Endocr Pract 2006;12(Suppl 1):60–2.

204. Stevens MJ. Oxidative-nitrosative stress as a contributing factor to cardiovascular disease in subjects with diabetes. Curr Vasc Pharmacol 2005;3(3):253–66.

205. Pacher P, Szabó C. Role of peroxynitrite in the pathogenesis of cardiovascular complications of diabetes. Curr Opin Pharmacol 2006;6(2):136–41.

206. Mason RP. Nitric oxide mechanisms in the pathogenesis of global risk. J Clin Hypertens (Greenwich) 2006;8(8 Suppl 2):31–8; quiz 40.

207. Förstermann U. Endothelial NO synthase as a source of NO and superoxide. Eur J Clin Pharmacol 2006;62(Suppl 1):5–12.

208. Radi R, Beckman JS, Bush KM, Freeman BA. Peroxynitrite-induced membrane lipid peroxidation: the cytotoxic potential of superoxide and nitric oxide. Arch Biochem Biophys 1991;288(2):481–7.

209. Wolin MS. Interactions of oxidants with vascular signaling systems. Arteriosclerosis, Thrombosis & Vascular Biology 2000;20(6):1430–42.

210. Wolin MS, Davidson CA, Kaminski PM, Fayngersh RP, Mohazzab HK. Oxidant–nitric oxide signalling mechanisms in vascular tissue. Biochemistry-Russia 1998;63(7):810–6.

211. Wolin MS, Gupte SA, Oeckler RA. Superoxide in the vascular system. J Vasc Res 2002;39(3):191–207.

212. Davidson CA, Kaminski PM, Wu M, Wolin MS. Nitrogen dioxide causes pulmonary arterial relaxation via thiol nitrosation and NO formation. Am J Physiol 1996;270(3 Pt 2):H1038–43.

213. Darley-Usmar V, White R. Disruption of vascular signalling by the reaction of nitric oxide with superoxide: implications for cardiovascular disease. Exp Physiol 1997;82(2):305–16.

214. Tannous M, Rabini RA, Vignini A, et al. Evidence for iNOS-dependent peroxynitrite production in diabetic platelets. Diabetologia 1999;42(5):539–44.

215. Ceriello A, Mercuri F, Quagliaro L, et al. Detection of nitrotyrosine in the diabetic plasma: evidence of oxidative stress. In: Diabetologia. 7 ed; 2001:834–8.

216. Mihm MJ, Jing L, Bauer JA. Nitrotyrosine causes selective vascular endothelial dysfunction and DNA damage. J Cardiovasc Pharmacol 2000;36(2):182–7.

217. Cosentino F, Eto M, De Paolis P, et al. High glucose causes upregulation of cyclooxygenase-2 and alters prostanoid profile in human endothelial cells: role of protein kinase C and reactive oxygen species (see comment). Circulation 2003;107(7):1017–23.

218. Zou M-H. Peroxynitrite and protein tyrosine nitration of prostacyclin synthase. Prostaglandins Other Lipid Mediat 2007;82(1–4):119–27.

219. Frank GD, Eguchi S, Motley ED. The role of reactive oxygen species in insulin signaling in the vasculature. Antioxidants & Redox Signaling 2005;7(7–8):1053–61.

220. Chang T, Wang R, Wu L. Methylglyoxal-induced nitric oxide and peroxynitrite production in vascular smooth muscle cells. Free Radic Biol Med 2005;38(2):286–93.

221. Touyz RM, Schiffrin EL. Reactive oxygen species in vascular biology: implications in hypertension. Histochem Cell Biol 2004;122(4):339–52.

222. Lefer DJ, Scalia R, Campbell B, et al. Peroxynitrite inhibits leukocyte–endothelial cell interactions and protects against ischemia-reperfusion injury in rats. J Clin Invest 1997;99(4):684–91.

223. Delyani JA, Nossuli TO, Scalia R, Thomas G, Garvey DS, Lefer AM. S-nitrosylated tissue-type plasminogen activator protects against myocardial ischemia/reperfusion injury in cats: role of the endothelium. J Pharmacol Exp Ther 1996;279(3):1174–80.

224. Moore TM, Khimenko PL, Wilson PS, Taylor AE. Role of nitric oxide in lung ischemia and reperfusion injury. Am J Physiol 1996;271(5 Pt 2):H1970–7.

225. Liu P, Xu B, Quilley J, Wong PYK. Peroxynitrite attenuates hepatic ischemia-reperfusion injury. Am J Physiol Cell Physiol 2000;279(6):C1970–7.

226. Vinten-Johansen J, Zhao Z-Q, Nakamura M, et al. Nitric oxide and the vascular endothelium in myocardial ischemia-reperfusion injury. Ann NY Acad Sci 1999;874(1):354–70.

227. Lelamali K, Wang W, Gengaro P, Edelstein C, Schrier RW. Effects of nitric oxide and peroxynitrite on endotoxin-induced leukocyte adhesion to endothelium. J Cell Physiol 2001;188(3):337–42.

228. Nossuli TO, Hayward R, Jensen D, Scalia R, Lefer AM. Mechanisms of cardioprotection by peroxynitrite in myocardial ischemia and reperfusion injury. Am J Physiol 1998;275(2 Pt 2):H509–19.

229. Villa LM, Salas E, Darley-Usmar VM, Radomski MW, Moncada S. Peroxynitrite induces both vasodilatation and impaired vascular relaxation in the isolated perfused rat heart. Proc Natl Acad Sci USA 1994;91(26):12383–7.

230. Lewis SJ, Graves JE, Bates JN, Kooy NW. Peroxynitrite elicits dysfunction of stereoselective s-nitrosocysteine recognition sites. J Cardiovasc Pharmacol 2005;46(5):637–45.

231. Benkusky NA, Lewis SJ, Kooy NW. Attenuation of vascular relaxation after development of tachyphylaxis to peroxynitrite in vivo. Am J Physiol 1998;275(2 Pt 2):H501–8.

232. Kooy NW, Lewis SJ. Elevation in arterial blood pressure following the development of tachyphylaxis to peroxynitrite. Eur J Pharmacol 1996;307(3):R5–7.

233. Benkusky NA, Lewis SJ, Kooy NW. Peroxynitrite-mediated attenuation of alpha- and beta-adrenoceptor agonist-induced vascular responses in vivo. Eur J Pharmacol 1999;364(2–3):151–8.

234. Dowell FJ, Martin W. The effects of peroxynitrite on rat aorta: interaction with glucose and related substances. Eur J Pharmacol 1997;338(1):43–53.

235. Wu M, Pritchard KA, Jr., Kaminski PM, Fayngersh RP, Hintze TH, Wolin MS. Involvement of nitric oxide and nitrosothiols in relaxation of pulmonary arteries to peroxynitrite. Am J Physiol 1994;266(5 Pt 2):H2108–13.

236. Li J, Li W, Altura BT, Altura BM. Peroxynitrite-induced relaxation in isolated canine cerebral arteries and mechanisms of action. Toxicol Appl Pharmacol 2004;196(1):176–82.

237. Li J, Li W, Altura BT, Altura BM. Peroxynitrite-induced relaxation in isolated rat aortic rings and mechanisms of action. Toxicol Appl Pharmacol 2005;209(3):269–76.

238. Halliwell B, Zhao K, Whiteman M. Nitric oxide and peroxynitrite. The ugly, the uglier and the not so good: a personal view of recent controversies. Free Radic Res 1999;31(6):651–69.

239. Royall JA, Kooy NW, Beckman JS. Nitric oxide-related oxidants in acute lung injury. New Horiz 1995;3(1):113–22.

240. Pryor WA, Squadrito GL. The chemistry of peroxynitrite: a product from the reaction of nitric oxide with superoxide (see comment). Am J Physiol 1995;268(5 Pt 1):L699–722.

241. Nossaman BD, Dabisch PA, Liles JT, et al. Peroxynitrite does not impair pulmonary and systemic vascular responses. Journal of Applied Physiology 2004;96(2):455–62.

242. Nossaman BD, Bivalacqua TJ, Champion HC, Baber SR, Kadowitz PJ. Analysis of vasodilator responses to peroxynitrite in the hindlimb vascular bed of the cat. J Cardiovasc Pharmacol 2007;50(4):358–66.

243. Mabley JG, Soriano FG. Role of nitrosative stress and poly(ADP-ribose) polymerase activation in diabetic vascular dysfunction. Curr Vasc Pharmacol 2005;3(3):247–52.

244. Arrick DM, Sharpe GM, Sun H, Mayhan WG. Diabetes-induced cerebrovascular dysfunction: role of poly(ADP-ribose) polymerase. Microvasc Res 2007;73(1):1–6.

245. Obrosova IG, Drel VR, Pacher P, et al. Oxidative-nitrosative stress and poly(ADP-ribose) polymerase (PARP) activation in experimental diabetic neuropathy: the relation is revisited. Diabetes 2005;54(12):3435–41.

246. Szabo. PARP as a drug target for the therapy of diabetic cardiovascular dysfunction. Drug News Perspect 2002;15(4):197–205.

247. Du Y, Miller CM, Kern TS. Hyperglycemia increases mitochondrial superoxide in retina and retinal cells. Free Radic Biol Med 2003;35(11):1491–9.

248. Lastra C de la, Villegas I, Sanchez-Fidalgo S. Poly(ADP-Ribose) polymerase inhibitors: New pharmacological functions and potential clinical implications. Curr Pharmaceutical Design 2007;13:933–62.

249. Szabó C. Roles of poly(ADP-ribose) polymerase activation in the pathogenesis of diabetes mellitus and its complications. Pharmacol Res 2005;52(1):60–71.

250. Soriano FG, Virág L, Szabó C. Diabetic endothelial dysfunction: role of reactive oxygen and nitrogen species production and poly(ADP-ribose) polymerase activation. J Mol Med 2001;79(8):437–48.

251. Davidson SM, Duchen MR. Effects of NO on mitochondrial function in cardiomyocytes: Pathophysiological relevance. Cardiovasc Res 2006;71(1):10–21.

252. McDaniel ML, Kwon G, Hill JR, Marshall CA, Corbett JA. Cytokines and nitric oxide in islet inflammation and diabetes. Proc Soc Exp Biol Med 1996;211(1):24–32.

253. Du X, Matsumura T, Edelstein D, et al. Inhibition of GAPDH activity by poly(ADP-ribose) polymerase activates three major pathways of hyperglycemic damage in endothelial cells. J Clin Invest 2003;112(7):1049–57.

254. Osawa T, Kato Y. Protective role of antioxidative food factors in oxidative stress caused by hyperglycemia. Ann NY Acad Sci 2005;1043(1):440–51.

255. Bonnefont-Rousselot D. Glucose and reactive oxygen species. Curr Opin Clin Nutr Metab Care 2002;5(5):561–8.

256. Rösen P, Du X, Tschöpe D. Role of oxygen derived radicals for vascular dysfunction in the diabetic heart: prevention by alpha-tocopherol? Mol Cell Biochem 1998;188(1–2):103–11.

257. Stoppa GR, Cesquini M, Roman EAFR, Ogo SH, Torsoni MA. Aminoguanidine prevented impairment of blood antioxidant system in insulin-dependent diabetic rats. Life Sci 2006;78(12):1352–61.

258. Sato T, Iwaki M, Shimogaito N, Wu X, Yamagishi S-I, Takeuchi M. TAGE (Toxic AGEs) Theory in diabetic complications. Curr Mol Med 2006;6:351–8.

259. Goldin A, Beckman JA, Schmidt AM, Creager MA. Advanced glycation end products: sparking the development of diabetic vascular injury. Circulation 2006;114(6):597–605.

260. Soro-Paavonen A, Forbes JM. Novel therapeutics for diabetic micro- and macrovascular complications. Curr Med Chem 2006;13(15):1777–88.

261. Chandra D, Jackson EB, Ramana KV, Kelley R, Srivastava SK, Bhatnagar A. Nitric oxide prevents aldose reductase activation and sorbitol accumulation during diabetes. Diabetes 2002;51(10):3095–101.

262. Ramana KV, Chandra D, Srivastava S, Bhatnagar A, Srivastava SK. Nitric oxide regulates the polyol pathway of glucose metabolism in vascular smooth muscle cells. FASEB J 2003;17(3):417–25.

263. Srivastava S, Tammali R, Chandra D, et al. Regulation of lens aldose reductase activity by nitric oxide. Exp Eye Res 2005;81(6):664–72.

264. Chung SSM, Ho ECM, Lam KSL, Chung SK. Contribution of polyol pathway to diabetes-induced oxidative stress. J Am Soc Nephrol 2003;14(90003):S233–6.

265. Morisco C, Lembo G, Trimarco B. Insulin resistance and cardiovascular risk: New insights from molecular and cellular biology. Trends Cardiovasc Med 2006;16(6):183–8.
266. Bansilal S, Farkouh ME, Fuster V. Role of insulin resistance and hyperglycemia in the development of atherosclerosis. Am J Cardiol 2007;99(4A):6B–14B.
267. Fujiwara T, Horikoshi H. Troglitazone and related compounds: therapeutic potential beyond diabetes. Life Sci 2000;67(20):2405–16.
268. Kakafika AI, Liberopoulos EN, Karagiannis A, Athyros VG, Mikhailidis DP. Dyslipidaemia, hypercoagulability and the metabolic syndrome. Curr Vasc Pharmacol 2006;4:175–83.
269. Kahn R. Metabolic syndrome: Is it a syndrome? Does it matter? Circulation 2007;115(13):1806–11.
270. Ukkola O, Santaniemi M. Adiponectin: a link between excess adiposity and associated comorbidities? J Mol Med 2002;80(11):696–702.
271. Ohashi K, Kihara S, Ouchi N, et al. Adiponectin replenishment ameliorates obesity-related hypertension. Hypertension 2006;47(6):1108–16.
272. Nishio K, Shigemitsu M, Kusuyama T, et al. Insulin resistance in nondiabetic patients with acute myocardial infarction. Cardiovasc Revasc Med 2006;7(2):54–60.
273. Musi N, Goodyear LJ. Insulin resistance and improvements in signal transduction. Endocrine 2006;29(1): 73–80.
274. Bluher M, Bullen JW, Jr, Lee JH, et al. Circulating adiponectin and expression of adiponectin receptors in human skeletal muscle: associations with metabolic parameters and insulin resistance and regulation by physical training. J Clin Endocrinol Metab 2006;91(6):2310–6.
275. Nomura S, Inami N, Kimura Y, et al. Effect of nifedipine on adiponectin in hypertensive patients with type 2 diabetes mellitus. J Hum Hypertens 2007;21(1):38–44.
276. Tan KCB, Xu A, Chow WS, et al. Hypoadiponectinemia is associated with impaired endothelium-dependent vasodilation. J Clin Endocrinol Metab 2004;89(2):765–9.
277. Blaschke F, Spanheimer R, Khan M, Law RE. Vascular effects of TZDs: new implications. Vascul Pharmacol 2006;45(1):3–18.
278. Stumvoll M. Thiazolidinediones – some recent developments. Expert Opin Invest Drugs 2003;12(7):1179–87.
279. Nishio K, Sakurai M, Kusuyama T, et al. A randomized comparison of pioglitazone to inhibit restenosis after coronary stenting in patients with type 2 diabetes. In: Diabetes Care. 1 ed; 2006:101–6.
280. Pfützner A, Marx N, Lübben G, et al. Improvement of cardiovascular risk markers by pioglitazone is independent from glycemic control: results from the pioneer study. J Am Coll Cardiol 2005;45(12):1925–31.
281. Martens FMAC, Visseren FLJ, de Koning EJ, Rabelink TJ. Short-term pioglitazone treatment improves vascular function irrespective of metabolic changes in patients with type 2 diabetes. J Cardiovasc Pharmacol 2005;46(6):773–8.
282. Schmieder RE. Endothelial dysfunction: how can one intervene at the beginning of the cardiovascular continuum? J Hypertens Suppl 2006;24(2):S31–5.
283. Nissen SE, Wolski K: Effect of rosiglitazone on the risk of myocardial infarction and death from cardiovascular causes. *N Engl J Med.* 2007;356:2457–2471.
284. Action to Control Cardiovascular Risk in Diabetes Study Group, Gerstein HC, Miller ME, Byington RP, Goff DC, Jr, Bigger JT, Buse JB, Cushman WC, Genuth S, Ismail-Beigi F, Grimm RH, Jr, Probstfield JL, Simons-Morton DG, Friedewald WT: Effects of intensive glucose lowering in type 2 diabetes. *N Engl J Med.* 2008;358:2545–2559.
285. Home PD, Pocock SJ, Beck-Nielsen H, Gomis R, Hanefeld M, Jones NP, Komajda M, McMurray JJ, RECORD Study Group: Rosiglitazone evaluated for cardiovascular outcomes–an interim analysis. *N Engl J Med.* 2007;357:28–38.

4 Free Fatty Acids, A Major Link Between Obesity, Insulin Resistance, Inflammation, and Atherosclerotic Vascular Disease

Guenther Boden, MD

CONTENTS

SUMMARY

Plasma free fatty acids (FFAs) are elevated in obesity. By causing insulin resistance in all major insulin targets including muscle, liver, and endothelial cells, FFAs contribute to the development of type 2 diabetes (T2DM), hypertension, dyslipidemia, disorders of blood coagulation and fibrinolysis, and nonalcoholic fatty liver disease (NAFLD). In pancreatic β-cells, FFAs potentiate glucose-stimulated insulin secretion precisely to the extent needed to compensate for the FFA-induced insulin resistance. This prevents T2DM in the majority of obese, insulin-resistant individuals. On the other hand, in people with inherited defects of β-cell function (pre-diabetics), this compensation fails and T2DM develops. The mechanism through which FFA induces insulin resistance is postulated to involve intracellular accumulation of triglycerides and diacylglycerol, activation of several serine/threonine kinases, resulting in reduction of tyrosine phosphorylation of the insulin receptor substrate (IRS) 1/2 and impairment of the IRS/phosphoinositol 3 kinase pathway of insulin signaling. Elevated plasma FFA levels also produce low-grade inflammation in skeletal muscle and liver via activation of the nuclear factor κB pathway which results in synthesis and release of proinflammatory and proatherogenic cytokines. Thus, elevated FFA levels, present in obese people or due to high fat feeding, cause insulin resistance in all major insulin targets and are a major cause for the development of T2DM. In addition, FFAs produce a state of low-grade inflammation, and increase hepatic production of very low density lipoprotein (VLDL), and via producing insulin resistance and hyperinsulinemia promote a state of increased blood coagulation and

From: *Contemporary Endocrinology: Cardiovascular Endocrinology: Shared Pathways and Clinical Crossroads*
Edited by: V. A. Fonseca © Humana Press, New York, NY

decreased fibrinolysis. All these effects contribute to the development of atherosclerotic vascular disease and NAFLD.

Key Words: Obesity, Insulin resistance, Inflammation, Type 2 diabetes, Hypertension, Dyslipidemia, Blood coagulation, Atherosclerotic vascular disease

INTRODUCTION

In the United States, two-thirds of the adult population is either overweight or obese *(1)*. Ominously, the largest rise in obesity during the last decade has been in children and young adults *(1)*. This development poses major public health concerns because obesity is associated with a number of serious health problems including type 2 diabetes (T2DM), hypertension, dyslipidemia, nonalcoholic fatty liver disease (NAFLD), and disorders of blood coagulation and fibrinolysis all of which are recognized as independent risk factors for atherosclerotic vascular disease (ASVD), including myocardial infarctions, strokes, and peripheral arterial disease *(2)*.

The understanding of why obesity is closely associated with these disorders was facilitated by the recognition *(1)* that fat was a metabolically active tissue which synthesizes and secretes a large number of biologically active substances which are collectively called adipokines, *(2)* that obesity causes insulin resistance *(3)* and that therefore practically all obese people are insulin resistant, albeit to varying degrees, and *(3)* that obesity is a low-grade inflammatory state (Reviewed in ref. *(4)*) (Figure 1).

Ad1: Blood levels of several of biologically active substances produced by adipose tissue (which are collectively call adipokines), including TNF-α, interleukin-6 (IL-6), and resistin are elevated in obesity and several have been postulated to be responsible for the obesity-associated increase of insulin resistance *(4)*. So far, however, a major role as a link between obesity and insulin resistance in human subjects has been established only for free fatty acids (FFAs). In addition, acute elevations of plasma FFAs have recently been shown to activate a major inflammatory pathway and to raise plasma adipokine levels (Reviewed in the section on FFA and Inflammation). Therefore, elevated plasma adipokine levels in obesity may be, at least in part, a consequence of elevated plasma FFA levels.

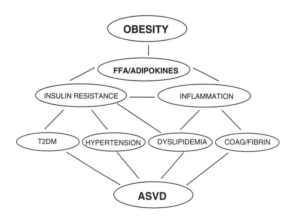

Fig. 1. Relationship between obesity, FFA, insulin resistance, inflammation and atherosclerotic vascular disease. Obesity causes insulin resistance and a state of low grade inflammation. Both contribute to the development of several disorders, including T2DM, hypertension, dyslipidemia and disorders of coagulation and fibrinolysis. All these disorders are independent risk factors for the development of atherosclerotic vascular disease. FFA: free fatty acids; T2DM: Type 2 diabetes mellitus; ASVD: atherosclerotic vascular disease.

Ad2: Insulin resistance is a key factor in the pathogenesis of T2DM and plays an important role in the development of hypertension, dyslipidemia, NAFLD, and disorders of coagulation and fibrinolysis *(5,6)*.

Ad3: The recognition that obesity is a low-grade inflammatory state was important because inflammation plays a pivotal role in the development of ASVD and NAFLD and, in addition, may contribute to insulin resistance *(7)*.

This chapter, therefore, focuses on the role of FFAs in the pathogenesis of insulin resistance/T2DM, hypertension, dyslipidemias, NAFLD, and ASVD.

FFA AND INSULIN RESISTANCE

The evidence for a causal role of FFAs in the development of insulin resistance in obese people can be summarized as follows: blood FFA levels are elevated in almost all obese people *(8)*, raising plasma FFA levels increases insulin resistance dose-dependently *(3,9)* while decreasing plasma FFA levels decreases insulin resistance *(10)*. It is not entirely clear why plasma FFA levels are elevated in obesity. Possible reasons include an increased release of FFAs from the enlarged adipose tissue, decreased uptake and utilization of FFAs *(11)*, and at a later stage, increased lipolysis due to developing insulin resistance in adipose tissue *(12)*. However, regardless of the reason why FFAs are elevated in obesity, it has been established that elevated blood FFA levels can inhibit insulin action in several target tissues including skeletal muscle, liver, and vascular endothelial cells.

Skeletal Muscle

Acute elevations of plasma FFAs (produced by i.v. infusion of heparinized triglyceride emulsions) produce dose-dependent inhibition of insulin-stimulated whole-body glucose uptake (>80% of which occurs in skeletal muscle) irrespective of gender, age, and the presence or absence of diabetes *(3)*. Under these conditions, insulin resistance develops with a delay of 2–4 h and disappears approximately 4 h after normalization of plasma FFA levels *(9)*.

Chronic elevations of plasma FFA levels, as found in obese individuals, also cause insulin resistance. This was demonstrated by lowering the chronically elevated FFA levels of obese diabetic and nondiabetic individuals into the normal range for 12 h *(10)*. This normalized insulin sensitivity in obese nondiabetic individuals and improved, but did not normalize, insulin sensitivity in obese diabetic patients *(10)*. This suggested that in obese nondiabetic subjects, high plasma FFA levels may have been the sole cause for their insulin resistance whereas in patients with T2DM, FFA was responsible for only part of their insulin resistance.

Liver

It has been well established that acute elevations of plasma FFA concentrations to levels frequently seen in obese individuals produce acute hepatic insulin resistance, that is, inhibit insulin's suppressive action on endogenous glucose production (EGP) *(13–16)*. Moreover, it has recently been shown that this is due primarily to FFA-induced inhibition of insulin suppression of glycogenolysis whereas FFAs have little acute effect on gluconeogenesis *(17)*.

Endothelial Cells

Insulin increases blood flow in arms and legs *(18)*. This effect is caused by an increase in peripheral vascular nitric oxide (NO) production *(19)*. FFAs inhibit the insulin-induced increase in venous NO and in peripheral blood flow *(20)*.

MECHANISM FOR FFA-INDUCED INSULIN RESISTANCE

Muscle

Whereas the precise mechanism by which obesity causes insulin resistance is still not completely understood, it has been established that FFAs can inhibit insulin action at the level of glucose transport and/or phosphorylation and that this inhibition is caused by a FFA-induced defect in insulin signaling *(21,22)*. Recently, an attractive mechanism has been proposed to explain how FFAs can inhibit insulin signaling. It is based on the finding that an increase in plasma FFA levels results in intramyocellular accumulation of triglycerides *(23)* and of several compounds involved in triglyceride synthesis including long-chain acyl-CoA and diacylglycerol (DAG) *(24)*. DAG is of particular interest in this respect because it is a potent allosteric activator of conventional and novel protein kinase C (PKC) isoforms *(25)*. Elevating FFA levels for 4 h has have been shown to increase total PKC activity and to activate the PKC-$\beta2$ and PKC-δ isoforms several fold in human skeletal muscle *(24)*. PKC is a serine/threonine kinase which is able to cause insulin resistance by decreasing tyrosine phosphorylation of the insulin receptor substrates (IRSs) 1/2 *(26)*. The issue, however, is complicated by the fact that IRS-1, for instance, has more than 40 serine/threonine consensus sites that can be phosphorylated. Therefore, other serine/threonine kinases, including c-Jun NH2 terminal kinase (JNK) and inhibitor of κB kinase-β (IKK-β) have been postulated to be involved in FFA-induced inhibition of insulin signaling and action *(27,28)* (Figure 2).

Liver

Acute elevations of plasma FFA concentrations produce acute hepatic insulin resistance, that is, inhibit insulin's suppressive action on EGP *(13–15)*. EGP consists of glucose derived from glycogenolysis and gluconeogenesis. It has recently been shown that acute elevations of plasma FFA levels produce hepatic insulin resistance primarily by inhibiting insulin-mediated suppression of glycogenolysis and have little acute effects on gluconeogenesis *(17)*. The mechanism by which FFAs cause hepatic insulin resistance has been directly addressed in two studies. Lam et al. *(29)* have shown that infusion of heparinized lipid (to increase plasma FFA levels) resulted in activation of PKC-δ in rat liver. In another study, euglycemic-hyperinsulinemic clamping with or without infusion of lipid/heparin (to raise or to lower plasma FFA levels) in male rats showed that the FFA-induced hepatic insulin resistance was associated with increased hepatic DAG content and increased activities of two serine/threonine kinases, namely, PKC-δ and IKK-β *(30)*. Thus, it appears that the mechanism by which FFAs cause insulin resistance in the liver appears to be similar to that in skeletal muscle.

Endothelial Cells

In endothelial cells, insulin increases peripheral vascular blood flow by simulating nitric oxide production *(18)*. FFAs inhibit the insulin-induced increase in peripheral venous NO and peripheral blood flow via two pathways. First, as outlined above, by reducing tyrosine phosphorylation of IRS-1/2, FFAs inhibit the PI3 kinase/AKT pathway which, aside from controlling

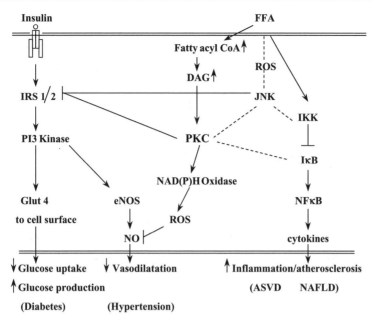

Fig. 2. Potential mechanisms of FFA-induced insulin resistance and inflammation. The key event is an increase in plasma FFA concentration. This leads to the accumulation of fatty acid CoA and DAG, and activation of PKC and other serine/threonine kinases including JNK and IKK in skeletal muscle, liver and vascular endothelial cells. It is assumed that activation of these kinases interrupts insulin signaling by serine phosphorylation of IRS 1/2, resulting in a decrease in tyrosine phosphorylation of IRS 1/2. In endothelial cells, PKC has been shown to activate NAD(P)H oxidase, which produces ROS and destroys NO. Elevation of plasma FFA levels also leads to the production of inflammatory and proatherogenic proteins through activation of the IKK/IκB-α/NFκB and JNK pathways. The broken lines indicate that activation of PKC by the IKK/ IκB-α/NFκB pathway and by ROS is a possibility that has not yet been demonstrated in human muscle or liver. Increased FFA-induced insulin resistance reduces glucose uptake in muscle and increases glucose production in the liver. Together, this results in hyperglycemia. FFA-mediated insulin resistance results in decreased NO and decreased vasodilatation in endothelial cells, which may contribute to the development of hypertension. In muscle and liver, FFA activation of the IKK/IκB-α/NFκB and JNK pathways results in low grade inflammation, which may promote ASVD and NAFLD. ASVD: atherosclerotic vascular disease; CoA: Coenzyme A; DAG: diacylgycerol; FFA: free fatty acids; IKK: inhibitor of κB kinases; IRS: insulin receptor substrate; JNK: c-jun N terminal kinase; NAD(P)H: nicotinamide adenine dinucleotide phosphate, reduced; NAFLD: non-alcoholic fatty liver disease; NFκB: nuclear factor κB; NO: nitric oxide; eNos: endothelial NO synthase; PI: phosphoinositide; PKC: protein kinase C; ROS: reactive oxygen species.

insulin-stimulated glucose uptake, is also needed to stimulate endothelial nitric oxide synthase (e-Nos) and thus the production of NO in endothelial cells *(19)*. Second, FFAs can reduce insulin-stimulated NO production by activating NADPH oxidase in a DAG/PKC-dependent manner *(31)*. Activation of NADPH oxidase leads to production of reactive-oxygen species (ROS) which results in destruction of NO *(31)* (Figure 2).

FFA AND INFLAMMATION

Obesity is now recognized as a low-grade inflammatory state associated with increased plasma levels of inflammatory cytokines. Many of those cytokines originate from the expanded adipose tissue and are collective called adipokines *(4)*. For instance, mice fed a high-fat diet developed hepatic insulin resistance and subacute hepatic inflammation with increased production and secretion of several inflammatory cytokines *(32)*. These studies left unanswered the question as to how the high-fat diet caused insulin resistance and the inflammatory state; other studies suggested that FFAs were the mediators *(24,30)*. In these studies, acute elevations of plasma FFA levels produced peripheral as well as hepatic insulin resistance which was associated with increased skeletal muscle and hepatic content of DAG, increased activities of two serine/threonine kinases (PKC and IKK), and activation of the proinflammatory nuclear factor (NF) κB pathway as well as increased expression of inflammatory cytokines, including TNF-α, IL1-β, and IL-6 and increased plasma levels of MCP-1 *(24,30)*. Moreover, infusion of heparinized lipid for 48 h has been shown in human muscle to increase expression of extracellular matrix-related genes in a pattern that was characteristic of an inflammatory response *(33)*. The concept emerging from these observations is that elevated plasma FFA levels, as result of either obesity or high-fat feeding, produce a state of insulin resistance and low-grade inflammation. Over time, this may result in T2DM and steatohepatitis and ASVD. In addition, it has been shown that in obesity, there is infiltration of macrophages into adipose tissue *(34,35)*. This macrophage infiltration is a late phenomenon and thus may not be an initial event but might contribute to chronic adipose tissue inflammation.

BLOOD COAGULATION/FIBRINOLYSIS

Coagulation

The tissue factor (TF) pathway is the primary physiological mechanism of initiation of blood coagulation *(36,37)*. Binding of native coagulation factor VII (FVII) to TF converts FVII to the activated form of FVIIa. The resulting TF–FVIIa complex then activates factors IX and X to factors IXa and Xa, respectively, leading to the formation of the prothrombinase complex and thrombin generation. The original concept that TF, present in the adventitia of normal blood vessels, initiates coagulation and thrombin formation only when the vessel wall is injured or plaques are fissured, has been broaden recently by the demonstration that there is, in addition, a circulating pool of TF in blood that is associated with cells and microparticles and is thrombogenic *(36–39)*. We have recently shown in nondiabetic volunteers that raising blood insulin and especially, raising blood insulin and blood glucose together to levels frequently seen in patients with T2DM, steeply increases circulating TF-procoagulant activity (TF-PCA) together with indicators of thrombin formation (prothrombin fragment 1+2 and thrombin–antithrombin complexes) *(40)*. As pointed out above, the increased plasma FFA levels in obesity cause insulin resistance. Insulin resistance, on the other hand, is associated with hyperinsulinemia in nondiabetic individuals and with hyperinsulinemia and hyperglycemia in patients with T2DM. Hence, our results suggested that FFA-induced insulin resistance, via its association with hyperinsulinemia in nondiabetic and hyperinsulinemia plus hyperglycemia in patients with T2DM, contributes to the hypercoagulable state in these individuals.

Fibrinolysis

Obesity, insulin resistance, and T2DM are also associated with impaired fibrinolysis *(41)*. Plasma concentration of plasminogen activator inhibitor 1 (PAI-1), which is the primary inhibitor of fibrinolysis, is increased in obese insulin-resistant individuals as well as in patients with T2DM *(42,43)* PAI-1 downregulates fibrinolysis by inhibiting the production of plasmin and thus promotes thrombosis and increases cardiovascular risks. PAI-1 is synthesized in endothelial cells and hepatocytes and is present in platelets and in plasma (Reviewed in ref. *(44))*. In vitro, PAI-1 secretion is stimulated by insulin in human adipocytes and by FFAs in hepatocytes. Hence, elevated plasma FFA levels, via producing insulin resistance and hyperinsulinemia (with or without hyperglycemia), promote a state characterized by increased tendency for thrombosis (see above) and decreased ability to lyse blood clots. Together this increases the risk for acute vascular events.

FFA AND LIPOPROTEINS

Hepatic overproduction of very low density lipoprotein (VLDL) is an important contributor to the dyslipidemia, that is, hypertriglyceridemia and low HDL levels, which is typically seen in obese insulin-resistant subjects and in patients with T2DM. Elevated plasma FFA levels resulting in increased hepatic FFA uptake are an important reason for the increased VLDL production (Reviewed in ref. *(45))*, and FFA have been shown to stimulate VLDL synthesis and secretion in cultured hepatocytes *(46,47)*. Nevertheless, increased hepatic FFA uptake is not the only cause for increased hepatic VLDL production. Equally important appears to be hepatic insulin resistance which can affect VLDL production through several mechanisms. For instance, insulin stimulates degradation of Apo B in hepatocytes *(48)* and inhibits the microsomal TG transfer protein (MTTP) and thus impairs maturing of pre-VLDL into VLDL ready for secretion *(49)*. Insulin resistance can be expected to have opposite effects. Hence, FFA may influence hepatic VLDL production not only by supplying a major substrate in increased quantity but in addition by interfering with the action of insulin which is a major inhibitor of VLDL production *(45)*.

LONG-TERM LOWERING OF PLASMA FFA LEVELS

It is generally accepted that elevated plasma FFA levels and insulin resistance are at the core of serious health problems associated with obesity. It follows, therefore, that elevated plasma FFA levels should be a target of therapy. Indeed, normalizing plasma FFA levels with acipimox, a nicotinic acid analogue, has been shown to improve insulin resistance in obese patients with T2DM *(50)* and in first-degree relatives of patients with T2DM *(51)*. It is, however, difficult to lower plasma FFA levels long-term with currently available drugs. The use of nicotinic acid or of long-acting nicotinic acid analogues is associated with rebound of plasma FFA to very high levels *(52)*. This renders these drugs unsuitable for long-term control of plasma FFA. Thiazolidinediones (TZDs) lower plasma FFA levels long-term and without rebound *(53–56)*. This effect, however, is modest (ranging from <10% to ~20%). Thus, TZD-induced lowering of plasma FFA levels is usually not sufficient to maximally improve insulin sensitivity in patients with T2DM. We have recently reported that therapy of patients with T2DM with a combination of a TZD (rosiglitazone) and a fibrate (fenofibrate) lowered plasma FFA levels more effectively than treatment with rosiglitazone alone and, in addition, tended to be more effective in lowering insulin resistance, blood sugar concentrations, and hemoglobin A1C *(57)*. Most interestingly, the rosiglitazone plus fenofibrate treatment completely prevented the water retention and weight gain associated with rosiglitazone treatment alone *(57)*. These preliminary results suggest that TZD plus fibrate may be a more suitable treatment than TZD alone to lower elevated plasma FFA levels long-term and without rebound and to improve insulin resistance, glucose tolerance, and glycemic control in obese patients with T2DM.

To make control of FFA levels a practical reality also requires ways to monitor plasma FFA concentrations. Whereas this is not yet possible on a routine basis, methods to allow episodic or continuous FFA measurements in blood or in interstitial fluids, similar to home glucose monitoring methods, are currently being developed by different companies.

ACKNOWLEDGMENTS

This work was supported by National Institutes of Health Grants R01-DK-58895, R01-HL-733267, and R01-DK-066003 and a Mentor-Based Training Grant from the American Diabetes Association.

REFERENCES

1. Mokdad AN, Bowman BA, Ford ES. The continuing epidemics of obesity and diabetes in the United States. JAMA 2001;286:1195–1200.
2. Bray GA. Medical consequences of obesity. J Clin Endocrinol Metab 1989;89:2583–2589.
3. Boden G. Role of fatty acids in the pathogenesis of insulin resistance and NIDDM. Diabetes 1997;46:3–10.
4. Tataranni PA, Ortega F. A burning question: does an adipokine-induced activation of the immune system mediate the effect of overnutrition on type 2 diabetes? Diabetes 2005;54:917–927.
5. Reaven GM. Role of insulin resistance in human disease. Diabetes 1988;37:1595–1607.
6. Ingelsson E, Sundstrom JA, Arnlov J, et al. Insulin resistance and risk of congestive heart failure. JAMA 2005;294:334–341.
7. Kershaw EE, Flier JS. Adipose tissue as an endocrine organ. J Clin Endocrinol Metab 2004;89:2548–2556.
8. Reaven GM, Hollenbeck C, Jeng C-Y, Wu MS, Chen YD. Measurement of plasma glucose, free fatty acid, lactate and insulin for 24 h in patients with NIDDM. Diabetes 1998;37:1020–1024.
9. Boden G, Jadali F, White J, et al. Effects of fat on insulin-stimulated carbohydrate metabolism in normal men. J Clin Invest 1991;88:960–966.
10. Santomauro AT, Boden G, Silva ME, et al. Overnight lowering of free fatty acids with acipimox improves insulin resistance and glucose tolerance in obese diabetic and nondiabetic subjects. Diabetes 1999;48:1836–1841.
11. Bjorntorp P, Bergman H, Varnauskas E. Plasma free fatty acid turnover in obesity. Acta Med Scand 1969;185:351–356.
12. Jensen MD, Haymond MW, Rizza RA, Cryer PE, Miles JM. Influence of body fat distribution on free fatty acid metabolism obesity. J Clin Invest 1989;83:1168–1173.
13. Ferrannini E, Barrett E, Bevilacqua S, DeFronzo R. Effect of fatty acids on glucose production and utilization in man. J Clin Invest 1993;72:1737–1747.
14. Bevilacqua S, Buzzigoli G, Bonadonna R, et al. Operation of Randle's cycle in patients with NIDDM. Diabetes 1990;39:383–389.
15. Fanelli C, Calderone S, Epifano I, et al. Demonstration of a critical role for free fatty acids in mediating counterregulatory stimulation in humans. J Clin Invest 1994;92:1617–1622.
16. Boden G, Chen X, Ruiz J, et al. Mechanisms of fatty acid-induced inhibition of glucose uptake. J Clin Invest 1994;93:2438–2446.
17. Boden G, Cheung P, Stein TP, Kresge K, Mozzoli M. FFA cause hepatic insulin resistance by inhibiting insulin suppression of glycogenolysis. Am J Physiol 2002;283:E12–E19.
18. Baron AD. Insulin resistance and vascular function. J Diabetes Complications 2002;16:92–102.
19. Zeng G, Nystrom FH, Ravichandran LV, et al. Roles for insulin receptor, PI3-kinase and Akt in insulin-signaling pathways related to production of nitric oxide in human vascular endothelial cells. Circulation 2000;101: L1539–L1545.
20. Steinberg HO, Tashoby M, Monestel R, et al. Elevated circulating free fatty acid levels impair endothelium-dependent vasodilation. J Clin Invest 1997;100:1230–1239.
21. Boden G, Chen X. Effects of fat on glucose uptake and utilization in patients with non-insulin-dependent diabetes. J Clin Invest 1995;96:1261–1268.
22. Dresner A, Laurent D, Marcucci M, et al. Effects of free fatty acids on glucose transport and IRS-1 associated phosphatidylinositol 3-kinase activity. J Clin Invest 1999;103:252–259.
23. Boden G, Lebed B, Schatz M, Homko C, Semieux S. Effects of acute changes of plasma free fatty acids on intramyocellular fat content and insulin resistance in healthy subjects. Diabetes 2001;50:1612–1617.
24. Itani SI, Ruderman NB, Schmieder F, Boden G. Lipid-induced insulin resistance in human muscle is associated with changes in diacylglycerol, protein kinase C, and IκB-α. Diabetes 2002;51:2005–2011.

25. Farese R. Diabetes Mellitus: a Fundamental and Clinical Text. LeRoith D, Taylor SI, Olefsky JM (Eds), Philadelphia, Lippincott, 2000;239–251.

26. Yu C, Chen Y, Cline GW, et al. Mechanism by which fatty acids inhibit activation of insulin receptor substrate-1 (IRS-1)-associated phosphatidylinositol 3-kinase activity in muscle. J Biol Chem 2002;277:50230–50236.

27. Hotamisligil GS. Role of endoplasmic reticulum stress and c-Jun NH2-terminal kinase pathways in inflammation and origin of obesity and diabetes. Diabetes 2005;54:S73–S78.

28. Ngyen MATA, Satoh H, Favelyukis S, et al. JNK and tumor necrosis factor-alpha mediate free fatty acid-induced insulin resistance in 3T3-L1 adipocytes. J Biol Chem 2005;280:35361–35371.

29. Lam TKT, Yoshii H, Haber A, et al. Free fatty acid-induced hepatic insulin resistance: a potential role for protein kinase C-delta. Am J Physiol 2002;283:E682–E691.

30. Boden G, She P, Mozzoli M, et al. Free fatty acids produce insulin resistance and activate the proinflammatory nuclear factor-kappaB pathway in rat liver. Diabetes 2005;54:3458–3465.

31. Inoguchi T, Li, P, Umeda F, et al. High glucose level and free fatty acid stimulate reactive oxygen species production through protein kinase C-dependent activation of NAD(P)H oxidase in cultured vascular cells. Diabetes 2000;49:1939–1945.

32. Cai D, Yuan M, Frantz DF, et al. Local and systemic insulin resistance resulting from hepatic activation of IKK-beta and NF-kappaB. Nat Med 2005;111:183–190.

33. Richardson DK, Kashyap S, Bajaj M, et al. Lipid infusion decreases the expression of nuclear encoded mitochondrial genes and increases the expression of extracellular matrix genes in human skeletal muscle. J Biol Chem 2005;280:10290–10297.

34. Xu H, Barnes GT, Yang Q, et al. Chronic inflammation in fat plays a crucial role in the development of obesity-related insulin resistance. J Clin Invest 2003;112:1821–1830.

35. Weisberg SP, McCann D, Desai M, et al. Obesity is associated with macrophage accumulation in adipose tissue. J Clin Invest 2003;112:1796–1808.

36. Rauch U, Nemerson Y. Tissue factor, the blood, and the arterial wall. Trends Cardiovasc Med 2000;10:139–143.

37. Mackman N. Role of tissue factor in hemostasis, thrombosis, and vascular development. Arterioscler Thromb Vasc Biol 2004;24:1015–1022.

38. Key NS, Slungaard A, Dandelet L, et al. Whole blood tissue factor procoagulant activity is elevated in patients with sickle cell disease. Blood 1998;91:4216–4223.

39. Chou J, Mackman N, Merrill-Skoloff G, Pedersen B, Furie BC, Furie B. Hematopoietic cell-derived microparticle tissue factor contributes to fibrin formation during thrombus propagation. Blood 2004;104:3190–3197.

40. Vaidyula VR, Rao AK, Mozzoli M, Homko C, Cheung P, Boden G. Effects of hyperglycemia and hyperinsulinemia on circulating tissue factor procoagulant activity and platelet CD40 ligand. Diabetes 2006;55:202–208.

41. Vague P, Juhan-Vague I, Aillaud MF, Badier C, Viard R, Alessi MC, et al. Correlation between blood fibrinolytic activity, plasminogen activator inhibitor level, plasma insulin level and relative body weight in normal and obese subjects. Metabolism 1986;35:250–253.

42. Pannacciulli N, De Mitrio R, Giorgino R, De Pergola G. Effect of glucose tolerance status on PAI-1 plasma levels in overweight and obese subjects. Obes Res 2002;10:717–725.

43. Festa A, D'Agostino R Jr, Tracy RP, Haffner SM. Elevated levels of acute-phase proteins and plasminogen activator inhibitor-1 predict the development of type 2 diabetes: the Insulin Resistance Atherosclerosis Study. Diabetes 2002;51:1131–1137.

44. Sobel BE, Schneider DJ. Platelet function, coagulopathy, and impaired fibrinolysis in diabetes. Cardiol Clin 2004;22:511–526.

45. Lewis GF, Carpentier A, Adeli K, Giacca A. Disordered fat storage and mobilization in the pathogenesis of insulin resistance and type 2 diabetes. Endocrine Reviews 2002;23:201–229.

46. White AI, Graham DL, LeGros J, Pease RJ, Scott J. Oleate-mediated stimulation of apolipoprotein B secretion from rat hepatoma cells. A function of the ability of apolipoprotein B to direct lipoprotein assembly and escape presecretory degradation. J Biol Chem 267:15657–15664, 1992.

47. Levinson M, Oswald B, Quarfordt S. Serum factors influencing cultured hepatocyte exogenous and endogenous triglyceride. Am J Physiol 1990;259:G15–G20.

48. Au CS, Wagner A, Chong T, Qiu W, Sparks JD, Adeli K. Insulin regulates hepatic apolipoprotein B production independent of the mass or activity of Akt1/PKBalpha. Metabolism 2004;53:228–235.

49. Brown AM, Gibbons GF. Insulin inhibits the maturation phase of VLDL assembly via a phosphoinositide 3-kinase-mediated event. Arterioscler Thromb Vasc Biol 2001;21:1656–1661.

50. Santomauro ATMG, Boden G, Silva M, et al: Overnight lowering of free fatty acids with acipimox improves insulin resistance and glucose tolerance in obese diabetic nondiabetic subjects. Diabetes 1999;48:1836–1841.

51. Bajaj M, Suraamornkul S, Kashyap S, Cusi K, Mandarino L, DeFronzo RA: Sustained reduction in plasma free fatty acid concentration improves insulin action without altering plasma adipocytokine levels in subjects with strong family history of type 2 diabetes. J Clin Endocrinol Metab 2004;89:4649–4655.

52. Chen X, Iqbal N, Boden G: The effects of free fatty acids on gluconeogenesis and glycogenolysis in normal subjects. J Clin Invest 1999;103:365–372.

53. Ghazzi MN, Perez JE, Antonucci TK, Driscoll JH, Huang SM, Faja BW, Whitcomb RW: Cardiac and glycemic benefits of troglitazone treatment in NIDDM: the Troglitazone Study Group. Diabetes 1997;46:433–439.

54. Maggs DG, Buchanan TA, Burant CF, Cline G, Gumbiner B, Hseuh WA, Inzucchi S, Kelley D, Nolan J, Olefsky JM, Polonsky KS, Silver D, Valiquett TR, Shulman GI: Metabolic effects of troglitazone monotherapy in type 2 diabetes mellitus. Ann Intern Med 1998;128:176–185.

55. Mayerson AB, Hundal RS, Dufour S: The effects of rosiglitazone on insulin sensitivity, lipolysis, and hepatic and skeletal muscle triglyceride content in patients with type 2 diabetes. Diabetes 2002;51:797–802.

56. Boden G, Cheung P, Mozzoli M, Fried SK: Effect of thiazolidinediones on glucose and fatty acid metabolism in patients with type 2 diabetes. Metabolism 2003;52:753–759.

57. Boden G, Homko C, Mozzoli M, Zhang M, Kresge K, Cheung P. Combined use of rosiglitazone and fenofibrate in patients with type 2 diabetes. Prevention of fluid retention. Diabetes 2007;56:248–255.

5 The Anti-Inflammatory and Antiatherogenic Effects of Insulin

Paresh Dandona, MD, PhD, Ajay Chaudhuri, MD, Husam Ghanim, PhD, and Priya Mohanty, MD

CONTENTS

SUMMARY

The concept that insulin affects carbohydrate, lipid, and protein metabolism and that its deficiency leads to diabetes mellitus has given this hormone a central position as a key metabolic regulator. However, its role as a vasoactive hormone and as an inhibitor of inflammation and oxidative stress has been revealed over the past decade and a half. These discoveries are relevant to the understanding of the role of oxidative stress and inflammation in the pathogenesis of insulin resistance and why obesity and type 2 diabetes are proinflammatory and proatherogenic states. A direct antiatherogenic effect of insulin has now been demonstrated in mice with experimental atherogenesis, and mice with an interference with insulin signal transduction have been shown to be proatherogenic. The recent discovery that glucose and macronutrient intake induce oxidative stress and inflammation have added a new dimension to understanding of why obesity and type 2 diabetes are proinflammatory and proatherogenic.

These data are now evolved enough for us to plan clinical strategies to use insulin as an anti-inflammatory agent in acute syndromes like acute myocardial infarction and in patients in surgical and medical intensive care units.

Key Words: Insulin, Glucose, Inflammation, Atherosclerosis

From: *Contemporary Endocrinology: Cardiovascular Endocrinology: Shared Pathways and Clinical Crossroads*
Edited by: V. A. Fonseca © Humana Press, New York, NY

ANTI-INFLAMMATORY EFFECTS OF INSULIN

The discovery of the anti-inflammatory effect of insulin can be traced back to the observation that insulin exerts a vasodilatory effect in arteries, veins, and capillaries (microcirculation) *(1,2)*. Since these reports also showed that this effect was due to nitric oxide (NO) generation from the endothelium, in vivo, a direct effect of insulin on NO release by the endothelium was investigated. The endothelium was shown to release NO in a dose-dependent fashion in response to insulin stimulation in human umbilical vein endothelial cells *(3,4)*. Furthermore, the expression of endothelial NO synthase (eNOS) in response to insulin also increased in a dose-dependent fashion in human aortic endothelial cells *(5)*.

Definitive experiments demonstrating the anti-inflammatory effects of insulin were first performed, in vitro, in human aortic endothelial cells. They showed that insulin suppressed the expression of the proinflammatory intracellular adhesion molecule-1, (ICAM-1), the chemokine, monocyte chemoattractant protein-1 (MCP-1), and the key proinflammatory transcription factor, nuclear factor kappa B (NFκB), in human aortic endothelial cells at physiologically relevant concentrations *(3,5,6)*. This was followed by the demonstration that insulin infusions given at a low dose (2 units per hour) to obese subjects suppressed reactive-oxygen species (ROS generation), $p47^{phox}$ expression (an indicator of NADPH oxidase action, the enzyme which generates the superoxide radical), NFκB binding, and increased inhibitor kappa B α (IκBα) expression by mononuclear cells (MNCs) *(7)*. In addition insulin causes an acute reduction in plasma concentrations of ICAM-1, MCP-1, and another proinflammatory transcription factor, early growth response-1 (Egr-1), tissue factor (TF), and plasminogen activator inhibitor 1 (PAI-1) *(8)*. Insulin has also been shown to suppress matrix metalloproteinase-9 (MMP-9) and vascular endothelial growth factor (VEGF), two key mediators involved in the spread of inflammation and in the increase of vascular permeability *(9,10)*.

In a study involving patients with acute myocardial infarction (AMI), insulin was also shown to suppress C-reactive protein (CRP) and serum amyloid A (SAA) by 40% within 24 h of the initiation of the insulin infusion while glucose concentrations were not allowed to change *(11)*. This effect of insulin was confirmed in hyperglycemic patients with myocardial infarction and has now also been confirmed in patients undergoing coronary artery bypass grafts in two studies *(12–14)*. While this effect of insulin was apparent even earlier at 12 h after the initiation of the infusion, the magnitude of the effect on CRP and SAA concentrations was similar to that (40%) observed in the earlier studies in spite of an overall increase in CRP and SAA concentrations which is 30 times greater than that observed in AMI *(11–13)*. One of the studies on CABG patients also demonstrated that the use of subcutaneously injected insulin to maintain normoglycemia was not able to cause a reduction in CRP concentrations *(12)*. Thus, it is likely that the anti-inflammatory effect of insulin is only exerted when insulin concentration is maintained at a high level using intravenous infusions supported by small amounts of glucose to prevent hypoglycemia. Treatment of AMI patients with insulin also suppresses PAI-1 and pro-MMP-1 *(11,15)*. In patients treated in an intensive care unit (ICU), insulin infusions have also been shown to suppress iNOS expression in the liver and reduce plasma concentrations of nitrite and nitrate, the two metabolites of NO *(16)*. The anti-inflammatory effect of insulin has also been shown in patients with burns *(17)*. Similar anti-inflammatory effects have been observed in animals with experimental burns *(18)*. More recently, data demonstrating interference by insulin on signal transduction by interleukin-6 (IL-6) on adipocytes, in vitro, has also been shown. Thus, the phosphorylation and activation of STAT-3 leads to its translocation into the nucleus and the transcriptional activation of genes

in subjects with type 2 diabetes and this effect has been reduced with the administration of antioxidants *(46)*.

The intake of saturated fat taken as cream (33 g fat = 300 Calories) also results in an increase in ROS generation by leukocytes and the occurrence of inflammation at the cellular and molecular level, similar to that described for glucose *(47)*. The infusion of triglyceride and heparin to raise the plasma concentration of free fatty acids (FFAs) from 200 to 300 μmol/l in normal subjects to 800–900 μmol/l, similar to that found in obese subjects, also leads to an increase in ROS generation, NFκB binding, and plasma concentration of MIF *(48)*. In addition, such an infusion is also known to cause acute insulin resistance. Calorie fast food meal also results in an increase in ROS generation, p47^{phox}, Iκ kinases α and β, an increase in NFκB binding, and a decrease in IκBα *(49)*. This inflammatory response lasts for more than 3 h. In the obese, the state of inflammation induced by a fast food meal is of a greater magnitude and lasts longer than that in normal subjects. This is probably due to the fact that the obese are in a proinflammatory oxidative stress *(50)* state even after fasting overnight and thus the effect of the fast food meal is additional. While discussing the proinflammatory effects of macronutrients, it is important to also investigate whether there are ways to avoid proinflammatory foods and to discover foods which are not likely to cause oxidative or inflammatory stress. Recent work has shown that orange juice, alcohol, and a meal rich in fruit and fiber are not likely to cause inflammatory or oxidative stress *(41,51,52)*. Thus, appropriate food choices can be made to avoid oxidative and inflammatory insults.

Just as macronutrient intake results in inflammation, its withdrawal or reduction results in a decrease in oxidative stress and inflammation. Thus, a reduction in caloric intake to 1000 calories per day in a group of obese patients resulted in a marked reduction in ROS generation, lipid peroxidation, protein carbonylation, and oxidative damage of the amino acid phenylalanine over the course of 4 weeks while subjects lost approximately 13 lbs in weight *(53)*. In a study involving normal subjects, a 48-h fast resulted in the reduction of ROS generation by leukocytes by 35% at 24 h and >50% at 48 h *(54)*. There was a concomitant decrease in the expression of p47^{phox}*(54)*. On the basis of these observations, one can conclude that macronutrient intake is probably the single most important contributor of oxidative stress, in vivo. These observations have been confirmed in the obese on the basis that dietary restriction led to a significant reduction in isoprostane excretion in the urine *(53)*. Long-term caloric restriction with weight loss also results in the fall of the proinflammatory cytokine, TNFα *(55)*. Weight loss and caloric restriction have also been shown to reduce other cytokines and CRP *(56)*.

CLINICAL IMPLICATIONS

In view of the rapidly developing data demonstrating an anti-inflammatory effect of insulin and a proinflammatory effect of glucose and FFAs and the relationship of clinical outcomes with indices of inflammation, it is clear that the maintenance of euglycemia with the help of insulin infusions is one potentially important strategy in the care of the critically ill, patients with cardiovascular disease including acute cardiac syndromes (AMI, ACS, and CABG surgery), stroke, and peripheral vascular disease (Figure 2). This area clearly needs further definitive investigation.

The published data demonstrate clearly that hyperglycemia worsens prognosis including mortality in ICU (surgical and medical) patients. It also causes a marked dose-dependent deterioration of morbidity and mortality in patients with AMI, stroke, and in all hospitalized patients. In patients with burns and those in ICUs, the control of hyperglycemia with insulin infusion improves clinical outcomes. The proinflammatory and pro-oxidant action of glucose

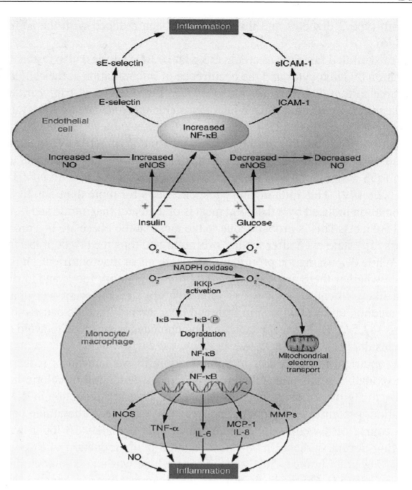

Fig. 2. The anti-inflammatory effect of insulin and the proinflammatory effect of glucose. Insulin suppresses ROS and O_2. generation and NADPH oxidase expression while glucose stimulates both. Within the macrophage, O_2. activates IKKbeta to enhance phosphorylation of IkappaB such that it undergoes proteosomal degradation, releasing NFκB to translocate into the nucleus. NFκB stimulates the transcription of genes encoding proinflammatory proteins including TNF alpha, IL-6, MCP-1, and MMPs. Within the endothelial cell insulin also induces eNOS expression in endothelial cells, which leads to controlled NO release and vasodilation, while glucose has the opposite effect. Glucose induces the expression of adhesion molecules ICAM-1 and E-selectin, while insulin suppreses their expression in the endothelial cell. (Adapted from reference *(53)*).

and the ROS suppressive and anti-inflammatory action of insulin are likely to play an important role in the pathogenesis and the treatment of these complications *(57)*. Regimes which infuse fixed doses of insulin with high rates of glucose are usually associated with hyperglycemia as observed in several studies with AMI patients. The induction of hyperglycemia may potentially neutralize the benefits of insulin and these regimes should, therefore, be avoided. We are currently conducting a study to test whether insulin infused to restore normoglycemia and then maintained at a low dose with a dextrose infusion titrated to prevent hypoglycemia, in AMI patients will provide cardioprotection and improve clinical outcomes. Such regimens will need to be tested in various clinical conditions in which such an approach is hypothesized to be beneficial.

REFERENCES

1. Grover A, Padginton C, Wilson MF, Sung BH, Izzo JL, Jr, Dandona P. Insulin attenuates norepinephrine-induced venoconstriction. An ultrasonographic study. Hypertension 1995;25:779–84.

2. Steinberg HO, Brechtel G, Johnson A, Fineberg N, Baron AD. Insulin-mediated skeletal muscle vasodilation is nitric oxide dependent. A novel action of insulin to increase nitric oxide release. J Clin Invest 1994;94:1172–9.

3. Aljada A, Saadeh R, Assian E, Ghanim H, Dandona P. Insulin inhibits the expression of intercellular adhesion molecule-1 by human aortic endothelial cells through stimulation of nitric oxide. J Clin Endocrinol Metab 2000;85:2572–5.

4. Zeng G, Quon MJ. Insulin-stimulated production of nitric oxide is inhibited by wortmannin. Direct measurement in vascular endothelial cells. J Clin Invest 1996;98:894–8.

5. Aljada A, Dandona P. Effect of insulin on human aortic endothelial nitric oxide synthase. Metabolism 2000;49:147–50.

6. Aljada A, Ghanim H, Saadeh R, Dandona P. Insulin Inhibits NFkappaB and MCP-1 expression in human aortic endothelial cells. J Clin Endocrinol Metab 2001;86:450–453.

7. Dandona P, Aljada A, Mohanty P, et al. Insulin inhibits intranuclear nuclear factor kappaB and stimulates IkappaB in mononuclear cells in obese subjects: evidence for an anti-inflammatory effect? J Clin Endocrinol Metab 2001;86:3257–65.

8. Aljada A, Ghanim H, Mohanty P, Kapur N, Dandona P. Insulin inhibits the pro-inflammatory transcription factor early growth response gene-1 (Egr)-1 expression in mononuclear cells (MNC) and reduces plasma tissue factor (TF) and plasminogen activator inhibitor-1 (PAI-1) concentrations. J Clin Endocrinol Metab 2002;87:1419–22.

9. Dandona P, Aljada A, Mohanty P, Ghanim H, Bandyopadhyay A, Chaudhuri A. Insulin suppresses plasma concentration of vascular endothelial growth factor and matrix metalloproteinase-9. Diabetes Care 2003;26:3310–4.

10. Weis S, Shintani S, Weber A, et al. Src blockade stabilizes a Flk/cadherin complex, reducing edema and tissue injury following myocardial infarction. J Clin Invest 2004;113:885–94.

11. Chaudhuri A, Janicke D, Wilson MF, et al. Anti-inflammatory and profibrinolytic effect of insulin in acute ST-segment-elevation myocardial infarction. Circulation 2004;109:849–54.

12. Koskenkari JK, Kaukoranta PK, Rimpilainen J, et al. Anti-inflammatory effect of high-dose insulin treatment after urgent coronary revascularization surgery. Acta Anaesthesiol Scand 2006;50:962–9.

13. Visser L, Zuurbier CJ, Hoek FJ, et al. Glucose, insulin and potassium applied as perioperative hyperinsulinaemic normoglycaemic clamp: effects on inflammatory response during coronary artery surgery. Br J Anaesth 2005;95:448–57.

14. Wong VW, McLean M, Boyages SC, Cheung NW. C-reactive protein levels following acute myocardial infarction: effect of insulin infusion and tight glycemic control. Diabetes Care 2004;27:2971–3.

15. Chaudhuri A, Janicke D, Wilson MF, Ghanim H, Aljada A, Dandona P. Free fatty acid suppressive, Pro- MMP-1 lowering and cardioprotective effect of insulin in STEMI. Diabetes 2005;54:A182:739-P.

16. Langouche L, Vanhorebeek I, Vlasselaers D, et al. Intensive insulin therapy protects the endothelium of critically ill patients. J Clin Invest 2005;115:2277–2286.

17. Herndon DN, Tompkins RG. Support of the metabolic response to burn injury. Lancet 2004;363:1895–902.

18. Jeschke MG, Einspanier R, Klein D, Jauch KW. Insulin attenuates the systemic inflammatory response to thermal trauma. Mol Med 2002;8:443–50.

19. Andersson CX, Sopasakis VR, Wallerstedt E, Smith U. Insulin antagonizes IL-6 signaling and is anti-inflammatory in 3T3-L1 adipocytes. JBC 2007;282:9430–9435.

20. Cheung NW, Wong VW, McLean M. The Hyperglycemia: Intensive Insulin Infusion in Infarction (HI-5) study: a randomized controlled trial of insulin infusion therapy for myocardial infarction. Diabetes Care 2006;29: 765–70.

21. Malmberg K, Ryden L, Efendic S, et al. Randomized trial of insulin–glucose infusion followed by subcutaneous insulin treatment in diabetic patients with acute myocardial infarction (DIGAMI study): effects on mortality at 1 year. J Am Coll Cardiol 1995;26:57–65.

22. Gao F, Gao E, Yue TL, et al. Nitric oxide mediates the antiapoptotic effect of insulin in myocardial ischemia-reperfusion: the roles of PI3-kinase, Akt, and endothelial nitric oxide synthase phosphorylation. Circulation 2002;105:1497–502.

23. Jonassen AK, Brar BK, Mjos OD, Sack MN, Latchman DS, Yellon DM. Insulin administered at reoxygenation exerts a cardioprotective effect in myocytes by a possible anti-apoptotic mechanism. J Mol Cell Cardiol 2000;32:757–64.

24. Zhang HX, Zang YM, Huo JH, et al. Physiologically tolerable insulin reduces myocardial injury and improves cardiac functional recovery in myocardial ischemic/reperfused dogs. J Cardiovasc Pharmacol 2006;48: 306–13.

25. Griselli M, Herbert J, Hutchinson WL, et al. C-reactive protein and complement are important mediators of tissue damage in acute myocardial infarction. J Exp Med 1999;190:1733–40.

26. Pepys MB, Hirschfield GM, Tennent GA, et al. Targeting C-reactive protein for the treatment of cardiovascular disease. Nature 2006;440:1217–21.

27. Bucciarelli-Ducci C, Bianchi M, De Luca L, et al. Effects of glucose–insulin–potassium infusion on myocardial perfusion and left ventricular remodeling in patients treated with primary angioplasty for ST-elevation acute myocardial infarction. Am J Cardiol 2006;98:1349–53.

28. Trovati M, Massucco P, Mattiello L, Mularoni E, Cavalot F, Anfossi G. Insulin increases guanosine-3′, 5′-cyclic monophosphate in human platelets. A mechanism involved in the insulin anti-aggregating effect. Diabetes 1994;43:1015–9.

29. Trovati M, Anfossi G, Massucco P, et al. Insulin stimulates nitric oxide synthesis in human platelets and, through nitric oxide, increases platelet concentrations of both guanosine-3′, 5′-cyclic monophosphate and adenosine-3′, 5′-cyclic monophosphate. Diabetes 1997;46:742–9.

30. Worthley MI, Holmes AS, Willoughby SR, et al. The deleterious effects of hyperglycemia on platelet function in diabetic patients with acute coronary syndromes: mediation by superoxide production, resolution with intensive insulin administration. J Am Coll Cardiol 2007;49:304–310.

31. Libby P, Simon DI. Inflammation and thrombosis: the clot thickens. Circulation 2001;103:1718–20.

32. Shamir R, Shehadeh N, Rosenblat M, et al. Oral insulin supplementation attenuates atherosclerosis progression in apolipoprotein E-deficient mice. Arterioscler Thromb Vasc Biol 2003;23:104–10.

33. Kubota T, Kubota N, Moroi M, et al. Lack of insulin receptor substrate-2 causes progressive neointima formation in response to vessel injury. Circulation 2003;107:3073–80.

34. Ross R. Atherosclerosis – an inflammatory disease. N Engl J Med 1999;340:115–26.

35. Dandona P, Aljada A, Mohanty P. The anti-inflammatory and potential anti-atherogenic effect of insulin: a new paradigm. Diabetologia 2002;45:924–30.

36. Han S, Liang CP, DeVries-Seimon T, et al. Macrophage insulin receptor deficiency increases ER stress-induced apoptosis and necrotic core formation in advanced atherosclerotic lesions. Cell Metab 2006;3:257–66.

37. Baumgartl J, Baudler S, Scherner M, et al. Myeloid lineage cell-restricted insulin resistance protects apolipoprotein E-deficient mice against atherosclerosis. Cell Metab 2006;3:247–56.

38. Nathan DM, Lachin J, Cleary P, et al. Intensive diabetes therapy and carotid intima-media thickness in type 1 diabetes mellitus. N Engl J Med 2003;348:2294–303.

39. Nathan DM, Cleary PA, Backlund JY, et al. Intensive diabetes treatment and cardiovascular disease in patients with type 1 diabetes. N Engl J Med 2005;353:2643–53.

40. Mohanty P, Hamouda W, Garg R, Aljada A, Ghanim H, Dandona P. Glucose challenge stimulates reactive oxygen species (ROS) generation by leucocytes. J Clin Endocrinol Metab 2000;85:2970–3.

41. Dhindsa S, Tripathy D, Mohanty P, et al. Differential effects of glucose and alcohol on reactive oxygen species generation and intranuclear nuclear factor-kappaB in mononuclear cells. Metabolism 2004;53:330–4.

42. Esposito K, Nappo F, Marfella R, et al. Inflammatory cytokine concentrations are acutely increased by hyperglycemia in humans: role of oxidative stress. Circulation 2002;106:2067–72.

43. Aljada A, Ghanim H, Mohanty P, Syed T, Bandyopadhyay A, Dandona P. Glucose intake induces an increase in activator protein 1 and early growth response 1 binding activities, in the expression of tissue factor and matrix metalloproteinase in mononuclear cells, and in plasma tissue factor and matrix metalloproteinase concentrations. Am J Clin Nutr 2004;80:51–7.

44. Mackman N. Role of tissue factor in hemostasis, thrombosis, and vascular development. Arterioscler Thromb Vasc Biol 2004;24:1015–22.

45. Steppich BA, Moog P, Matissek C, et al. Cytokine profiles and T cell function in acute coronary syndromes. Atherosclerosis 2007;190:443–51.

46. Ceriello A, Giacomello R, Stel G, et al. Hyperglycemia-induced thrombin formation in diabetes. The possible role of oxidative stress. Diabetes 1995;44:924–8.

47. Mohanty P, Ghanim H, Hamouda W, Aljada A, Garg R, Dandona P. Both lipid and protein intakes stimulate increased generation of reactive oxygen species by polymorphonuclear leukocytes and mononuclear cells. Am J Clin Nutr 2002;75:767–72.

48. Tripathy D, Mohanty P, Dhindsa S, et al. Elevation of free fatty acids induces inflammation and impairs vascular reactivity in healthy subjects. Diabetes 2003;52:2882–7.

49. Aljada A, Mohanty P, Ghanim H, et al. Increase in intranuclear nuclear factor κB and decrease in inhibitor κB in mononuclear cells after a mixed meal: evidence for a proinflammatory effect. Am J Clin Nutr 2004;79: 682–690.

50. Ghanim H, Aljada A, Hofmeyer D, Syed T, Mohanty P, Dandona P. Circulating mononuclear cells in the obese are in a proinflammatory state. Circulation 2004;110:1564–71.

51. Mohanty P, Daoud N, Ghanim H, et al. Absence of oxidative stress and inflammation following the intake of a 900 kcalorie meal rich in fruit and fiber. Diabetes 2004;53:A405.

52. Ghanim H, Mohanty P, Pathak R, Chaudhuri A, Sia CL, Dandona P. Orange juice or fructose intake does not induce oxidative and inflammatory Response. Diabetes Care 2007.

53. Dandona P, Mohanty P, Ghanim H, et al. The suppressive effect of dietary restriction and weight loss in the obese on the generation of reactive oxygen species by leukocytes, lipid peroxidation, and protein carbonylation. J Clin Endocrinol Metab 2001;86:355–362.

54. Dandona P, Mohanty P, Hamouda W, et al. Inhibitory effect of a two day fast on reactive oxygen species (ROS) generation by leucocytes and plasma ortho-tyrosine and meta-tyrosine concentrations. J Clin Endocrinol Metab 2001;86:2899–902.

55. Dandona P, Weinstock R, Thusu K, Abdel-Rahman E, Aljada A, Wadden T. Tumor necrosis factor-alpha in sera of obese patients: fall with weight loss. J Clin Endocrinol Metab 1998;83:2907–10.

56. Dandona P, Aljada A, Chaudhuri A, Mohanty P, Garg R. Metabolic syndrome: a comprehensive perspective based on interactions between obesity, diabetes, and inflammation. Circulation 2005;111:1448–1454.

57. Dandona P, Mohanty P, Chaudhuri A, Garg R, Aljada A. Insulin infusion in acute illness. J Clin Invest 2005;115:2069–72.

6 Insulin Sensitizers and Cardiovascular Disease

Tina K. Thethi, MD, Shipra Singh, Vivian Fonseca, MD

CONTENTS

SUMMARY

Type 2 diabetes mellitus (DM) is a progressive disease caused by insulin resistance (IR) in the skeletal muscle, adipose tissue, and liver in conjunction with impaired pancreatic secretion. Epidemiologic studies have shown IR to be an independent risk factor for cardiovascular disease (CVD). Insulin resistance contributes to the development of atherosclerosis through multiple other well-established risk factors such as hypertension, dyslipidemia, and hypercoagulabilty. Endothelial dysfunction is a central cause of many vascular diseases, including atherosclerosis and diabetic microangiopathy and many of the components of the IR syndrome affect the integrity of the endothelial function. Metformin inhibits hepatic gluconeogenesis and improves peripheral insulin sensitivity, possibly by reducing body weight and has been suggested to decrease cardiovascular

From: *Contemporary Endocrinology: Cardiovascular Endocrinology: Shared Pathways and Clinical Crossroads*
Edited by: V. A. Fonseca © Humana Press, New York, NY

events in patients with type 2 DM independent of glycemic control. Thiazolidinediones (TZDs) decrease IR primarily at the level of the muscles, thereby increasing glucose uptake and decreasing plasma glucose and may improve insulin sensitivity by decreasing the plasma free fatty acid concentration (FFA). The TZDs act on the endothelium by way of various mechanisms and also affect the modulation of various cytokines. Recently, metformin also was shown to improve endothelial function. Several long-term studies are currently undergoing to evaluate the long-term effects on cardiovascular outcomes, as well as long-term glycemic control in high risk patients.

Key Words: Type 2 diabetes mellitus, Insulin resistance, Insulin sensitizers, Cardiovascular disease, Endothelial function

INTRODUCTION
Insulin Sensitizers: An Overview

Type 2 diabetes mellitus (DM) is a progressive disease caused by insulin resistance (IR) in the skeletal muscle, adipose tissue, and liver in conjunction with impaired pancreatic secretion *(1)*. Hyperinsulinemia reflects IR. Epidemiologic studies have shown IR to be an independent risk factor for cardiovascular disease (CVD) *(2)*. Correction of underlying IR in the management of type 2 DM is important and may decrease the risk for CVD. IR contributes to the development of atherosclerosis through multiple other well-established risk factors such as hypertension, dyslipidemia, and hypercoagulability *(3)*. Patients with type 2 DM have increased relative risk of CVD when compared to patients who do not have type 2 DM *(4)*. Morbidity and mortality in type 2 DM is associated with cardiovascular events. In patients with established CVD, subsequent cardiovascular event rate *(5)* and morbidity and mortality are significantly greater than in those without DM. Advances in the field of cardiology have led to significant reduction in the cardiovascular mortality in patients without diabetes. However, the reduction has been modest and not statistically significant in those with DM *(6)*.

IR contributes to hyperglycemia in type 2 DM and is responsible for a multitude of other metabolic abnormalities, such as high level of plasma triglycerides (TGs), low level of high-density lipoprotein (HDL) cholesterol, hypertension, abnormal fibrinolysis, and is associated with coronary heart disease *(7,8)*. This cluster of abnormalities has been recognized as the IR syndrome or the metabolic syndrome *(9,10)*.

In the obesity substudy in the UKPDS, patients with type 2 DM treated with Metformin had a 30% reduction in CVD events and mortality compared with those who received conventional treatment *(11)*. These results are controversial due to the small number of patients. Metformin inhibits hepatic gluconeogenesis and improves peripheral insulin sensitivity, possibly by reducing body weight and has been suggested to decrease cardiovascular events in patients with type 2 DM independent of glycemic control *(11)*.

Thiazolidinediones (TZDs) are a class of drugs used widely for the treatment of type 2 DM. They decrease IR primarily at the level of the muscles, thereby increasing glucose uptake and decreasing plasma glucose *(12,13)*. To a lesser degree, they also decrease glucose production by the liver *(14)*. TZDs may improve insulin sensitivity by decreasing the plasma free fatty acid concentration (FFA) *(15)*. Due to the involvement of the FFAs in glucose and lipid metabolism *(16)*, they have deleterious effects on the vasculature *(17)*. Thus, reduction in the plasma FFA level may have a beneficial effect on CVD.

As IR plays a pivotal role in CVD, it has been proposed that drugs that directly improve insulin sensitivity, such as TZDs, may correct other abnormalities of the IR syndrome in addition to improving hyperglycemia *(18)*. The purpose of this chapter is to review the effects of the insulin sensitizers on CVD.

EFFECTS OF INSULIN SENSITIZERS ON LIPID METABOLISM

Nearly 30%–50% of the patients with type 2 DM have lipid abnormalities *(5)*. The characteristic pattern of dyslipidemia in patients with type 2 DM and IR include decreased HDL cholesterol (HDL-C); elevated TG levels; and an increase in small, dense low-density lipoprotein (LDL) particles, which are more atherogenic. Metformin modestly decreases LDL and increases HDL and has variable effects on TGs *(19)*. In combination with a sulfonylurea or as monotherapy, it has recently been shown to decrease some of the nontraditional cardiac risk factors, including remnant lipoprotein cholesterol *(20)*.

The effects of TZDs on lipid metabolism are more complex *(21,22)*. In patients with type 2 DM, the LDL particles tend to be smaller and dense and therefore more atherogenic. TZD monotherapy has been associated with a modest (8%–10%) increase in LDL levels. There is little change in the apolipoprotein B levels and a marked shift from small and dense to large and fluffy LDL phenotype. They also increase HDL significantly, especially in patients who had diabetes and HDL levels less than 35 mg/dl. Type 2 DM is also associated with increased TG-rich particles, which trigger inflammation by activating the nuclear factor κB (NFκB) *(23)*. The effects of TZDs on TGs however are variable and correlate with the baseline TG level. All of the TZDs increase HDL-C levels, although only pioglitazone and troglitazone have been shown to decrease TG consistently *(24,25)*.

Low HDL-C is also one of the components of the lipid abnormalities seen in type 2 DM and IR. This results in a reduction in the activity of the protective effect of reverse cholesterol transport pathway *(26)*. Visceral adiposity causes enhanced lipolysis *(27)* and increased FFA flux into the portal system. Increased FFA flow into the liver may induce hepatic IR, decrease insulin clearance, and enhance lipid synthesis.

Metformin reduces basal and postprandial hyperglycemia by about 25% in patients when given alone or with other therapies *(28)*. A randomized, double-blind, active-controlled, fixed dose, phase III clinical trial was conducted to evaluate the efficacy, tolerability, and safety of the extended release of metformin in comparison to the immediate release form of metformin *(29)*. Changes in the concentrations of total cholesterol, HDL cholesterol, LDL cholesterol, and TGs from baseline to specified times during the study were some of the secondary parameters. Eligible study patients were randomly assigned to receive 1500 mg extended-release metformin daily, 1500 mg extended-release metformin twice daily, 2000 mg extended-release metformin daily, or 1500 mg immediate-release metformin twice daily together with appropriate placebo tablets to maintain the study blind. Total, LDL, and HDL cholesterol levels were similar at baseline and endpoint in all treatment groups, except for significant differences among treatment groups for final LDL cholesterol and TGs. The 2000 mg extended-release metformin treatment group had the lowest mean concentrations for the LDL cholesterol ($P = 0.015$) and TGs ($P = 0.03$) while the immediate-release metformin treatment group had the lowest mean concentrations for TGs ($P = 0.030$).

INSULIN SENSITIZERS AND HYPERTENSION

There is evidence to suggest that IR contributes to hypertension *(30–32)*. If this is the case, then improving insulin sensitivity should in turn help lower blood pressure. The effect of TZDs on blood pressure has been examined in several clinical and experimental settings. Rosiglitazone treatment added onto the patient's usual antihypertensive regimen resulted in blood pressure control and improved IR *(33)*. Raji et al. *(33)* evaluated the effect of rosiglitazone on IR and blood pressure in patients who had essential hypertension. There were significant, albeit small, decreases in mean 24-h systolic blood pressure. The decline in systolic blood pressure correlated with the improvement in insulin sensitivity as measured by the clamp method.

Treatment of nondiabetic, hypertensive patients with rosiglitazone improved insulin sensitivity, reduced systolic and diastolic blood pressure, and induced favorable changes in markers of cardiovascular risk (33,34). A decrease in systolic blood pressure in nondiabetic, hypertensive patients has also been reported with the use of pioglitazone by Scherbaum and colleagues (35). Similar results have been obtained with rosiglitazone (36). Metformin however has not been shown to have any intrinsic effect on blood pressure (37).

Improved insulin sensitivity which promotes insulin-mediated vasodilatation may be a potential mechanism for TZD-mediated decrease in blood pressure. Alternative hypotheses for the decrease in blood pressure include inhibition of intracellular calcium and myocyte contractility (38,39) and endothelin-1 expression and secretion. In contrast to TZDs, metformin's effect on blood pressure is at best minimal, and even that is controversial.

ROLE OF INSULIN SENSITIZERS IN ENDOTHELIAL FUNCTION AND VASCULAR REACTIVITY

Vascular endothelium is involved in the regulation of vascular tone, vessel permeability, and angiogenesis. Various vasodilatory and vasoconstrictor factors, most notably nitric oxide and endothelin-1, are determinants of vascular tone (40,41). The endothelium plays a crucial role in the maintenance of vascular tone, permeability, and blood fluidity. Endothelial dysfunction is a central cause of many vascular diseases, including atherosclerosis and diabetic microangiopathy. Many of the components of the IR syndrome such as hypertension, dyslipidemia, and hyperglycemia affect the integrity of the endothelial function (42).

Vascular disease is present before diabetes, as evident by the 2–3-fold increased death rate from coronary artery disease in the pre-diabetic state (43). Endothelial dysfunction, a precursor of atherosclerosis, is present in both pre-diabetes and diabetes (44,45). Quinones et al. (46) hypothesized that coronary vasomotor dysfunction is present before carbohydrate abnormalities develop in persons with IR, possibly even before the onset of the metabolic syndrome as defined by the National Cholesterol Education Program (10). To test this hypothesis, they used positron emission tomography to noninvasively measure coronary blood flow in insulin-sensitive versus insulin-resistant patients without glucose intolerance or other cardiovascular risk factors associated with endothelial dysfunction. The study subjects were aged Mexican-Americans, 50 with IR and 22 without IR. Twenty five insulin-resistant patients received 3 months of treatment with TZD. Myocardial blood flow was measured by using positron emission tomography at rest, during cold pressor test (largely endothelium dependent), and after dipyridamole administration (largely vascular smooth muscle-dependent). Myocardial blood flow responses to dipyridamole were similar in the insulin-sensitive and insulin-resistant groups. In response to the cold pressor test, myocardial blood flow response increased by 14.4% in the insulin-resistant subjects, and by 47.6% in the insulin-sensitive subjects from their resting values. During therapy with TZD, a subgroup of insulin-resistant patients showed improvement in insulin sensitivity, fasting plasma insulin levels, and normalization of the myocardial blood flow responses to cold pressor test. This beneficial effect was completely lost after the TZD therapy was discontinued, indicating that the normalization resulted from TZD treatment. However, the mechanisms by which TZDs normalize coronary flow response to cold pressor test are not understood. These results suggest an association between IR and abnormal coronary vasomotor function and place an emphasis on the importance of early identification of IR as a risk factor for endothelial dysfunction. However, the results of this study need to be interpreted with caution, as it was limited by a small number of subjects.

Another study has shown that IR is a major contributor toward endothelial dysfunction in type 2 DM. Pistrosch et al. *(47)* showed that IR is related to endothelial dysfunction, independent of glycemic control. Endothelial IR may be an aspect of IR, in general. They showed that IR and endothelial dysfunction are amenable to treatment with rosiglitazone, with up to 60% reduction in IR. Results from their study also suggest that rosiglitazone may improve non-nitric oxide/prostacyclin-related endothelium-dependent vasodilatation. Improvement in vascular reactivity in obese, nondiabetic patients after treatment with rosiglitazone has also been was reported *(48)*. This was associated with beneficial changes in several markers of inflammation and endothelial activation.

The effect of pioglitazone on the endothelial function has been assessed. Asnani et al. *(49)* conducted a randomized, double-blind, placebo-controlled trial involving 20 patients with type 2 DM being treated with insulin. Study subjects received either pioglitazone 30 mg or placebo for 4 months. Endothelial function as assessed by FMD (see Fig. 1) showed significant improvement ($10.1 \pm 4.0\%$ to $14.6 \pm 6.2\%$, $P = 0.036$) in the pioglitazone group as compared to the placebo group ($P = 0.705$). In the pioglitazone group there was a trend toward improvement in the nitroglycerin-induced dilatation (NID). Addition of pioglitazone to insulin therapy in patients with type 2 DM improved vascular function.

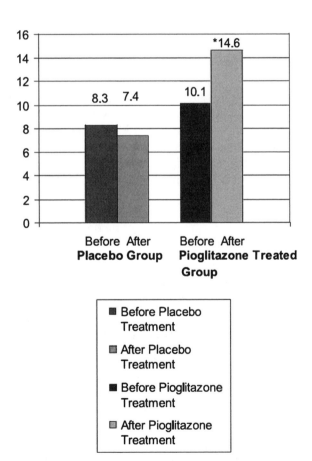

Fig. 1.   Effect of pioglitazone compared to placebo on flow-mediated dilatation. *p value = 0.04.

Source: Adapted with Permission from Metabolic Syndrome and Related Disorders, Volume 4, Number 3, 2006, Mary Ann Leibert, Inc.

The TZDs act on the endothelium by way of various mechanisms, including increased nitric oxide synthesis. They also affect the modulation of various cytokines, including adhesion molecules that are involved in the process of atherosclerosis *(50–52)*. Recently, metformin also was shown to improve endothelial function. Mather et al. *(53)* studied subjects with type 2 DM, but without the other cardiovascular risk factors seen in the metabolic syndrome. Patients who received metformin 500 mg twice daily showed statistically significant improvement in acetylcholine-stimulated flows in comparison to placebo ($P=0.0027$). However, the effect was modest in comparison to TZDs.

INSULIN SENSITIZERS AND VASCULAR WALL ABNORMALITIES

Carotid intimal-medial complex thickness is an indicator of early atherosclerosis and is associated with IR *(54,55)*. B-mode ultrasound is a noninvasive modality of measuring carotid intimal-medial complex thickness. This measurement may serve as a surrogate marker for atherosclerotic events. Patients who have increased intimal-medial complex thickness have a greater rate of cardiovascular events over time *(55)*. Treatment with troglitazone significantly decreased intima-media thickness in patients who had type 2 DM *(54)*. Koshiyama and associates *(56)* recently reported a significant decrease in the intima-media thickness in patients who had type 2 DM when treated with pioglitazone. It is possible that the effects of TZDs are directly cellular on the atherosclerotic process and not linked to the effects on IR.

The CHICAGO (Carotid Intima-Media Thickness in Atherosclerosis Using Pioglitazone) *(57)* trial was a randomized, prospective, double-blind, comparator-controlled, multicenter trial conducted in a multiracial and multiethnic population at 28 clinical sites in Chicago. It was done to evaluate the effect of pioglitazone versus glimiperide (active comparator) on changes in carotid artery intima-media thickness (CMIT) of the common carotid artery in patients with type 2 DM. Pioglitazone was used in the doses of 15–45 mg/day and glimiperide was used in the dose of 1–4 mg/day. The main outcome measure was the absolute change from baseline to final visit in mean posterior-wall CIMT of the left and right common carotid arteries. Over a treatment period of 18 months, in patients with type 2 DM, pioglitazone slowed progression of CIMT compared to glimiperide. At week 72, the primary endpoint of progression of mean CIMT was –0.001 mm with pioglitazone and +0.012 mm with glimiperide. The difference was –0.013 mm, with 95% confidence interval, –0.024 to –0.002, and P value= 0.02. However, the authors do acknowledge that TZDs may cause acute changes in intravascular volume and affect vascular tone. Such changes are also seen as a result of antihypertensive therapy. The effect of antihypertensive therapy on CIMT has been studied by Zanchetti et al. *(58)*. They conclude that only 1% of CIMT change could be attributed to overall change in carotid artery diameter.

INSULIN SENSITIZERS AND FIBRINOLYSIS AND COAGULATION

Atherosclerosis and CVD are associated with decreased fibrinolytic activity, and elevated plasma plasminogen activator inhibitor type 1 (PAI-1) *(59,60)*. PAI-1 is the primary inhibitor of endogenous tissue plasminogen activator. Patients who have type 2 DM and IR but no DM also have elevated levels of PAI-1. Increased PAI-1 levels are now recognized as an integral part of the IR syndrome and correlate significantly with plasma insulin. Impaired fibrinolysis is also noted in other insulin-resistant states, such as polycystic ovary syndrome *(61)*. Fonseca and colleagues *(62)* have demonstrated a decrease in plasma PAI-1 levels in patients with DM who were treated with a TZD. This observation has been confirmed in several studies *(63–65)*. The postulated mechanism for the effect of the TZDs is by activation of PPAR-γ and subsequent suppression of PAI-1.

INSULIN SENSITIZERS AND ALBUMINURIA

Urinary microalbuminuria is routinely monitored in patients with DM and is recognized as a marker of CVD and diabetic nephropathy *(66)*. Strict glycemic control and use of angiotensin-converting enzyme (ACE) or angiotensin receptor blocker (ARB) inhibitors are the modalities currently available for reducing microalbuminuria *(67)*. In a 52-week open trial of patients who had type 2 DM, who were given either rosiglitazone or glyburide, rosiglitazone significantly reduced urinary albumin:creatinine ratio compared to the baseline values *(68)*. PPAR-γ receptors are expressed in mesangial cells of animal models and inhibit mesangial cell proliferation and angiontensin II-induced PAI-1 expression *(69)*. Consequently, the effect of TZDs on microalbuminuria may represent yet another element to consider in selecting antihyperglycemic agents that may have an additive benefit to ACE or ARB inhibitors in reducing microalbuminuria. The subsequent impact of TZDs on the course and progression of diabetic nephropathy however is not known.

EFFECT OF INSULIN SENSITIZERS ON CONGESTIVE HEART FAILURE, LEFT VENTRICULAR MASS, AND TYPE 2 DIABETES

Ghazzi et al. *(24)* investigated whether patients who had type 2 diabetes who were treated with troglitazone 800 mg daily (a dosage larger than used in clinical practice) or glyburide developed any cardiac mass increase or functional impairment. Two-dimensional echocardiography and pulsed Doppler demonstrated that troglitazone and glyburide did not change left ventricular mass index significantly over 48 weeks. Similar studies performed with rosiglitazone and pioglitazone also did not demonstrate any affect on cardiac mass or function *(35,70)*.

Nonetheless, advanced heart failure (New York Heart Association class III and IV) is a contraindication for the use of TZDs due to the expansion of plasma volume *(71)*. Physicians need to be cognizant of certain points when prescribing TZDs. Congestive heart failure (CHF) was not seen frequently in trials using TZDs. The prevalence of CHF was less than 1% for rosiglitazone monotherapy or when rosiglitazone was added to sulfonylurea or metformin. Also important to note is the fact that the prevalence was similar to that observed during treatment with a placebo *(72)*. The incidence of CHF rose to 2% and 3% when rosiglitazone, 4 mg/day or 8 mg/day, respectively, were added to insulin therapy of the study population, compared to 1% in the group that was treated with insulin alone *(72)*. Pre-existing microvascular and cardiovascular comorbidity was more prevalent in those clinical trials in which rosiglitazone was added to insulin therapy than in those trials in which rosiglitazone was used alone and compared with placebo or combined with metformin or sulfonylureas. The patients who developed CHF on rosiglitazone plus insulin were older and had diabetes of longer duration.

The data on pioglitazone are similar *(73)*. In a placebo-controlled trial, 2 of 191 patients (1.1%) who received 15 mg of pioglitazone plus insulin and 2 of 188 (1.1%) patients who received 30 mg of pioglitazone plus insulin developed CHF, compared with none of the 187 patient who received insulin alone. All four of these patients had underlying coronary artery disease. It is unlikely, however, that the drugs differ with regard to the risk of CHF because they incur similar degrees of volume expansion. To summarize, the prevalence of CHF in TZD-treated patients is low but is definitely greater in patients who already are treated with insulin and receive larger dosages of the TZD and have other risk factors for CHF.

In several clinical trials, PPAR-α agents have reduced cardiovascular events or demonstrated slowing of the progression of atherogenesis *(43,74,75)*. As mentioned above, PPAR-γ agonist are known to increase insulin sensitivity and are widely used in the treatment of type

2 DM. Muraglitazar is a dual PPAR agonist targeting both the α and the γ families. Review of the clinical trials showed that muraglitazar was associated with an excess incidence of CHF *(76)*. In comparison to placebo, the relative risk for adjudicated CHF was 7.43 ((0.97–56.8), $P = 0.053$). The exact mechanism responsible for the increased cardiovascular toxicity observed with muraglitazar is uncertain. Interaction with other medications should certainly be entertained as a possibility.

Diabetes Reduction Assessment with ramipril and rosiglitazone medication (DREAM) *(36)* is a double-blind, randomized placebo-controlled clinical trial that studied the effects of ramipril and/or a TZDs on the development of diabetes or death which was the primary outcome. The study population had 5269 adults more than 30 years of age with impaired fasting glucose and/or impaired glucose tolerance and no previous CVD. The primary outcome of diabetes or death was significantly lower in the rosiglitazone group than in the placebo group (Hazard ration (HR) 0.40, 95% CI 0.35–0.46; $p < 0.0001$). Significantly larger number of study subjects receiving rosiglitazone regressed to normo glycemia as compared to placebo (HR 1.71, 157–1.87; $P<0.001$).

An international, multicenter, double-blind, randomized, controlled clinical trial, A Diabetes outcome progression trial (ADOPT) *(77)*, compared the efficacy of rosiglitazone, glyburide, and metformin as initial treatment in subjects recently diagnosed with type 2 DM. The cumulative incidence of monotherapy failure at 5 years was 15% with rosiglitazone, 21% with metformin, and 34% with glyburide. This translated into a risk reduction of 32% for rosiglitazone in comparison to metformin and 63% in comparison to glyburide ($P < 0.001$ for both comparisons). The risk of cardiovascular events including CHF was lower with glyburide when compared to rosiglitazone ($P < 0.05$). The risk was similar for metformin and rosiglitazone.

Metformin is also contraindicated in patients who have CHF. Diabetes management in patients who have CHF can be particularly difficult, probably related to the IR that is caused by sympathetic overactivity and the use of diuretics that can worsen hyperglycemia and often requires insulin therapy. A study by Masoudi et al. *(73)* showed that the use of metformin and TZDs has increased rapidly among Medicare beneficiaries who have diabetes and heart failure, despite the warnings against this practice from the US Food and Drug Administration.

OUTCOME STUDIES FOR PREVENTION OF MACROVASCULAR COMPLICATIONS IN TYPE 2 DM

Several large human trials have been initiated using PPAR agonists in varied settings such as pre-diabetes to late-stage diabetes, to study their role in prevention of primary and secondary cardiovascular events *(78)*. First such trial was the PROactive study, whose results are being discussed below *(79)*.

PROactive was a prospective, randomized, controlled trial in 5238 patients with type 2 DM, with evidence of CVD. The subjects were randomized to either pioglitazone titrated to 45 mg/daily or matching placebo. Those receiving pioglitazone were receiving it in addition to their usual glucose-lowering medications. This was done to assess the pure effect of pioglitazone, independent of its glucose-lowering effects. The primary composite endpoint consisted of all-cause mortality, nonfatal myocardial infarction, stroke, acute coronary syndrome, revascularization, or amputation. The main secondary endpoint (see Fig. 2) included death from any cause, nonfatal myocardial infarction (excluding silent myocardial infarction), or stroke (see Fig. 3). The results revealed pioglitazone to have only a modest, and not statistically significant 10% reduction in the risk of the primary composite endpoint, but a significant reduction by 16% of some of the secondary endpoint. Despite the negative result on the primary endpoint,

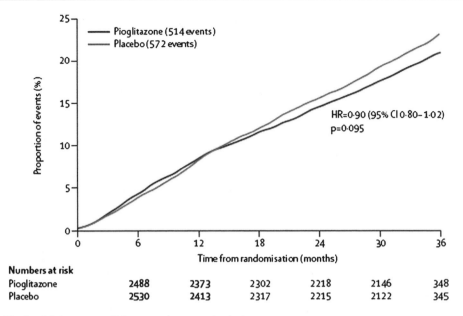

Fig. 2.   Kaplan-Meler curve of time to primary endpoint*
*Death from any cause, non-fatal myocardial infraction (including silent myocardial infarction) stroke, acute coronary syndrome, leg amputation, coronary revascularisation, or revascularisation of the leg.

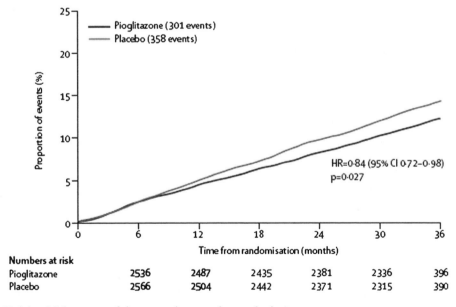

Fig. 3.   Kalplan-Meler curve of time to main secondary endpoint*
*Death from any cause, non-fatal myocardial infarction (excluding silent myocardial infarction), or stroke.

the secondary endpoints were significantly reduced. Pioglitazone reduced mortality, myocardial infarction, and stroke.

The study had major limitations. First of all, the study subjects comprised mainly of Caucasian subjects who were probably less insulin resistant than the United States population and other countries. Cigarette smoking rates were relatively high, and rate of statin use for subjects with established macrovascular disease was relatively low. The rate of recruitment was higher than expected as well, which led to the study being concluded earlier than was anticipated. The Kaplan–Meier curves of the time to primary endpoint start to separate only after 18 months. The 36-month result of the trial might not have been able to detect a true difference. This could be explained based on the slow onset action of TZDs, which may be related to their primary mechanism of action. The chosen secondary endpoints certainly are important in diabetes.

The positive effects of pioglitazone may be tempered by an increase in the incidence of CHF in patients who received treatment with pioglitazone. This is a well-recognized side effect of pioglitazone, especially when patients are on combination therapy with insulin and TZDs in high doses. Pioglitazone is currently not approved in a dose of 45 mg/day in combination therapy. So, the question arises as to whether the results of the trial would have been different if pioglitazone would have been used in a 30 mg/day dose. Patients with NYHA class II–IV heart failure were excluded from the study, when the drug is actually approved for use in patients with NYHA class II CHF. The validity of the hospitalization and the mortality related to CHF comes into question if one considers the inclusion of NYHA class II CHF patients in the trial. The mortality from heart failure however was not increased, suggestive of the fact that heart failure associated with the use of TZDs is easily manageable *(72)*. Improvement in liver function tests was seen during the duration of the trial with the use of pioglitazone.

It is possible that subjects in this study had disease too advanced to benefit from therapy. Though data is awaited from other ongoing studies to address certain key questions, the PROactive trial has provided the impetus for further investigation and at the same time supports the concept of treating IR to reduce mortality and myocardial infarction.

The UKPDS among other things has shown that intensive treatment with metformin results in significant reduction in macrovascular endpoints and mortality in individuals with newly diagnosed type 2 DM compared with intensive treatment with insulin or sulphonylurea therapy despite similar glycemic control *(37)*. When added on to a regimen consisting of maximum sulfonylurea dose in patients with type 2 DM, metformin decreased fasting plasma glucose concentrations by mean (95% CI) –0.47 (–0.82 to –0.13) mmol/l over 3 years as compared to an increase of 0.44 (0.07–0.81) mmol/l on sulfonylurea alone ($P < 0.00001$) *(80)*. However, metformin-associated effects on systolic and diastolic blood pressure and HDL cholesterol are small and statistically not significant *(37)*.

ONGOING STUDIES

In the last decade, there has been a surge in mortality attributable to diabetes, despite the overall decrease in mortality attributable to coronary artery disease in patients without diabetes. The prevalence of diabetes in the United States is enormous and is rapidly increasing. IR with or without overt type 2 DM has emerged as a major determinant of accelerated coronary artery disease and its sequelae. Patients with diabetes have a less favorable outcome to percutaneous coronary interventions in comparison to their nondiabetic counterparts. These considerations have led to the initiation of the Bypass Angioplasty Revascularization Investigation 2 Diabetes

(BARI 2D) trial *(81,82)*. It is designed to determine whether treatment targeting IR can arrest or retard progression of coronary artery disease compared with treatment targeted to the same level of glycemic control with an insulin-providing approach *(81,82)*. This study is currently underway.

As discussed in this chapter, studies suggest that TZDs play a vital role in improving some cardiovascular risk factors and surrogate markers in type 2 DM. Use of TZDs may also cause fluid retention that may lead to cardiac failure in some patients. Rosiglitazone Evaluated for Cardiac Outcomes and Regulation of Glycemia in Diabetes (RECORD) *(83)* is a 6-year randomized, open-label study involving patients with type 2 DM with HbA1c 7.1%–9.0% on metformin or sulphonylurea alone. This study which is currently undergoing, aims to evaluate the long-term effects on cardiovascular outcomes, as well as long-term glycemic control in patients with type 2 DM.

CONCLUSION

Type 2 DM is a progressive disease with IR as one of the pivotal underlying mechanisms involved. IR contributes to hyperglycemia in type 2 DM and is responsible for a multitude of metabolic abnormalities. Patients with type 2 DM have an increased relative risk for CVD with higher morbidity and mortality when compared to those without type 2 DM. TZDs are high-affinity ligands for the peroxisome proliferators-activated receptor (PPAR)-γ, a member of the nuclear receptor family that mediates their insulin-sensitizing effect *(84)*. They are effective in reducing blood glucose, insulin, and TG levels in both insulin-resistant animal models and type 2 DM patients *(85–87)*. In clinical trials, TZDs have been shown to favorably affect the various metabolic abnormalities and the surrogate markers of CVD. They have also been shown to delay the progress to diabetes and cause regression to normo glycemia in subjects with impaired fasting glucose and impaired glucose tolerance. They do however carry the risk of CHF.

Metformin, a biguanide ameliorates hyperglycemia by improvement in peripheral insulin sensitivity, reducing gastrointestinal glucose absorption and decreasing hepatic glucose production *(88)*. In clinical trials, metformin monotherapy has been shown to be beneficial in patients recently diagnosed with type 2 DM compared to placebo. The benefit applies also when metformin is added on to sulfonylurea therapy. Insulin sensitizers have become a very important cornerstone of treatment of type 2 DM.

ACKNOWLEDGMENTS

Diabetes research at Tulane University Health Sciences Center is supported in part by Susan Harling Robinson Fellowship in Diabetes Research and the Tullis-Tulane Alumni Chair in Diabetes.

REFERENCES

1. DeFronzo RA. Pathogenesis of type 2 (non-insulin dependent) diabetes mellitus: a balanced overview. *Diabetologia*. 1992;35:389–397.
2. Despres JP, Lamarche B, Mauriege P et al. Hyperinsulinemia as an independent risk factor for ischemic heart disease. *N Engl J Med*. 1996;334:952–957.
3. Alexander CM, Landsman PB, Teutsch SM, Haffner SM. NCEP-defined metabolic syndrome, diabetes, and prevalence of coronary heart disease among NHANES III participants age 50 years and older. *Diabetes*. 2003;52:1210–1214.
4. Kannel WB, McGee DL. Diabetes and cardiovascular disease. The Framingham study. *JAMA*. 1979;241: 2035–2038.

5. Haffner SM. Management of dyslipidemia in adults with diabetes. *Diabetes Care*. 1998;21:160–178.

6. Gu K, Cowie CC, Harris MI. Diabetes and decline in heart disease mortality in US adults. *JAMA*. 1999;281: 1291–1297.

7. Davidson MB. Is treatment of insulin resistance beneficial independent of glycemia? *Diabetes Care*. 2003;26:3184–3186.

8. Reaven GM. Banting lecture 1988. Role of insulin resistance in human disease. *Diabetes*. 1988;37:1595–1607.

9. Reaven GM, Lithell H, Landsberg L. Hypertension and associated metabolic abnormalities – the role of insulin resistance and the sympathoadrenal system. *N Engl J Med*. 1996;334:374–381.

10. Executive Summary of the Third Report of The National Cholesterol Education Program (NCEP) Expert Panel on Detection, Evaluation, And Treatment of High Blood Cholesterol In Adults (Adult Treatment Panel III). *JAMA*. 2001;285:2486–2497.

11. Effect of intensive blood-glucose control with metformin on complications in overweight patients with type 2 diabetes (UKPDS 34). UK Prospective Diabetes Study (UKPDS) Group. *Lancet*. 1998;352:854–865.

12. Martens FM, Visseren FL, Lemay J, de Koning EJ, Rabelink TJ. Metabolic and additional vascular effects of thiazolidinediones. *Drugs*. 2002;62:1463–1480.

13. Wagstaff AJ, Goa KL. Rosiglitazone: a review of its use in the management of type 2 diabetes mellitus. *Drugs*. 2002;62:1805–1837.

14. Inzucchi SE, Maggs DG, Spollett GR et al. Efficacy and metabolic effects of metformin and troglitazone in type II diabetes mellitus. *N Engl J Med*. 1998;338:867–872.

15. Olefsky JM. Treatment of insulin resistance with peroxisome proliferator-activated receptor gamma agonists. *J Clin Invest*. 2000;106:467–472.

16. Boden G, Lebed B, Schatz M, Homko C, Lemieux S. Effects of acute changes of plasma free fatty acids on intramyocellular fat content and insulin resistance in healthy subjects. *Diabetes*. 2001;50:1612–1617.

17. Steinberg HO, Paradisi G, Hook G, Crowder K, Cronin J, Baron AD. Free fatty acid elevation impairs insulin-mediated vasodilation and nitric oxide production. *Diabetes*. 2000;49:1231–1238.

18. Parulkar AA, Pendergrass ML, Granda-Ayala R, Lee TR, Fonseca VA. Nonhypoglycemic effects of thiazolidine-diones. *Ann Intern Med*. 2001;134:61–71.

19. Kirpichnikov D, McFarlane SI, Sowers JR. Metformin: an update. *Ann Intern Med*. 2002;137:25–33.

20. Abbasi F, Chu JW, McLaughlin T, Lamendola C, Leary ET, Reaven GM. Effect of metformin treatment on multiple cardiovascular disease risk factors in patients with type 2 diabetes mellitus. *Metabolism*. 2004;53: 159–164.

21. Freed MI, Ratner R, Marcovina SM, et al. Effects of rosiglitazone alone and in combination with atorvastatin on the metabolic abnormalities in type 2 diabetes mellitus. *Am J Cardiol*. 2002;90:947–952.

22. Rosenblatt S, Miskin B, Glazer NB, Prince MJ, Robertson KE. The impact of pioglitazone on glycemic control and atherogenic dyslipidemia in patients with type 2 diabetes mellitus. *Coron Artery Dis*. 2001;12:413–423.

23. Dichtl W, Nilsson L, Goncalves I, et al. Very low-density lipoprotein activates nuclear factor-kappaB in endothelial cells. *Circ Res*. 1999;84:1085–1094.

24. Ghazzi MN, Perez JE, Antonucci TK, et al. Cardiac and glycemic benefits of troglitazone treatment in NIDDM. The Troglitazone Study Group. *Diabetes*. 1997;46:433–439.

25. Suter SL, Nolan JJ, Wallace P, Gumbiner B, Olefsky JM. Metabolic effects of new oral hypoglycemic agent CS-045 in NIDDM subjects. *Diabetes Care*. 1992;15:193–203.

26. Gotto AM, Jr, Brinton EA. Assessing low levels of high-density lipoprotein cholesterol as a risk factor in coronary heart disease: a working group report and update. *J Am Coll Cardiol*. 2004;43:717–724.

27. Matsuzawa Y, Funahashi T, Nakamura T. Molecular mechanism of metabolic syndrome X: contribution of adipocytokines adipocyte-derived bioactive substances. *Ann N Y Acad Sci*. 1999;892:146–154.

28. Howlett HC, Bailey CJ. A risk–benefit assessment of metformin in type 2 diabetes mellitus. *Drug Saf*. 1999;20:489–503.

29. Schwartz S, Fonseca V, Berner B, Cramer M, Chiang YK, Lewin A. Efficacy, tolerability, and safety of a novel once-daily extended-release metformin in patients with type 2 diabetes. *Diabetes Care*. 2006;29:759–764.

30. DeFronzo RA. Insulin resistance: a multifaceted syndrome responsible for NIDDM, obesity, hypertension, dyslipidaemia and atherosclerosis. *Neth J Med*. 1997;50:191–197.

31. Ferrannini E, Natali A. Essential hypertension, metabolic disorders, and insulin resistance. *Am Heart J*. 1991;121:1274–1282.

32. Natali A, Ferrannini E. Hypertension, insulin resistance, and the metabolic syndrome. *Endocrinol Metab Clin North Am*. 2004;33:417–429.

33. Raji A, Seely EW, Bekins SA, Williams GH, Simonson DC. Rosiglitazone improves insulin sensitivity and lowers blood pressure in hypertensive patients. *Diabetes Care*. 2003;26:172–178.

34. Bennett SM, Agrawal A, Elasha H, et al. Rosiglitazone improves insulin sensitivity, glucose tolerance and ambulatory blood pressure in subjects with impaired glucose tolerance. *Diabet Med.* 2004;21:415–422.
35. Scherbaum W GB. Pioglitazone reduces blood pressure in patients with type-2 diabetes mellitus. Diabetes [50(Suppl)], A462. 2001. Ref Type: Generic.
36. Gerstein HC, Yusuf S, Bosch J et al. Effect of rosiglitazone on the frequency of diabetes in patients with impaired glucose tolerance or impaired fasting glucose: a randomised controlled trial. *Lancet.* 2006;368:1096–1105.
37. Wulffele MG, Kooy A, de ZD, Stehouwer CD, Gansevoort RT. The effect of metformin on blood pressure, plasma cholesterol and triglycerides in type 2 diabetes mellitus: a systematic review. *J Intern Med.* 2004;256:1–14.
38. Morikang E, Benson SC, Kurtz TW, Pershadsingh HA. Effects of thiazolidinediones on growth and differentiation of human aorta and coronary myocytes. *Am J Hypertens.* 1997;10:440–446.
39. Song J, Walsh MF, Igwe R et al. Troglitazone reduces contraction by inhibition of vascular smooth muscle cell Ca^{2+} currents and not endothelial nitric oxide production. *Diabetes.* 1997;46:659–664.
40. Blackman DJ, Morris-Thurgood JA, Atherton JJ, et al. Endothelium-derived nitric oxide contributes to the regulation of venous tone in humans. *Circulation.* 2000;101:165–170.
41. Sobel BE. Coronary artery disease and fibrinolysis: from the blood to the vessel wall. *Thromb Haemost.* 1999;82 Suppl 1:8–13.
42. Tooke J. The association between insulin resistance and endotheliopathy. *Diabetes Obes Metab.* 1999;1 Suppl 1:S17–S22.
43. DECODE Study Group, the European Diabetes Epidemiology Group. Glucose tolerance and cardiovascular mortality: comparison of fasting and 2-hour diagnostic criteria. *Arch Intern Med.* 2001;161:397–405.
44. Steinberg HO, Chaker H, Leaming R, Johnson A, Brechtel G, Baron AD. Obesity/insulin resistance is associated with endothelial dysfunction. Implications for the syndrome of insulin resistance. *J Clin Invest.* 1996;97: 2601–2610.
45. Williams SB, Cusco JA, Roddy MA, Johnstone MT, Creager MA. Impaired nitric oxide-mediated vasodilation in patients with non-insulin-dependent diabetes mellitus. *J Am Coll Cardiol.* 1996;27:567–574.
46. Quinones MJ, Hernandez-Pampaloni M, Schelbert H, et al. Coronary vasomotor abnormalities in insulin-resistant individuals. *Ann Intern Med.* 2004;140:700–708.
47. Pistrosch F, Passauer J, Fischer S, Fuecker K, Hanefeld M, Gross P. In type 2 diabetes, rosiglitazone therapy for insulin resistance ameliorates endothelial dysfunction independent of glucose control. *Diabetes Care.* 2004;27:484–490.
48. Mohanty P, Aljada A, Ghanim H et al. Evidence for a potent antiinflammatory effect of rosiglitazone. *J Clin Endocrinol Metab.* 2004;89:2728–2735.
49. Asnani S, Kunhiraman B, Jawa A, Akers D, Lumpkin D, Fonseca V. Pioglitazone restores endothelial function in patients with type 2 diabetes treated with insulin. *Metabolic Syndrome and Related Disorders.* 2006;4:179–184. 2006. Ref Type: Generic
50. Cominacini L, Garbin U, Pasini AF et al. The expression of adhesion molecules on endothelial cells is inhibited by troglitazone through its antioxidant activity. *Cell Adhes Commun.* 1999;7:223–231.
51. Ohta MY, Nagai Y, Takamura T, Nohara E, Kobayashi K. Inhibitory effect of troglitazone on TNF-alpha-induced expression of monocyte chemoattractant protein-1 (MCP-1) in human endothelial cells. *Diabetes Res Clin Pract.* 2000;48:171–176.
52. Yoshimoto T, Naruse M, Shizume H, et al. Vasculo-protective effects of insulin sensitizing agent pioglitazone in neointimal thickening and hypertensive vascular hypertrophy. *Atherosclerosis.* 1999;145:333–340.
53. Mather KJ, Verma S, Anderson TJ. Improved endothelial function with metformin in type 2 diabetes mellitus. *J Am Coll Cardiol.* 2001;37:1344–1350.
54. Minamikawa J, Tanaka S, Yamauchi M, Inoue D, and Koshiyama H. Potent inhibitory effect of troglitazone on carotid arterial wall thickness in type 2 diabetes. *J Clin Endocrinol Metab.* 1998;83:1818–1820. Ref Type: Generic.
55. O'Leary DH, Polak JF, Kronmal RA, Manolio TA, Burke GL, Wolfson SK, Jr. Carotid-artery intima and media thickness as a risk factor for myocardial infarction and stroke in older adults. Cardiovascular Health Study Collaborative Research Group. *N Engl J Med.* 1999;340:14–22.
56. Koshiyama H, Shimono D, Kuwamura N, Minamikawa J, Nakamura Y. Rapid communication: inhibitory effect of pioglitazone on carotid arterial wall thickness in type 2 diabetes. *J Clin Endocrinol Metab.* 2001;86: 3452–3456.
57. Mazzone T, Meyer PM, Feinstein SB et al. Effect of pioglitazone compared with glimepiride on carotid intima-media thickness in type 2 diabetes: a randomized trial. *JAMA.* 2006;296:2572–2581.
58. Zanchetti A, Bond MG, Hennig M et al. Calcium antagonist lacidipine slows down progression of asymptomatic carotid atherosclerosis: principal results of the European Lacidipine Study on Atherosclerosis (ELSA), a randomized, double-blind, long-term trial. *Circulation.* 2002;106:2422–2427.

59. Davidson MB. Clinical implications of insulin resistance syndromes. *Am J Med*. 1995;99:420–426.

60. Nagi DK, Yudkin JS. Effects of metformin on insulin resistance, risk factors for cardiovascular disease, and plasminogen activator inhibitor in NIDDM subjects. A study of two ethnic groups. *Diabetes Care*. 1993;16: 621–629.

61. Ehrmann DA, Schneider DJ, Sobel BE, et al. Troglitazone improves defects in insulin action, insulin secretion, ovarian steroidogenesis, and fibrinolysis in women with polycystic ovary syndrome. *J Clin Endocrinol Metab*. 1997;82:2108–2116.

62. Fonseca VA, Reynolds T, Hemphill D, et al. Effect of troglitazone on fibrinolysis and activated coagulation in patients with non-insulin-dependent diabetes mellitus. *J Diabetes Complications*. 1998;12:181–186.

63. Kato K, Satoh H, Endo Y, et al. Thiazolidinediones down-regulate plasminogen activator inhibitor type 1 expression in human vascular endothelial cells: A possible role for PPARgamma in endothelial function. *Biochem Biophys Res Commun*. 1999;258:431–435.

64. Kruszynska YT, Yu JG, Olefsky JM, Sobel BE. Effects of troglitazone on blood concentrations of plasminogen activator inhibitor 1 in patients with type 2 diabetes and in lean and obese normal subjects. *Diabetes*. 2000;49: 633–639.

65. Zirlik A, Leugers A, Lohrmann J et al. Direct attenuation of plasminogen activator inhibitor type-1 expression in human adipose tissue by thiazolidinediones. *Thromb Haemost*. 2004;91:674–682.

66. Mattock MB, Morrish NJ, Viberti G, Keen H, Fitzgerald AP, Jackson G. Prospective study of microalbuminuria as predictor of mortality in NIDDM. *Diabetes*. 1992;41:736–741.

67. Imano E, Kanda T, Nakatani Y et al. Effect of troglitazone on microalbuminuria in patients with incipient diabetic nephropathy. *Diabetes Care*. 1998;21:2135–2139.

68. Bakris G, Viberti G, Weston WM, Heise M, Porter LE, Freed MI. Rosiglitazone reduces urinary albumin excretion in type II diabetes. *J Hum Hypertens*. 2003;17:7–12.

69. Nicholas SB, Kawano Y, Wakino S, Collins AR, Hsueh WA. Expression and function of peroxisome proliferator-activated receptor-gamma in mesangial cells. *Hypertension*. 2001;37:722–727.

70. Zanchetti A, Bond MG, Hennig M et al. Calcium antagonist lacidipine slows down progression of asymptomatic carotid atherosclerosis: principal results of the European Lacidipine Study on Atherosclerosis (ELSA), a randomized, double-blind, long-term trial. *Circulation*. 2002;106:2422–2427.

71. Nichols GA, Hillier TA, Erbey JR, Brown JB. Congestive heart failure in type 2 diabetes: prevalence, incidence, and risk factors. *Diabetes Care*. 2001;24:1614–1619.

72. Nesto RW, Bell D, Bonow RO et al. Thiazolidinedione use, fluid retention, and congestive heart failure: a consensus statement from the American Heart Association and American Diabetes Association. *Diabetes Care*. 2004;27:256–263.

73. Masoudi FA, Wang Y, Inzucchi SE, et al. Metformin and thiazolidinedione use in Medicare patients with heart failure. *JAMA*. 2003;290:81–85.

74. Frick MH, Elo O, Haapa K, et al. Helsinki Heart Study: primary-prevention trial with gemfibrozil in middle-aged men with dyslipidemia. Safety of treatment, changes in risk factors, and incidence of coronary heart disease. *N Engl J Med*. 1987;317:1237–1245.

75. Rubins HB, Robins SJ, Collins D, et al. Gemfibrozil for the secondary prevention of coronary heart disease in men with low levels of high-density lipoprotein cholesterol. Veterans Affairs High-Density Lipoprotein Cholesterol Intervention Trial Study Group. *N Engl J Med*. 1999;341:410–418.

76. Nissen SE, Wolski K, Topol EJ. Effect of muraglitazar on death and major adverse cardiovascular events in patients with type 2 diabetes mellitus. *JAMA*. 2005;294:2581–2586.

77. Kahn SE, Haffner SM, Heise MA et al. Glycemic durability of rosiglitazone, metformin, or glyburide monotherapy. *N Engl J Med*. 2006;355:2427–2443.

78. Jawa AA, Fonseca VA. Role of insulin secretagogues and insulin sensitizing agents in the prevention of cardiovascular disease in patients who have diabetes. *Cardiol Clin*. 2005;23:119–138.

79. Dormandy JA, Charbonnel B, Eckland DJ, et al. Secondary prevention of macrovascular events in patients with type 2 diabetes in the PROactive Study (PROspective pioglitAzone Clinical Trial In macroVascular Events): a randomised controlled trial. *Lancet*. 2005;366:1279–1289.

80. UKPDS 28: a randomized trial of efficacy of early addition of metformin in sulfonylurea-treated type 2 diabetes. U.K. Prospective Diabetes Study Group. *Diabetes Care*. 1998;21:87–92.

81. Frye RL. Optimal care of patients with type 2 diabetes mellitus and coronary artery disease. *Am J Med*. 2003;115 Suppl 8A:93S–98S.

82. Sobel BE, Frye R, Detre KM. Burgeoning dilemmas in the management of diabetes and cardiovascular disease: rationale for the Bypass Angioplasty Revascularization Investigation 2 Diabetes (BARI 2D) Trial. *Circulation*. 2003;107:636–642.

83. Home PD, Pocock SJ, Beck-Nielsen H et al. Rosiglitazone Evaluated for Cardiac Outcomes and Regulation of Glycaemia in Diabetes (RECORD): study design and protocol. *Diabetologia*. 2005;48:1726–1735.

84. Yang C, Chang TJ, Chang JC, et al. Rosiglitazone (BRL 49653) enhances insulin secretory response via phosphatidylinositol 3-kinase pathway. *Diabetes*. 2001;50:2598–2602.

85. Chaiken RL, Eckert-Norton M, Pasmantier R et al. Metabolic effects of darglitazone, an insulin sensitizer, in NIDDM subjects. *Diabetologia*. 1995;38:1307–1312.

86. Day C. Thiazolidinediones: a new class of antidiabetic drugs. *Diabet Med*. 1999;16:179–192.

87. Saltiel AR, Olefsky JM. Thiazolidinediones in the treatment of insulin resistance and type II diabetes. *Diabetes*. 1996;45:1661–1669.

88. Davidson MB, Peters AL. An overview of metformin in the treatment of type 2 diabetes mellitus. *Am J Med*. 1997;102:99–110.

7 Screening for Cardiovascular Disease in Symptomatic and Asymptomatic Patients with Diabetes Mellitus

Paolo Raggi, MD and Leslee J. Shaw, PhD

Contents

SUMMARY

The growing incidence of diabetes mellitus and the continuing epidemic of cardiovascular disease associated with this ailment have induced numerous investigators to seek evidence of pre-clinical disease besides trying to diagnose advanced stages of disease. Although many of the techniques used in the general population to diagnose obstructive coronary artery disease have proven of value, it appears that the overall diagnostic accuracy of these methodologies may be lower in diabetic patients. Furthermore, in the presence of normal results the short-term event rate is considerably higher in a diabetic patient than in the general population. In this chapter, we discuss the current evidence surrounding some of the most popular techniques to diagnose coronary artery disease as well as some emerging techniques for detection of subclinical atherosclerosis.

Key Words: Atherosclerosis, Coronary artery disease, Computed tomography imaging, Diabetes mellitus, Echocardiography, Prognosis, Stress testing

From: *Contemporary Endocrinology: Cardiovascular Endocrinology: Shared Pathways and Clinical Crossroads*
Edited by: V. A. Fonseca © Humana Press, New York, NY

CORONARY ARTERY DISEASE IN DIABETES MELLITUS

The incidence of type-2 diabetes mellitus is rapidly increasing throughout the world. A sedentary lifestyle and the increasing population age and obesity are the most probable culprits for this escalation (1,2). In 1995, the prevalence of diabetes in United States adults over the age of 20 was estimated to be 4%. Today 6.3% of the population is estimated to suffer from diabetes (~90% type-2), though as many as 5.2 million are not aware of being affected by the disease (3–6).

Diabetes has long been recognized as an independent risk factor for cardiovascular disease (CVD) both at the microvascular and macrovascular level (7). Additionally, diabetic patients suffer a poorer prognosis than nondiabetic individuals once a primary event has occurred. In fact, after suffering a first myocardial infarction (MI) diabetic patients have more frequent recurrent events and die from sudden death more often than nondiabetic patients (8). Similarly, after a percutaneous coronary angioplasty diabetic patients require recurrent procedures more frequently and suffer a MI or die more often than nondiabetic subjects (9–11). This has resulted in a lack of decreased mortality for coronary heart disease in diabetic patients while such trend has been recorded in the general population in the past several decades (12). Hence, early detection of coronary artery disease (CAD) and aggressive primary prevention are the only pathways that may potentially improve the life expectancy of these patients.

Nonetheless, the diagnosis of CAD remains difficult especially in its early and pre-clinical phases, although physicians face several challenges even in the establishment of the diagnosis of critical CAD. One of the main issues with all and any of the technologies used to diagnose CAD, is what is known as verification bias. Indeed, test characteristics are often assessed in patients with an abnormal test (e.g., an abnormal stress nuclear test) who are then submitted to another test (coronary angiography) to confirm or exclude disease. This approach can only provide the sensitivity, specificity, etc., of a "positive test" not necessarily of the specific test as a whole. There are further substantial limitations of the electrocardiographic stress test (EST) that one should consider. In a study where verification bias was eliminated, the sensitivity of EST was low (40–50%), although the specificity was high (85%) (13). This suggests that EST may be a good test for subjects with low pre-test probability of disease (to exclude disease) but not for subjects with high pre-test probability. Nonetheless, EST results appear to yield prognostic information. In the Milano Study on Atherosclerosis and Diabetes (MiSAD, (14)) a negative EST predicted an event rate as low as 0.97/100 person-years, while an abnormal EST result was associated with an event rate of 3.85/100 person-years ($p<0.001$). Other, nonischemic data acquired during an EST also carry substantial prognostic information. Exercise duration (cardiorespiratory fitness) (15), and heart rate recovery (speed of heart rate returning to normal after exercise interruption) (16) have been associated with an unfavorable outcome.

Given the difficulties inherent with the current technological approaches, the implementation of accurate, often complementary, imaging techniques may be helpful to establish a diagnosis of CAD, especially for the detection of early stages of disease.

STRESS ECHOCARDIOGRAPHY

Stress echocardiography can be performed either on an exercise treadmill or a bicycle ergometer (ESE) or with pharmacological agents such as dobutamine. Since diabetic patients are often unable to exercise, pharmacological stress echocardiography is a frequently employed, safe, and sensitive alternative (17). Myocardial ischemia is diagnosed when stress induces new

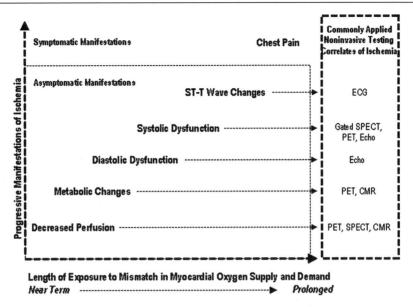

ECG=Electrocardiogram, SPECT=Single Photon Emission Computed Tomography, PET=Positron Emission Tomography, Echo=Echocardiogram, CMR=Cardiovascular Magnetic Resonance Imaging

Fig. 1. The "ischemic cascade" showing the progression of events occurring during myocardial ischemia identified through a variety of noninvasive tests.

or worsening hypokinesia, akinesia, or dyskinesia in one or more segments of the left ventricular myocardium. Since wall motion abnormalities occur much before the occurrence of chest pain or electrocardiographic abnormalities (Fig. 1), this is a sensitive method to detect myocardial ischemia.

Due to poor acoustic windows, patient habitus, excessive respiratory motion, and limited technical experience of the operator, about 10% of the stress echocardiography tests are nondiagnostic. In comparison, the nondiagnostic rate for stress nuclear testing varies between 1% and 2%. However, stress echocardiography offers the advantage of easy portability, lower cost, and no radiation exposure compared to nuclear stress testing.

The diagnostic accuracy for obstructive CAD of stress echocardiography in diabetic patients is probably slightly lower than that reported in nondiabetic subjects *(17–19)*. According to a summary statement of the American College of Cardiology *(20)* the average sensitivity and specificity of stress echocardiography is 86% and 81%, respectively, in the general population. The test seemed to perform slightly worse in the few studies conducted in the diabetic population.

Penfornis et al. *(21)* performed three tests in 56 asymptomatic diabetic subjects: electrocardiographic stress testing, dobutamine stress echocardiography (DSE), and exercise Thallium-201 single photon emission computed tomography (SPECT). All patients had a long history of diabetes (>15 years for type-1 diabetic patients and >5 years for type-2 diabetic patients), carried at least three other risk factors for CAD, and had no resting electrocardiographic abnormalities. The investigators reported a positive predictive value (to detect >50% luminal stenosis at angiography) of 69%, 75%, and 60% for DSE, SPECT, and exercise electrocardiography, respectively. Hence, DSE and SPECT demonstrated similar, albeit not excellent, diagnostic capabilities and both were superior to electrocardiographic stress testing.

Hennessy et al. *(22)* performed DSE in 52 symptomatic diabetic patients and reported the following test characteristics: sensitivity 82%, specificity 54%, positive predictive value 54%, and negative predictive value 50%, confirming the lower accuracy in this population compared to the general population *(20)*.

Nonetheless, stress echocardiography carries important prognostic information in diabetic patients. Marwick et al. conducted a multicenter study *(23)*, with 937 predominantly type-2 diabetic patients who underwent ESE or DSE for evaluation of known or suspected CAD. The primary endpoint was all-cause mortality. Resting or stress-induced wall motion abnormalities were associated with a high mortality rate (45–50%) both in patients with and without prior CAD (Fig. 2). In multivariable models, the strongest predictor of mortality was a referral for pharmacological stress testing, rather than ESE, followed by the demonstration of ischemia during stress, presence of heart failure, and age. Hence, the inability to exercise was an important predictor of an unfavorable outcome. Additionally, the authors demonstrated that the presence of inducible ischemia on a stress echocardiogram adds incremental prognostic information for the prediction of all-cause death to a model based on clinical variables alone (age, heart failure, previous MI, and referral for pharmacological stress test). Similar results were reported in other studies that examined the value of stress echocardiography both for the prediction of all-cause mortality and specific cardiovascular events *(19,24–27)*. For example, McCully et al. *(27)* performed ESE in 1874 patients, of which 206 were diabetic. All patients studied in the report demonstrated good exercise tolerance, but had an abnormal echocardiographic response during stress. At the end of 3 years of follow-up, the event rate for cardiac death and MI was 2% yearly. Diabetes mellitus, stress-induced left ventricular dysfunction, and prior MI were independent predictors of outcome *(27)*.

Although the above results are important, another noticeable finding deserves remarking upon. Both Marwick et al. *(23)* and Kamalesh et al. *(28)* reported that the mortality rate for patients with a negative stress echocardiogram averages 4% per year in the first five years of follow up. This is a much higher rate than that of nondiabetic subjects with a negative stress echocardiogram (~1% per year). Hence, three important lessons could be learned from these

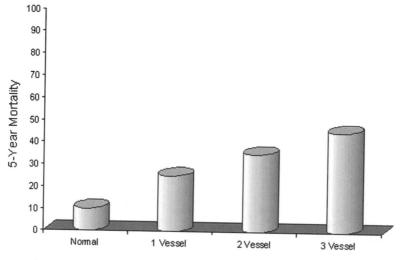

Fig. 2. 5-Year cardiac mortality according to number of vascular territories with inducible wall motion abnormalities in 937 diabetic patients (modified from Marwick et al. *(23)*).

studies. First, the strongest predictor of death in diabetic subjects with either a positive or a negative stress test is a referral for pharmacological rather than exercise stress test, underlying the importance of limited exercise tolerance in the prognosis of diabetic patients with suspected CAD. Further, the greater event rate in the presence of a negative stress echocardiogram for diabetic than nondiabetic subjects is probably related to the large number of comorbidities and the greater deconditioning demonstrated by diabetic patients. Furthermore, the high event rate despite a negative stress echocardiogram underlines the importance of not relying solely on tests for obstructive CAD to fully appreciate risk in diabetic patients. As discussed later in this chapter, techniques employed to directly visualize the atherosclerotic plaque burden may offer an opportunity to refine risk stratification in these patients.

Newer techniques for detection of CAD have also been explored in diabetic patients. Intravascular echocontrast, consisting of lipid shelled microbubbles of an inert gas (typically perfluorocarbon) can be used to assess myocardial perfusion under stress and at rest *(29,30)* (*see* Fig. 3 and Color Plate 2). With this technique, also known as myocardial contrast echocardiography (MCE), assessment of CAD is done in a manner similar to nuclear stress imaging. However, a much greater degree of expertise is required for stress echo perfusion imaging at this stage of technology development and physician training. Scognamiglio et al. *(31)* performed dypiridamole stress MCE in 1899 asymptomatic type-2 diabetic patients among whom a majority (1121 patients) had at least two other risk factors for CAD. The incidence of abnormal MCE was similar between patients with one or fewer associated risk factors compared to those with two or more risk factors ($\sim$60% for each). Nonetheless, the coronary anatomy on invasive angiography was very different with the latter group showing more frequent multivessel, as well as disseminated disease, and complete coronary occlusion (33.3% vs. 7.6%, 55% vs. 18%, 31% vs. 3.8%, respectively, $P<0.001$ each). As a consequence, 45% of the diabetic patients with multiple risk factors could not be revascularized. The authors concluded that the then current ADA recommendation to pursue the diagnosis of CAD in patients with two or more risk factors would bring to the identification of advanced disease, with a diminished

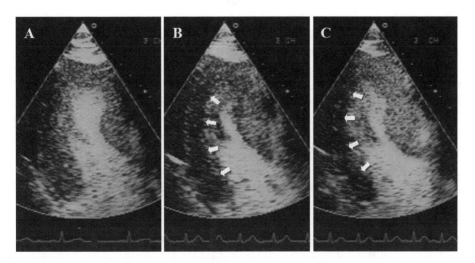

Fig. 3. Example of myocardial perfusion performed by echocardiography after intravascular injection of echocontrast (microbubbles). The arrows point at an area of decreased perfusion of the inferior wall of the myocardium during dobutamine stress (panels B and C) (courtesy of Dr. Sanjiv Kaul, Oregon Health and Science University, Portland, OR). (*see* Color Plate 2)

effectiveness of medical intervention as compared to a more aggressive strategy that involves testing earlier in the course of the disease process.

Stress echocardiography has been employed for purposes other than the primary diagnosis of CAD in diabetic populations. It appears to constitute an optimal risk-stratification screening test prior to intra-abdominal organ transplant in diabetic subjects (32), it has been used to exclude restenosis after the performance of coronary angioplasty (33) and it provides accurate information on residual myocardial viability post MI (34,35).

In summary, stress echocardiography is a safe and broadly available technique and, although slightly less sensitive than stress nuclear testing, it demonstrates a higher specificity than nuclear techniques with a lower operational cost. There remain some limitations to stress echocardiography such as the need for highly trained and qualified echocardiographers and physicians and the lower overall accuracy in the diabetic than in the general population.

NUCLEAR STRESS MYOCARDIAL PERFUSION IMAGING

Technical Considerations

In the past three decades, nuclear myocardial perfusion imaging (MPI) has become one of the most useful and informative noninvasive tools to define the presence and assess the prognosis of obstructive CAD. The overall reported sensitivity and specificity of this test for detection of critical luminal stenoses in the general population are 88% and 74%, respectively (36). Obstructive CAD is demonstrated by detecting a reduced uptake of a radiotracer (defined as a perfusion abnormality) in one or more areas of the myocardium perfused by a coronary artery with a critical (>50%) luminal stenosis (see Fig. 4 and Color Plate 3) (37). A perfusion defect is induced after the performance of a stress test by the induction of a demand/supply imbalance in the area perfused by a vessel with a fixed luminal obstruction. The obstruction does not allow sufficient increase in flow in relation to the increased oxygen demand imposed by the stress conditions. The area of abnormality may partially or completely normalize during rest (partially or completely reversible perfusion defect) or persist unchanged (fixed perfusion defect). Reversible defects indicate the presence of ischemia in viable myocardium, while a fixed defect is mostly indicative of a prior MI and scar. However, with more sophisticated techniques it is often possible to demonstrate that even areas apparently dead contain islands of viable myocardium. Scoring systems are available to assess the extent and severity of perfusion abnormalities, although in clinical practice physicians tend to use a simplified approach that takes into consideration myocardial sections corresponding to major vascular territories (i.e., left anterior descending, right coronary, and left circumflex distributions). Recent advances in computer technology have rendered possible the analysis of rest and stress-induced left ventricular ejection fraction and wall motion abnormalities (see Fig. 5 and Color Plate 4) in combination with assessment of regional myocardial perfusion (38). The combination of all of these techniques provides a comprehensive examination of the extent and severity of myocardial perfusion and ventricular function.

The most frequently employed radiopharmaceutical agents are Thallium-201 or Technetium-99m-based tracers (Tc-99m Sestamibi or Tc-99m Tetrofosmin) for the performance of SPECT imaging. Positron emission tomography imaging (PET) is performed using a variety of tracers although the most frequently used one for perfusion purposes is Rubidium 82. Each of these tracers has different pharmacodynamic and pharmacokinetic characteristics. Thallium-201 has a long half-life (~73 h), a lower peak emission rate (70–90 keV) than Technetium-99m, and recirculates in and out of viable cells utilizing potassium channels (37,39). Due to its rapid

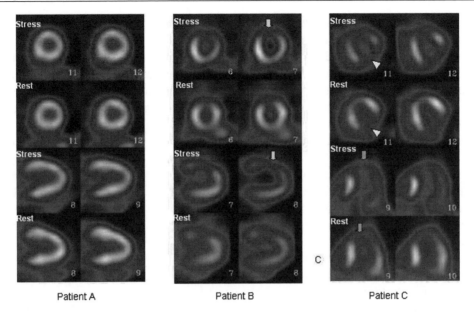

Patient A   Patient B   Patient C

Fig. 4. Examples of nuclear myocardial perfusion imaging of the left ventricular myocardium. Patient A shows a homogeneous distribution of the radioactive tracer both at rest and during stress. Patient B shows a moderate size defect in the anterior wall of the left ventricle (yellow arrows) during stress (top row images). The defect disappears (i.e., is reversible) during rest (bottom row images). Patient C demonstrates a large and fixed perfusion defect of the infero-lateral wall (white arrow heads) and a partially reversible defect of the apex of the left ventricle (green arrows). (*see* Color Plate 3)

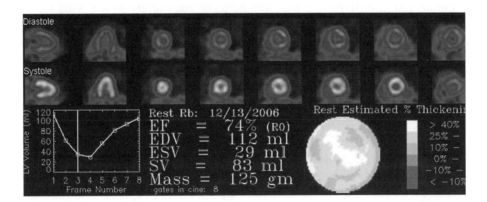

Fig. 5. An example of assessment of left ventricular function on position emission tomography imaging. The calculated left ventricular ejection fraction is 74%. The top row shows diastolic images of the left ventricle (the chamber is larger and the walls are thinner) while the bottom row shows systolic frames (the chamber is almost virtual and the walls are thick). (*see* Color Plate 4)

redistribution, imaging must begin right after the injection of the tracer at peak exercise to detect stress-induced perfusion defects. Because of latent recirculation across the membrane of viable myocardial cells, delayed imaging (usually 3–4 h from stress imaging) may demonstrate tracer uptake where it may not have been detected during stress. Technetium-99m has a higher peak emission rate (140 keV) and a shorter half-life (∼6.5 h) than Thallium-201. It recirculates minimally in and out of viable cells and remains essentially trapped in the location of initial uptake giving an instantaneous impression of the perfusion status at the time of injection. Due to its lack of redistribution, Technetium-99m-based tracers must be injected a peak exercise and reinjected at rest to compare stress and rest images (37,40). Rubidium-82 is a positron-emitting tracer with a very short half-life (1–2 min) and biological properties similar to those of Thallium-201 (and potassium). It is used for imaging with PET scanners and due to this extremely short half-life it must be injected at rest and again after stress. For this reason, stress testing in PET imaging can only be performed pharmacologically by means of adenosine infusion (see below).

Nuclear images are typically reconstructed utilizing a tomographic technique (Figs. 4 and 5) known as SPECT for Thallium-201 and Technitium-99m tracers or PET for Rubidium-82. With SPECT and PET it is possible to segment the left ventricle in several slices oriented along three orthogonal planes in space with superior spatial resolution and diagnostic quality compared to the original planar imaging that has currently become obsolete.

Stress testing can be performed by either treadmill or bicycle exercise or, as discussed with stress echocardiography, by means of pharmacological stress agents. Diabetic patients frequently demonstrate poor exercise tolerance and are affected by peripheral vascular disease and cardiomyopathy that hinder their ability to achieve an optimal exercise workload. Hence, pharmacological stress testing is frequently employed as an alternative to exercise stress testing to risk stratify diabetic patients for CAD. The most frequently employed pharmacological stress agents with MPI are vasodilatory agents (dipyridamole or adenosine) (41), while inotropic agents such as dobutamine are employed less frequently. With vasodilatory agents the purpose is to induce a regional myocardial blood flow maldistribution, favoring territories perfused by patent coronary arteries capable of vasodilation in response to pharmacological stimulation, over territories perfused by a coronary artery with a fixed stenosis (41). Inotropic agents increase heart rate and contractility and perfusion abnormalities are created by increasing oxygen demand and induction of ischemia in segments of the myocardium perfused by stenosed coronary arteries that cannot supply as much oxygen as required to sustain the stress (42).

Clinical Applications

CAD is often silent in diabetic patients and typically in advanced stages of development by the time it manifests (43). Hence, several investigators have utilized stress testing to detect silent ischemia (SI). Abnormal results have been reported in as low as 12% and as high as 50% of asymptomatic diabetic individuals submitted to screening for SI (44–51). This wide variation in test results is likely due to the different interpretation criteria used by the investigators and, above all, the pretest probability of disease of the patients tested. Of interest, male gender has been identified by several authors as a variable independently associated with SI on exercise electrocardiography in type-2 diabetes (44,45,48). Senior et al. (51) tested 60 consecutive type-1 diabetic patients prior to islet cell transplantation, and found that exercise stress testing with electrocardiography is highly specific (97%) but very insensitive (17%) for prediction of obstructive CAD. Rutter et al. (50) performed treadmill EST in 43 type-2 diabetes mellitus patients with microalbuminuria and 43 without microalbuminuria, and found SI in 52% of the patients. In multivariable models, SI emerged as the strongest predictor of cardiovascular events. Cosson et al. (52) performed both treadmill electrocardiographic stress testing and nuclear perfusion imaging in 262 asymptomatic patients with long-standing diabetes mellitus (mean 12 years) and followed them for an average of 3 years after screening. The electrocardiographic response was abnormal in approximately 21% of the patients and an abnormal stress test result was a univariate predictor of events. Furthermore, the exercise stress test had a high negative predictive value (97%).

The addition of MPI to plain electrocardiographic stress testing confirmed the high prevalence of SI (varying between 20% and 40%) in asymptomatic diabetic patients. In the DIAD study *(53)*, 1124 type-2 diabetic patients were enrolled at 14 sites in the US and Canada. Of the 1124 patients, 502 underwent an adenosine-Tc-99m sestamibi stress test and the remaining did not. In the imaging cohort, 22% of the individuals showed abnormal MPI results although only 1 every 18 subjects (5.5%) showed a moderate-to-severe perfusion defect indicative of poor prognosis. Since the entry criteria required an established diagnosis of diabetes mellitus type-2, a normal electrocardiogram and no known CAD, the authors concluded that screening should be considered even in the absence of a minimum of two other risk factors as recommended in the consensus statement of the ADA *(54)*. Indeed, the results of the DIAD trial indicate that as many as 41% of type-2 diabetic patients would go undetected for silent CAD if the ADA recommendations for screening were followed strictly *(54)*. Of interest, in the DIAD trial there was no association between the inducibility of perfusion abnormalities and traditional or emerging (such as CRP) risk factors.

Similarly, De Lorenzo et al. *(55)* submitted 180 asymptomatic adult-onset diabetic patients to stress MPI for the detection of unsuspected obstructive CAD. A positive test result was reported in 26% of the subjects. During a follow-up of approximately 2 years, 34 patients suffered cardiac events: 7 cardiac deaths, 6 nonfatal MIs, 10 coronary artery by-pass surgeries, and 11 percutaneous angioplasties. Male gender and perfusion abnormalities on MPI were independent predictors of cardiac events. Abnormal MPI results added incremental prognostic value to clinical variables and exercise stress test variables for prediction of hard events (MI and cardiac death; chi-square 5.4; $p = 0.001$) and total events (chi-square 7.4; $p = 0.0001$). In patients with normal MPI the hard event and total event rate were 2% and 5% respectively, compared to 9% and 38% in those with abnormal MPI.

Faglia et al. *(14)* reported the 5-year follow-up results of the MISAD (Milan Study on Atherosclerosis and Diabetes) study. The investigators performed electrocardiographic exercise stress tests in 925 asymptomatic type-2 diabetic patients, followed by a nuclear stress test when the former was abnormal. 735 patients were followed for 5 years; among these 638 had undergone a normal exercise stress test, 45 had an abnormal EST with normal MPI, and the remaining 52 had both an abnormal EST and an abnormal MPI. The total event rate was significantly higher in those with any abnormal stress test of any type compared to those with normal results (21% vs. 5%; $P<0.0001$). On multivariable analyses, an abnormal MPI was the strongest predictor of events (hazard ratio: 5.47, $P < 0.001$), followed by diabetic retinopathy and diabetes duration. In the study by Valensi et al. *(56)*, 370 asymptomatic patients with a minimum of two or more risk factors for CAD were submitted to either exercise or dipyridamole MPI and were followed for an average of 38 ± 23 months. SI was present in 35% of the subjects screened and was strongly associated with the occurrence of hard events (hazard ratio: 3, CI: 1.53–5.87). Hence, it seems quite clear that the occurrence of cardiovascular events is linked to the presence of SI in asymptomatic diabetic patients, and that the presence of pre-clinical CAD can be accurately investigated by means of MPI.

The utility of MPI has also been reviewed extensively in patients with known or suspected CAD. The importance of symptoms in determining the results of MPI and influencing outcome was tested in a large group ($N = 1737$) of diabetic patients submitted to dual-isotope nuclear stress testing by Zellweger and colleagues *(57)*. Dual-isotope imaging (thallium for rest and technetium for stress imaging) was introduced several years ago to improve the signal-to-noise ratio and, ultimately, the accuracy of nuclear stress testing. Objective evidence of CAD was found in 39% of asymptomatic patients, compared to 44% of those with angina and 51% of those with dyspnea. During a 2-year follow-up, the annual event rate was highest in patients with abnormal MPI results and dyspnea as a main symptom (13.2% vs. 7.7% normal MPI with dyspnea), followed by angina (5.6% vs. 3.2% normal MPI with angina) and no symptoms (3.6% vs. 2.2% normal MPI and no symptoms). MPI added incremental predictive value to pre-test clinical information (increase in global chi-square from 52 to 98, $P < 0.0001$).

Kang et al. published two series (58,59) analyzing the contribution of MPI to the diagnosis and management of CAD in diabetic patients. In a smaller series inclusive of 203 diabetic and 260 nondiabetic patients (58), they demonstrated similar sensitivity (86% for each) and specificity of MPI (56% and 46%, respectively) in diabetic and nondiabetic patients. The sensitivity was high in both patient groups but the specificity was only moderate and lower than that reported in the general population (36). In the second series (59) the authors addressed the question of the incremental prognostic information provided by MPI over clinical data for prediction of events in 1271 diabetic and 5862 nondiabetic patients. During an average follow-up of 24 months, diabetic patients suffered a higher rate of hard events (4.3% vs. 2.3%, $P < 0.001$) and combined events (hard events plus revascularizations, 9% vs. 5.3%, $P < 0.001$) than nondiabetic subjects. As shown by others, findings on MPI added significantly ($P < 0.001$) to the prognostic value provided by clinical and historical data.

Two groups of investigators reviewed the impact of abnormal stress MPI results on all-cause mortality in diabetic patients. In a large multicenter study, Giri et al. (60) assessed the value of MPI as a risk-stratification tool in symptomatic diabetic and nondiabetics patients. The investigators prospectively followed 8411 patients (20% diabetics) for an average of 2.5 years after a baseline MPI. Primary endpoints were the occurrence of cardiac death and nonfatal MI or the performance of revascularization procedures. An abnormal MPI result was a significant predictor of cardiac death and MI in both diabetic and nondiabetic subjects (Table 1). Using a simple scoring system reflecting the extent of myocardial ischemia by number of vascular territories, the total number of ischemic territories (ranging from none to 3) was associated with a stepwise increment in the death rate of both diabetic and nondiabetic subjects. In diabetic patients, however, even ischemia in a single vessel territory increased the risk of death in a very significant way compared to nondiabetic individuals. Regardless of risk factors, in diabetic patients the presence of multivessel ischemia was the strongest predictor of total coronary events, whereas the presence of multiple fixed defects was the strongest predictor of cardiac

Table 1

Kaplan–Meier 3-year rates of cardiac death or nonfatal myocardial infarction according to number of vascular territories with inducible ischemia on myocardial perfusion SPECT for patients with and without diabetes stratified by sex

	Death / Myocardial Infarction		
	0-Vessel Ischemia	1-Vessel Ischemia	≥2-Vessel Ischemia
Diabetic Women	3.5%	27.5%	40.0%
Non-Diabetic Women	4.5%	15.0%	22.5%
Diabetic Men	13.7%	23.0%	21.0%
Non-Diabetic Men	6.2%	12.0%	15.0%

death. The authors further described that a normal MPI is associated with a very good event-free survival both in subjects with and without diabetes in the short range. Nonetheless, the so-called "protective effect" of a normal MPI study in diabetic patients appeared to expire after about 2 years from testing when events started occurring very rapidly. Therefore, the authors recommended retesting diabetic patients sooner than the rest of the population in the presence of a normal MPI due to faster disease progression. Notably, diabetic women showed the worst outcome for any given extent of reversible myocardial ischemia in this study. Elhendy et al. *(61)* performed stress MPI in 297 diabetic patients with known or suspected CAD. The incidence of abnormal MPI was exceedingly high (~60%) and the death rate at the end of 2 years approached 27%. The annual mortality rate was 2.5% in subjects with normal MPI, 4.5% in patients with fixed perfusion defects, and 6% in patients with ischemia. Age, congestive heart failure, peripheral artery disease, and ischemia on stress MPI were independent predictors of death.

In a single-center study, Berman et al. *(62)* reported on the incremental prognostic value for cardiac events of adenosine stress MPI in 6173 consecutively tested diabetic and nondiabetic patients. For the nondiabetic patients, a normal, mildly abnormal, and moderately-to-severely abnormal SPECT study was associated with cardiac death rates ranging from 0.8% to 6.1% per year of follow-up (Fig. 6). Though event rates were similar for nondiabetic men and women, diabetic women with perfusion defects demonstrated higher death rates than diabetic men (Fig. 6). For diabetic women, event rates were 1.5%, 3.3%, 4.1%, and 8.5% for normal, mildly abnormal, moderately abnormal, and severely abnormal MPI results, respectively ($p <$ 0.0001). By comparison, the event rates ranged from 0.8% to 6% for diabetic men with normal-to-severely abnormal nuclear scans ($p < 0.0001$). The higher event rate in diabetic women with provocative ischemia echoed the results of the previous study by Giri et al. *(60)*. The reasons for the more unfavorable outcome for diabetic women than men are poorly understood but appear to be related to their advanced age and greater clustering of risk factors *(63)*. In the study by Berman et al. *(62)*, the cardiac death rate was higher for insulin-requiring diabetic patients than non-insulin-dependent diabetic patients in the presence of a normal MPI and, obviously higher

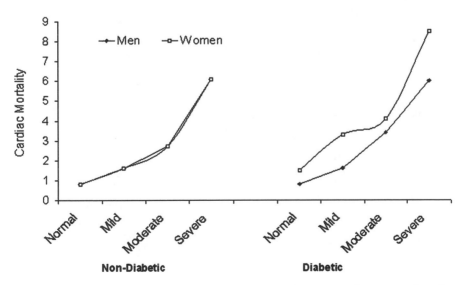

Fig. 6. Cardiac mortality in diabetic and nondiabetic women and men according to severity of myocardial perfusion defects ranging from low to severely abnormal (modified from Berman D, et al. *(62)*).

than that of nondiabetic subjects. Thus, in the setting of a normal MPI the death rate increased from approximately 0.6% for nondiabetic subjects to 1.8% for non-insulin requiring, to 2.5% for insulin-requiring diabetic patients, respectively. In contrast, in the setting of an abnormal study, the annual cardiac death rates were approximately twofold higher for insulin-dependent diabetic patients compared with non-insulin-requiring diabetic patients and nondiabetic subjects alike. These findings should alert the clinician as to the serious risk posed by diabetes even in the absence of inducible perfusion defects and the need for further investigation of the vascular health status of these individuals.

COMPUTED TOMOGRAPHY FOR CORONARY ARTERY CALCIUM SCREENING

Technical Considerations

Traditional noninvasive imaging methods used to diagnose the presence of CAD (electrocardiographic or pharmacological stress testing with and without imaging) are germane to the diagnosis of obstructive luminal disease, with very important consequences for revascularization therapy. However, the presence of an extensive atherosclerotic plaque burden in the vessel wall, even in the absence of obstructive disease, is associated with the occurrence of acute coronary events *(64,65)*. Hence, recently there has been an emerging interest in diagnosing atherosclerosis prior to the development of symptoms of CAD.

Cardiac computed tomography has been used to assess the extent of coronary artery calcium (CAC) (Fig. 7) in asymptomatic and symptomatic patients for the purpose of stratifying subjects

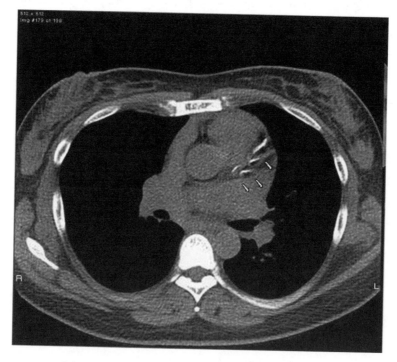

Fig. 7. Coronary artery calcium on an axial computed tomography image of the chest. Calcium deposits are present along the left anterior descending coronary artery and its branches (white arrows).

for risk of cardiac events. Calcium is deposited in the atherosclerotic plaque since the early stages of development and grows in parallel with the growth of the plaque *(66)*. The deposition of crystals of hydroxyapatite (calcium-phosphate crystals similar to bone) is not due to simple precipitation of crystals in solution, but is under the control of active processes of calcification similar to bone formation *(67–69)*. The processes are governed by vascular cells that turn into osteoblast-like cells and utilize enzymes normally found in bone and necessary for the normal process of remodeling of bone *(69)*. The initiating event of such a cascade is not known though multiple noxious stimuli (oxidized lipids, inflammatory stimuli, hyperphosphatemia, vitamin D, endproducts of glycation, etc.) are capable of inducing a phenotypic transformation of vascular smooth muscle cells into noncontractile and bone-like cells *(70–78)*.

Calcium accumulation in the coronary arteries can be detected and precisely quantified with computerized tomography technologies utilizing high imaging speed. The speed of imaging is necessary to prevent image blurring due to continuous cardiac motion. The first CT developed for this purpose was the electron beam tomography (EBT) scanner, followed more recently by multidetector CTs with simultaneous acquisition of multiple sections. In either case the extent of calcification is measured by means of a calcium score calculated by the computer software on the basis of plaque size and density *(79)*. There is a modest relationship between calcium score and coronary artery lumen stenosis on angiography, with a greater likelihood of stenosis as the calcium score increases *(80–83)*. It should be remembered that this correlation is not perfect (R-value ~50%) and the use of CAC screening for the prediction of coronary artery stenosis is therefore not recommendable. On the contrary, the main purpose of CAC screening is to detect vessel wall atherosclerosis, which appears to hasten the occurrence of coronary events even in the absence of luminal stenoses *(64,65)*.

Clinical Applications

A large body of evidence has been accumulated demonstrating the utility of CAC screening in nondiabetic populations. In such populations the presence of CAC poses a significantly increased risk of events proportional to the extent of calcification and it adds incremental prognostic value to traditional risk factors for the prediction of hard cardiovascular events *(84–86)*. The evidence surrounding the utility of CAC screening in diabetes mellitus patients, however, is still preliminary and actively being investigated.

Patients suffering from diabetes type-2 have been shown to harbor larger amounts of CAC than nondiabetic patients with the metabolic syndrome *(87)* and subjects of similar age and otherwise similar risk factor profile *(87,88)*. Furthermore, the amount of coronary calcium in patients with type-2 diabetes is similar to that of patients with established CAD but without diabetes, confirming the clinical notion that diabetes mellitus should be considered a CVD risk equivalent. Interestingly, diabetic women harbor as much CAC as diabetic men, again confirming the clinical evidence that diabetes mellitus negates the well-known advantage of women over men in prevalence and extent of atherosclerosis *(89,90)*. Hoff et al. *(91)* utilized a large database to calculate the age and gender normative (percentile) distribution of calcium scores in asymptomatic (self-reported) diabetic individuals. They showed that younger diabetic individuals have a plaque burden comparable to that of older nondiabetic individuals. Hence, diabetes mellitus not only negates the gender advantage but levels age differences as far as atherosclerosis progression. However, there may be an important racial and genetic influence on prevalence and extent of CAC. In fact, Hispanic patients living in the US affected by type-2 diabetes mellitus show lower CAC and aortic calcification scores than nonHispanic whites their counterpart *(92)*. Furthermore, Wagenknecht et al. *(93)* showed that there is a large component of heritability to the variance of CAC in patients affected by type-2 diabetes mellitus.

Olson et al. *(94)* investigated the presence of CAC as well as the association with a history of CAD in patients with diabetes mellitus type-1. They recruited 302 subjects (146 men and 156 women) with a history of MI, angina, or evidence of ischemia on stress testing or surface electrocardiograms. Patients were participants in the Pittsburgh Epidemiology of Diabetes Complications (EDC) study, a 10-year prospective follow-up study of risk factors for complications of type-1 diabetes diagnosed before the age of 17. EBT imaging showed that the prevalence of CAC increased with age (from 11% before age 30 to 88% in individuals aged 50–55 years or older). CAC was detected in all patients 50 and older with established CAD. Of the subjects who were free of clinical CAD, 5% had a CAC score $\geq$400 (indicative of a large atherosclerosis burden) *(80)*, as did 25% of the subjects with angina/ischemia and 80% of the patients with MI or luminal stenosis on invasive angiography. CAC showed a sensitivity of 84% and 71% for clinical CAD in men and women, respectively, and 100% sensitivity for MI and obstructive CAD. In multivariable regression analyses CAC was independently correlated with MI or obstructive CAD in both sexes and was the strongest independent correlate in men.

In the Coronary Artery Calcification in Type 1 Diabetes (CACTI) study *(95)*, type-1 diabetic subjects showed a high prevalence and severity of coronary calcifications again with a disappearance of the known difference between men and women. The authors suggested that insulin resistance, associated with an android deposition of fat, may be related to the increased prevalence of CAC in women with type-1 diabetes mellitus. Interestingly, the increased prevalence of CAC in women affected by type-1 diabetes mellitus is not associated with traditional risk factors for atherosclerosis nor the size and concentration of lipoproteins, while it may be related to the extent of inflammation *(96)*.

Limited data exist on outcome related to CAC in diabetic patients. The potential impact of CAC as a predictor of events was analyzed in a small study by Hosoi et al. *(97)*. The authors studied a cohort of 101 diabetic and 181 nondiabetic patients who presented to the emergency department with angina pectoris and electrocardiographic findings suggestive of myocardial ischemia. Coronary angiography was performed in all patients and CAC imaging was performed within 2 weeks of angiography. In the absence of coronary artery stenoses, CAC was more extensive in diabetic patients than nondiabetic subjects. In contrast, no significant difference in CAC burden was found between diabetic and nondiabetic patients in the presence of coronary luminal obstruction. In diabetic patients, a CAC score $\geq$90 was associated with an equal sensitivity and specificity of 75% for coronary obstruction, whereas a CAC score >200 was associated with a sensitivity of 64% and a specificity of 83%. The authors concluded that CAC in symptomatic diabetic subjects is predictive of the severity of coronary stenosis and the potential need for revascularization. In a subsequent publication, Wong et al. *(98)* confirmed this opinion by performing CAC screening and stress MPI in 1043 patients, 313 of whom were affected by either diabetes mellitus ($N = 140$) or the metabolic syndrome ($N = 173$). In patients with a CAC score below 100, the prevalence of stress-induced MPI abnormalities was very low ($\sim$2%). However, in the presence of a metabolic disorder (diabetes mellitus or the metabolic syndrome) a CAC score between 100 and 399 or greater than 400 was associated with a greater incidence of ischemia than in patients without a metabolic disease (13% vs. 3.6%, $p < 0.02$, and 23.4% vs. 13.6%, $p = 0.03$, respectively). The odds of MPI ischemia were 4.3-fold greater per standard deviation of log-CAC score ($p < 0.001$) and twofold greater in the presence of metabolic abnormalities ($p<0.01$). Similarly, Anand et al. performed sequential CAC and MPI in 180 type-2 diabetic patients. The incidence of myocardial ischemia was directly related to

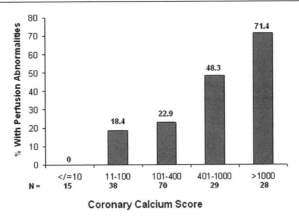

Fig. 8. Frequency of ischemia on a nuclear myocardial perfusion study according to coronary artery calcium score in 180 type-2 diabetic patients (modified from Anand et al. *(99)*).

the CAC score (Fig. 8). For type-2 diabetic patients with a CAC score of 0, 11–100, 101–400, 401–1,000, and >1,000, the incidence of myocardial ischemia on stress MPI was 0%, 18%, 23%, 48%, and 71%, respectively. Thus, although direct imaging with MPI was not successful in identifying a large group of at-risk diabetics, as noted in the DIAD study *(53)*, sequential imaging strategies involving the use of a CT-derived CAC score provided an effective means of identifying a large percentage of patients with inducible ischemia. In summary, based on the Wong *(98)* and Anand data *(99)*, type-2 diabetic patients with a CAC score >100 are expected to have an increased frequency of ischemia on MPI.

Two outcome studies addressed the question of whether CAC constitutes a risk for events in asymptomatic patients but came to opposite conclusions. The South Bay Heart Watch (SBHW) was a prospective cohort study designed to determine the relation between radiographically detectable CAC and cardiovascular outcome in high-risk asymptomatic adults *(100)*. A total of 1312 asymptomatic subjects ≥45 years old with cardiac risk factors were recruited via mass-mailing advertisement in the Los Angeles area; of these 19% were diabetic patients. In a subanalysis of the main database after a mean follow-up of 6 years, Qu et al. *(100)* found an increased risk of cardiovascular events (death, MI, stroke, and revascularizations) in diabetic patients compared to nondiabetic subjects in the presence of CAC. However, the risk did not increase in a statistically significant way as the CAC score increased. Raggi et al. *(101)* utilized data from a database of 10,377 asymptomatic individuals (903 diabetic patients), followed for an average of 5 years after having been referred by a primary care physician for a CAC screening test. The primary endpoint of the study was all-cause mortality. The authors showed that the risk of all-cause mortality was higher in diabetic patients than nondiabetic subjects for any degree of calcification and the risk increased as the calcium score increased (Fig. 9). Additionally, the absence of CAC predicted a low short-term risk of death (~1% at 5 years) for both diabetic patients and nondiabetic subjects (Fig. 9). Hence, both the presence and absence of CAC were important modifiers of risk even in the presence of established risk factors for atherosclerosis such as diabetes mellitus. This suggests that there is a great heterogeneity among diabetes mellitus patients as well as any other risk cohort and that risk stratification may be of benefit even in patients considered to be at high-risk of atherosclerosis complications.

Of interest, in the study by Giri et al. *(60)* diabetic patients with a normal stress MPI had a fourfold higher morbidity and mortality during follow-up than nondiabetic subjects with normal

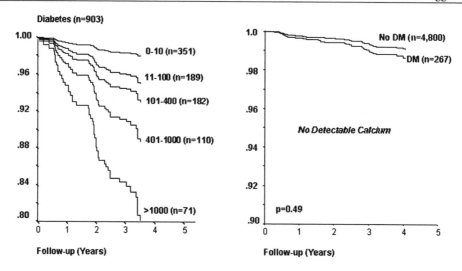

Fig. 9. Prognostic significance of coronary calcium scores in diabetes mellitus. In panel A the all-cause mortality of diabetic patients increases as the coronary artery calcium scores increase. In panel B, however, the overall mortality is similar for diabetic and nondiabetic patients with no coronary artery calcium (i.e., atherosclerosis) (modified from Raggi et al. *(101)*).

stress MPI scans, while in the study by Raggi et al. *(101)* patients with no or minimal calcium had the same outcome independent of the presence of diabetes.

The preceding discussion suggests that an approach to the diagnosis of CAD that combines different techniques may be very helpful to the practicing physician faced with the dilemma of accurate patient risk assessment.

CURRENT RECOMMENDATIONS

There are currently almost 16 million patients with known diabetes mellitus in the United States alone. Of these, 3.5 million are known to have CAD. Who should be screened among the 12.5 million asymptomatic diabetic patients with subclinical CAD? Until recently the standing recommendations of the ADA and American College of Cardiology (ACC) could have been summarized as shown in *see* Fig. 10 and Color Plate 5. According to these 1998 guidelines, stress testing with or without imaging (i.e., functional stress testing) should be performed in symptomatic patients and in asymptomatic subjects with abnormal resting electrocardiograms, patients with two or more risk factors for CAD, patients with peripheral or carotid artery disease, or those beginning a vigorous exercise program *(54)*. Consideration should be given to testing diabetic patients over age 35 with evidence of autonomic neuropathy and patients with microalbuminuria, as these two markers of disease have been associated with a high risk of cardiovascular events. Nonetheless, in January 2007 the ADA issued new standard of care relating to screening for CAD in diabetes *(102)*. Symptomatic diabetic patients, with either typical or atypical symptoms, and those with abnormal resting electrocardiogram, remain candidates for stress testing *(102)*. In the new paradigm (shown in Fig. 11 and Color Plate 6), however, asymptomatic patients are candidates for stress testing only in the presence of prior history of peripheral or carotid artery disease, or when planning to begin a vigorous exercise program having followed a sedentary lifestyle and being older than 35 years. Since the vast majority of patients with diabetes have at least two other risk factors, the ADA considered it impractical to recommend screening according to this criterion any longer *(102)*.

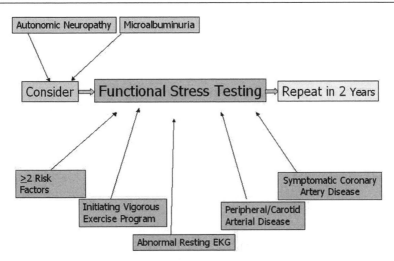

Fig. 10. Guidelines proposed in 1998 by the American Diabetic Association on performance of exercise stress testing, with or without an imaging modality associated with it, in diabetic patients (modified from reference *(54)*). (*see* Color Plate 5)

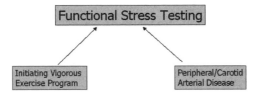

Fig. 11. New standard of care from the American Diabetic Association on performance of exercise stress testing, with or without an imaging modality associated with it, in asymptomatic diabetic patients (modified from reference *(102)*). (*see* Color Plate 6)

Furthermore, concludes the statement, there is no current evidence that testing in asymptomatic patients with risk factors improves survival. There are at least two relevant comments with respect to this new ADA position: evidence needs to build up and avoiding (or recommending against) testing is going to delay the necessary acquisition of data. Screening in itself (the act of acquiring pictures) cannot be charged with the task "of saving lives" as this is the responsibility of the treating physician acting on the basis of the results of a test.

Of interest, older guidelines of the AHA resemble the recent ADA statement. In fact, they recommended against routine testing in asymptomatic diabetic patients *(103)*. This position was guided by the interpretation of diabetes mellitus as a cardiovascualr disease equivalent that mandates aggressive therapy irrespective of findings on noninvasive imaging and the absence of solid data to demonstrate an improved outcome with interventional techniques in asymptomatic diabetic subjects. Finally, the French Diabetes Association *(104)* recommends stress testing in patients with peripheral vasculopathy, proteinuria and/or multipe risk factors for CVD or in patients over the age of 65.

CONCLUSIONS

Although every diabetic patient should be treated aggressively and considered at very high risk for CAD, each patient should be considered and treated as an individual and not as part of a group given the heterogeneity among this patient population. To improve the cardiovascular prognosis it may become necessary to start testing diabetic patients with comorbidities more aggressively. The responsibility for treatment will then fall upon the physician ordering the test which, as discussed above, should not be charged with the task of saving lives. As a guide to choosing the right patient for testing, one could use clinical indicators of risk such as poor exercise tolerance, autonomic dysfunction, microalbuminuria, retinopathy, sex, and insulin dependence. Nonetheless, as correctly stated in the recent ADA standard of care release *(102)*, much of the evidence to support a more aggressive screening program is still lacking.

Among the available noninvasive tests to diagnose obstructive CAD, both stress echocardiography and SPECT imaging have been shown to accurately risk stratify patients for major adverse events. The extent and severity of perfusion and wall motion abnormalities are at the core of effective risk stratification. A normal stress test confers a good prognosis though inferior to that of a normal stress test in a nondiabetic subject. This fact associated with the more rapid development of symptoms in diabetic patients (about 2 years) with a normal test indicates the need for "tested" diabetic patients to undergo more frequent retesting than nondiabetic individuals. Furthermore, the occurrence of a substantial number of events in the presence of a normal stress test raises the question of whether direct plaque imaging, such as measurement of atherosclerotic plaque burden with computed tomography for CAC or carotid intima-media thickness, may improve risk prediction. The role of these techniques in diabetes mellitus is awaiting further clarification. Nonetheless, these methodologies allow a refinement of risk assessment in the general population and may eventually become useful in the diabetic population as well.

REFERENCES

1. Grundy SM, Benjamin IJ, Burke GL, et al. Diabetes and cardiovascular disease: A statement for healthcare professionals from the American Heart Association. *Circulation*. 1999;100:1134–1146.
2. Grundy SM, Benjamin IJ, Burke GL, et al. Diabetes mellitus: A major risk factor for cardiovascular disease: A joint editorial statement by the American Diabetes Association; the National Heart, Lung, and Blood Institute; the Juvenile Diabetes Foundation International; the National Institute of Diabetes and Digestive and Kidney Diseases; and the American Heart Association. *Circulation*.1999;100:1132–1133.
3. Diabetes Statistics. National Diabetes Information Clearinghouse. Bethesda, MD: National Institute of Diabetes and Digestive and Kidney Diseases, NIH publication. 1999: 99–326.
4. Nesto RW, Peter L. Diabetes mellitus and the cardiovascular system. In: Braunwald E, Zipes DP, Libby P eds. Heart Disease: A Textbook of Cardiovascular Medicine. Saunders Co: Philadelphia. 2001: 2133–2150.
5. King H, Aubert RE, Herman WH. Global Burden of Diabetes, 1995–2025: Prevalence, numerical estimates, and projections. *Diabetes Care*. 1998;21:1414–1431.
6. Venkat Narayan KM, Boyle JP, Thompson TJ, et al. Lifetime risk for diabetes mellitus in the United States. *JAMA*. 2003;290:1884–1890.
7. Haffner SM, Stern MP, Hazuda HP, et al. Cardiovascular risk factors in confirmed prediabetic individuals. Does the clock for coronary heart disease start ticking before the onset of clinical diabetes? *JAMA*. 1990;263: 2893–2898.
8. Miettinen H, Lehto S, Veikko S, et al. Impact of diabetes on mortality after the first myocardial infarction. *Diabetes Care*. 1998;21:69–75.
9. Norhammar A, Malmberg K, Diderholm E, et al. Diabetes mellitus: the major risk factor in unstable coronary artery disease even after consideration of the extent of coronary artery disease and benefits of revascularization. *J Am Coll Cardiol*. 2004;43:585–591.
10. Mehran R, Dangas GD, Kobayashi Y, et al. Short- and long-term results after multivessel stenting in diabetic patients. *J Am Coll Cardiol*. 2004;43:1348–1354.
11. The BARI Investigators. Influence of diabetes on 5-year mortality and morbidity in a randomized trial comparing CABG and PTCA in patients with multivessel disease: The Bypass Angioplasty Revascularization Investigation (BARI). *Circulation*. 1997;96:1761–1769.
12. Gu K, Cowie CC, Harris MI. Diabetes and decline in heart disease mortality in US adults. *JAMA*. 1999;281:1291–1297.

13. Froelicher VF, Lehmann KG, Thomas R, Goldman S, Morrison D, Edson R, Lavori P, Myers J, Dennis C, Shabetai R, Do D, Froning J. The electrocardiographic exercise test in a population with reduced workup bias: diagnostic performance, computerized interpretation, and multivariable prediction. Veterans Affairs Cooperative Study in Health Services #016 (QUEXTA) Study Group. Quantitative Exercise Testing and Angiography. *Ann Int Med.* 1998;128:965–974.

14. Faglia E, Favales F, Calia P, Paleari F, Segalini G, Gamba PL, Rocca A, Musacchio N, Mastropasqua A, Testori G, Rampini P, Moratti F, Braga A, Morabito A. Milan Study on Atherosclerosis and Diabetes (Mi SAD). Cardiac events in 735 type 2 diabetic patients who underwent screening for unknown asymptomatic coronary heart disease: 5-year follow-up report from the Milan Study on Atherosclerosis and Diabetes (MiSAD). *Diabetes Care.* 2002;25:2032–2036.

15. Wei M, Gibbons LW, Kampert JB, Nichaman MZ, Blair SN. Low cardiorespiratory fitness and physical inactivity as predictors of mortality in men with type 2 diabetes. *Ann Intern Med.* 2000;132;605–611.

16. Cheng YJ, Lauer MS, Earnest CP, Church TS, Kampert JB, Gibbons LW, Blair SN. Heart rate recovery following maximal exercise testing as a predictor of cardiovascular disease and all-cause mortality in men with diabetes. *Diabetes Care.* 2003;26;2052–2057.

17. Elhendy A, van Domburg RT, Poldermans D, et al. Safety and feasibility of dobutamine-atropine stress echocardiography for the diagnosis of coronary artery disease in diabetic patients unable to perform an exercise stress test. *Diabetes Care .* 1998;21:1797–1802.

18. Gaddi O, Tortorella G, Picano E, et al. Diagnostic and prognostic value of vasodilator stress echocardiography in asymptomatic Type 2 diabetic patients with positive exercise thallium scintigraphy: a pilot study. *Diabet Med.* 1999;16:762–766.

19. Bigi R, Desideri A, Cortigiani L, et al. Stress echocardiography for risk stratification of diabetic patients with known or suspected coronary artery disease. *Diabetes Care.* 2001;24:1596–1601.

20. Cheitlin MD, Armstrong WF, Aurigemma GP, et al. ACC/AHA/ASE 2003 guideline update for the clinical application of echocardiography – summary article: a report of the American College of Cardiology/American Heart Association Task Force on Practice Guidelines (ACC/AHA/ASE Committee to Update the 1997 Guidelines for the Clinical Application of Echocardiography). *J Am Coll Cardiol.* 2003;42:954–970.

21. Penfornis A, Zimmermann C, Boumal D, et al. Use of dobutamine stress echocardiography in detecting silent myocardial ischaemia in asymptomatic diabetic patients: a comparison with thallium scintigraphy and exercise testing. *Diabet Med.* 2001;18:900–905.

22. Hennessy TG, Codd MB, Hennessy MS, et al. Comparison of dobutamine stress echocardiography and treadmill exercise electrocardiography for detection of coronary artery disease. *Coron Artery Dis.* 1997;8:171–174.

23. Marwick TH, Case C, Sawada S, et al. Use of stress echocardiography to predict mortality in patients with diabetes and known or suspected coronary artery disease. *Diabetes Care.* 2002;25:1042–1048.

24. Elhendy A, Arruda AM, Mahoney DW, et al. Prognostic stratification of diabetic patients by exercise echocardiography. *J Am Coll Cardiol.* 2001;37:1551–1557.

25. Sozzi FB, Elhendy A, Roelandt JR, et al. Prognostic value of dobutamine stress echocardiography in patients with diabetes. *Diabetes Care.* 2003;26(4):1074–1078.

26. D'Andrea A, Severino S, Caso P, et al. Prognostic value of pharmacological stress echocardiography in diabetic patients. *Eur J Echocardiogr.* 2003;4:202–208.

27. McCully RB, Roger VL, Mahoney, et al. DW Outcome after abnormal exercise echocardiography for patients with good exercise capacity: prognostic importance of the extent and severity of exercise-related left ventricular dysfunction. *J Am Coll Cardiol.* 2002;39:1345–1352.

28. Kamalesh M, Matorin R, Sawada S. Prognostic value of a negative stress echocardiographic study in diabetic patients. *Am Heart J.* 2002;143:163–168.

29. Villanueva FS, Wagner WR, Vannan MA, Narula J. Targeted ultrasound imaging using microbubbles. *Cardiology Clinics.* 2004;22:283–298, vii.

30. Kang DH, Kang SJ, Song JM, Choi KJ, Hong MK, Song JK, Park SW, Park SJ. Efficacy of myocardial contrast echocardiography in the diagnosis and risk stratification of acute coronary syndrome. *Am J Card.* 2005;96: 1498–1502.

31. Scognamiglio R, Negut C, Ramondo A, Tiengo A, Avogaro A. Detection of coronary artery disease in asymptomatic patients with type 2 diabetes mellitus. *J Am Coll Cardiol.* 2006;47:66–71.

32. Bates JR, Sawada SG, Segar DS, et al. Evaluation using dobutamine stress echocardiography in patients with insulin-dependent diabetes mellitus before kidney and/or pancreas transplantation. *Am J Cardiol.* 1996;77: 175–179.

33. Takeuchi M, Miura Y, Toyokawa T, et al. The comparative diagnostic value of dobutamine stress echocardiography and thallium stress tomography for detecting restenosis after coronary angioplasty. *J Am Soc Echocardiogr.* 1995;5:696–702.

34. Bigi R, Desideri A, Bax JJ, et al. Prognostic interaction between viability and residual myocardial ischemia by dobutamine stress echocardiography in patients with acute myocardial infarction and mildly impaired left ventricular function. *Am J Cardiol.* 2001;87:283–288.

35. Picano E, Sicari R, Landi P, et al. Prognostic value of myocardial viability in medically treated patients with global left ventricular dysfunction early after an acute uncomplicated myocardial infarction: a dobutamine stress echocardiographic study. *Circulation.* 1998;98:1078–1084.

36. Klocke FJ, Baird MG, Lorell BG, et al. ACC/AHA/ASNC guidelines for the clinical use of cardiac radionuclide imaging – executive summary: a report of the American College of Cardiology/American Heart Association Task Force on Practice Guidelines (ACC/AHA/ASNC Committee to Revise the 1995 Guidelines for the Clinical Use of Cardiac Radionuclide Imaging). *Circulation.* 2003;108:1404–1418.

37. Cullom SJ. Principles of cardiac SPECT imaging. In: DePuey EG, Garcia EV, Berman DA eds. Cardiac SPECT Imaging. 2nd ed. Lippincott, Williams and Wilkins: Philadelphia, PA. 2001:3–16.

38. Germano G, Kiat H, Kavanagh PB, et al. Automatic quantification of ejection fraction from gated myocardial perfusion SPECT. *J Nucl Med.* 1995;36:2138–2147.

39. Sharir T, Berman DS, Lewin HC, et al. Incremental prognostic value of rest-redistribution (201) Tl single-photon emission computed tomography. *Circulation.* 1999;100:1964–1970.

40. Taillefer R, Primeau M, Costi P, Lambert et al. Technetium-99m-sestamibi myocardial perfusion imaging in detection of coronary artery disease: comparison between initial (1-hour) and delayed (3-hour) postexercise images. *J Nucl Med.* 1991;32:1961–1965.

41. Taillefer R, Amyot R, Turpin S, et al. Comparison between dipyridamole and adenosine as pharmacologic coronary vasodilators in detection of coronary artery disease with thallium 201 imaging. *J Nucl Cardiol.* 1996;3:204–211.

42. Calnon DA, Glover DK, Beller GA, et al. Effects of dobutamine stress on myocardial blood flow, 99mTc sestamibi uptake, and systolic wall thickening in the presence of coronary artery stenoses: implications for dobutamine stress testing. *Circulation.* 1997;96:2353–2360.

43. Alexander CM, Landsman PB, Teutsch SM. Diabetes mellitus, impaired fasting glucose, atherosclerotic risk factors, and prevalence of coronary heart disease. *Am J Cardiol.* 2000;86:897–902.

44. Unknown. Prevalence of unrecognized silent myocardial ischemia and its association with atherosclerotic risk factors in noninsulin-dependent diabetes mellitus. Milan Study on Atherosclerosis and Diabetes (MiSAD) Group. *Am J Cardiol.* 1997;79:134–139.

45. Koistinen MJ, Huikuri HV, Pirttiaho H, et al. Evaluation of exercise electrocardiography and thallium tomographic imaging in detecting asymptomatic coronary artery disease in diabetic patients. *Br Heart J.* 1990;63:7–11.

46. Janand-Delenne B, Savin B, Habib G, et al. Silent myocardial ischemia in patients with diabetes: who to screen. *Diabetes Care.* 1999;22:1396–400.

47. May O, Arildsen H, Damsgaard EM, et al. Prevalence and prediction of silent ischaemia in diabetes mellitus: a population-based study. *Cardiovasc Res.* 1997;34:241–247.

48. Naka M, Hiramatsu K, Aizawa T, et al. Silent myocardial ischemia in patients with non-insulin-dependent diabetes mellitus as judged by treadmill exercise testing and coronary angiography. *Am Heart J.* 1992;123:46–53.

49. Koistinen MJ. Prevalence of asymptomatic myocardial ischaemia in diabetic subjects. *BMJ.* 1990;301:92–95.

50. Rutter MK, Wahid ST, McComb JM, Marshall SM. Significance of silent ischemia and microalbuminuria in predicting coronary events in asymptomatic patients with type 2 diabetes. *J Am Coll Cardiol.* 2002 Jul 3;40(1):56–61.

51. Senior PA, Welsh RC, McDonald CG, Paty BW, Shapiro AM, Ryan EA. Coronary artery disease is common in nonuremic, asymptomatic type 1 diabetic islet transplant candidates. *Diabetes Care.* 2005 Apr;28(4):866–72.

52. Cosson E, Paycha F, Paries J, Cattan S, Ramadan A, Meddah D, Attali JR, Valensi P. Detecting silent coronary stenoses and stratifying cardiac risk in patients with diabetes: ECG stress test or exercise myocardial scintigraphy? *Diabet Med.* 2004 Apr;21(4):342–348.

53. Wackers FJ, Young LH, Inzucchi SE, et al. Detection of silent myocardial ischemia in asymptomatic diabetic subjects: the DIAD study. *Diabetes Care.* 2004;27:1954–1961.

54. American Diabetes Association Consensus development conference on the diagnosis of coronary heart disease in people with diabetes: Miami, Florida. *Diabetes Care.* 1998; 21:1551–1559.

55. De Lorenzo A, Lima RS, Siqueira-Filho AG, Prevalence and prognostic value of perfusion defects detected by stress technetium-99m sestamibi myocardial perfusion single-photon emission computed tomography in asymptomatic patients with diabetes mellitus and no known coronary artery disease. *Am J Cardiol.* 2002;90:827–832.

56. Valensi P, Paries J, Brulport-Cerisier V, Torremocha F, Sachs RN, Vanzetto G, Cosson E, Lormeau B, Attali JR, Marechaud R, Estour B, Halimi S. Predictive value of silent myocardial ischemia for cardiac events in diabetic patients: influence of age in a French multicenter study. *Diabetes Care*. 2005 Nov;28(11): 2722–7.

57. Zellweger MJ, Hachamovitch R, Kang X, Hayes SW, Friedman JD, Germano G, Pfisterer ME, Berman DS. Prognostic relevance of symptoms versus objective evidence of coronary artery disease in diabetic patients. *Eur Heart J*. 2004 Apr;25(7):543–550.

58. Kang X, Berman DS, Lewin H, et al. Comparative ability of myocardial perfusion single-photon emission computed tomography to detect coronary artery disease in patients with and without diabetes mellitus. *Am Heart J*. 1999;137:949–957.

59. Kang X, Berman DS, Lewin HC, et al. Incremental prognostic value of myocardial perfusion single photon emission computed tomography in patients with diabetes mellitus. *Am Heart J*. 1999;138:1025–1032.

60. Giri S, Shaw LJ, Murthy DR, et al. Impact of diabetes on the risk stratification using stress single-photon emission computed tomography myocardial perfusion imaging in patients with symptoms suggestive of coronary artery disease. *Circulation*. 2002;105:32–40.

61. Elhendy A, Huurman A, Schinkel AF, Bax JJ, van Domburg RT, Valkema R, Biagini E, Poldermans D. Association of ischemia on stress (99m)Tc-tetrofosmin myocardial perfusion imaging with all-cause mortality in patients with diabetes mellitus. *J Nucl Med*. 2005 Oct;46(10):1589–1595.

62. Berman DS, Kang X, Hayes SW, et al. Adenosine myocardial perfusion single-photon emission computed tomography in women compared with men: Impact of diabetes mellitus on incremental prognostic value and effect on patient management. *J Am Coll Cardiol*. 2003;41:1125–1133.

63. Shaw LJ, Iskandrian AE. Prognostic value of gated myocardial perfusion SPECT. *J Nucl Cardiol*. 2004;11: 171–185.

64. Naghavi M, Libby P, Falk E, et al. From vulnerable plaque to vulnerable patient: a call for new definitions and risk assessment strategies: Part I. *Circulation*. 2003;108:1664–1672.

65. Virmani R, Kolodgie FD, Burke AP, et al. Lessons from sudden coronary death: a comprehensive morphological classification scheme for atherosclerotic lesions. *Arterioscler Thromb Vasc Biol*. 2000;20:1262–1275.

66. Stary HC. The development of calcium deposits in atherosclerotic lesions and their persistence after lipid regression. *Am J Cardiol*. 2001;88:16E–19E.

67. Tintut Y, Demer LL. Recent advances in multifactorial regulation of vascular calcification. *Curr Opin Lipidol*. 2001;12:555–560.

68. Watson KE, Demer LL. The atherosclerosis–calcification link? *Curr Opin Lipidol*. 1996;7:101–104.

69. Bostrom KI. Cell differentiation in vascular calcification. *Z Kardiol*. 2000;89:69–74.

70. Parhami F, Basseri B, Hwang J, Tintut Y, Demer LL. High-density lipoprotein regulates calcification of vascular cells. *Circ Res*. 2002;91:570–576.

71. Parhami F, Morrow AD, Balucan J, et al. Lipid oxidation products have opposite effects on calcifying vascular cell and bone cell differentiation. A possible explanation for the paradox of arterial calcification in osteoporotic patients. *Arterioscler Thromb Vasc Biol*. 1997;17:680–687.

72. Tintut Y, Patel J, Parhami F. Tumor necrosis factor-alpha promotes in vitro calcification of vascular cells via the CAMP pathway. *Circulation*. 2000;102:2636–2642.

73. Shioi A, Katagi M, Okuno Y, et al. Induction of bone-type alkaline phosphatase in human vascular smooth muscle cells: roles of tumor necrosis factor-alpha and oncostatin M derived from macrophages. *Circ Res*. 2002;91:9–16.

74. Kizu A, Shioi A, Jono S, et al. Statins inhibit in vitro calcification of human vascular smooth muscle cells induced by inflammatory mediators. *J Cell Biochem* . 2004 Sep 9 [Epub ahead of print].

75. Jono S, McKee MD, Murry CE, et al. Phosphate regulation of vascular smooth muscle cell calcification. *Circ Res*. 2000;87:E10–E7.

76. Jono S, Nishizawa Y, Shioi A, Morii H. 1,25-Dihydroxyvitamin D3 increases in vitro vascular calcification by modulating secretion of endogenous parathyroid hormone-related peptide. *Circulation*. 1998;98: 1302–1306.

77. Towler DA, Bidder M, Latifi T, et al. Diet-induced diabetes activates an osteogenic gene regulatory program in the aortas of low density lipoprotein receptor-deficient mice. *J Biol Chem*. 1998;273:27–34.

78. Mori S, Takemoto M, Yokote K, et al. Hyperglycemia-induced alteration of vascular smooth muscle phenotype. *J Diabetes Complications*. 2002;16:65–68.

79. Agatston AS, Janowitz AS, Hildner FJ, et al. Quantification of coronary artery calcium using ultrafast computed tomography. *J Am Coll Cardiol*. 1990;15:827–832.

80. Rumberger JA, Brundage BH, Rader DJ, et al. Electron beam computed tomographic coronary calcium scanning: a review and guidelines for use in asymptomatic persons. *Mayo Clin Proc*. 1999;74:243–252.

81. Bielak LF, Rumberger JA, Sheedy PF 2nd, et al. Probabilistic model for prediction of angiographically defined obstructive coronary artery disease using electron beam computed tomography calcium score strata. *Circulation.* 2000;102:380–385.

82. Rumberger JA, Sheedy PF, Breen JF, et al. Electron beam computed tomographic coronary calcium score cutpoints and severity of associated angiographic lumen stenosis. *J Am Coll Cardiol.* 1997;29:1542–1549.

83. Budoff MJ, Diamond GA, Raggi P, et al. Continuous probabilistic prediction of angiographically significant coronary artery disease using electron beam tomography. *Circulation.* 2002;105:1791–1796.

84. Raggi P, Callister TQ, Cooil B, et al. Identification of patients at increased risk of first unheralded acute myocardial infarction by electron-beam computed tomography. *Circulation.* 2000;101:850–855.

85. Shaw LJ, Raggi P, Schisterman E, et al. Prognostic value of cardiac risk factors and coronary artery calcium screening for all-cause mortality. *Radiology.* 2003;228: 826–833.

86. Greenland P, LaBree L, Azen SP, et al. Coronary artery calcium score combined with Framingham score for risk prediction in asymptomatic individuals. *JAMA.* 2004;29:210–215.

87. Wong ND, Sciammarella MG, Polk D, Gallagher A, Miranda-Peats L, Whitcomb B, Hachamovitch R, Friedman JD, Hayes S, Berman DS. The metabolic syndrome, diabetes, and subclinical atherosclerosis assessed by coronary calcium. *J Am Coll Cardiol.* 2003 May 7;41(9):1547–1553.

88. Schurgin S, Rich S, Mazzone T. Increased prevalence of significant coronary artery calcification in patients with diabetes. *Diabetes Care.* 2001;24:335–338.

89. Mielke CH, Shields JP, Broemeling LD. Coronary artery calcium, coronary artery disease, and diabetes. *Diabetes Res Clin Pract.* 2001;53:55–61.

90. Khaleeli E, Peters SR, Bobrowsky K, et al. Diabetes and the associated incidence of subclinical atherosclerosis and coronary artery disease: Implications for management. *Am Heart J.* 2001;14:637–644.

91. Hoff JA, Quinn L, Sevrukov A, et al. The prevalence of coronary artery calcium among diabetic individuals without known coronary artery disease. *J Am Coll Cardiol.* 2003;41:1008–1012.

92. Reaven PD, Sacks J. Investigators for the Veterans Affairs Cooperative Study of Glycemic Control and Complications in Diabetes Mellitus Type 2. Reduced coronary artery and abdominal aortic calcification in Hispanics with type 2 diabetes. *Diabetes Care.* 2004 May;27(5):1115–1120.

93. Wagenknecht LE, Bowden DW, Carr JJ, Langefeld CD, Freedman BI, Rich SS. Familial aggregation of coronary artery calcium in families with type 2 diabetes. *Diabetes.* 2001 Apr;50(4):861–866.

94. Olson JC, Edmundowicz D, Becker DJ, et al. Coronary calcium in adults with type 1 diabetes: a stronger correlate of clinical coronary artery disease in men than in women. *Diabetes.* 2000;49:1571–1578.

95. Dabelea D, Kinney G, Snell-Bergeon JK, et al. The Coronary Artery Calcification in Type 1 Diabetes Study. Effect of type 1 diabetes on the gender difference in coronary artery calcification: a role for insulin resistance? The Coronary Artery Calcification in Type 1 Diabetes (CACTI) Study. *Diabetes.* 2003;52:2833–2839.

96. Colhoun HM, Schalkwijk C, Rubens MB, et al. C-reactive protein in type 1 diabetes and its relationship to coronary artery calcification. *Diabetes Care.* 2002;25:1813–1817.

97. Hosoi M, Sato T, Yamagami K, et al. Impact of diabetes on coronary stenosis and coronary artery calcification detected by electron-beam computed tomography in symptomatic patients. *Diabetes Care.* 2002;25: 696–701.

98. Wong ND, Rozanski A, Gransar H, Miranda-Peats R, Kang X, Hayes S, Shaw L, Friedman J, Polk D, Berman DS. Metabolic syndrome and diabetes are associated with an increased likelihood of inducible myocardial ischemia among patients with subclinical atherosclerosis. *Diabetes Care.* 2005;28(6):1445–1450.

99. Anand DV, Lim E, Hopkins D, Corder R, Shaw LJ, Sharp P, Lipkin D, Lahiri A. Risk stratification in uncomplicated type 2 diabetes: prospective evaluation of the combined use of coronary artery calcium imaging and selective myocardial perfusion scintigraphy. *Eur Heart J.* 2006;27:713–21. [Epub 2006 Feb 23].

100. Qu W, Le TT, Azen SP, et al. Value of coronary artery calcium scanning by computed tomography for predicting coronary heart disease in diabetic subjects. *Diabetes Care.* 2003;26:905–910.

101. Raggi P, Shaw LJ, Berman DS, et al. Prognostic value of coronary artery calcium screening in subjects with and without diabetes. *J Am Coll Cardiol.* 2004;43:1663–1669.

102. American Diabetes Association. Standards of medical care in diabetes – 2006. *Diabetes Care.* 2007;30:S4–S41.

103. Grundy SM, Garber A, Goldberg R, et al. Prevention Conference VI: Diabetes and Cardiovascular Disease: Writing Group IV: lifestyle and medical management of risk factors. *Circulation.* 2002;105:e153–e158.

104. Passa P, Drouin P, Issa-Sayegh M, et al. Coronary disease and diabetes. *Diabetes Metab.* 1995;21:446–451.

II ENDOCRINE HYPERTENSION AND CARDIOVASCULAR EVENTS

8 Renin-Angiotensin System

L. Romayne Kurukulasuriya, MD, FACE and James Sowers, MD, FACE, FACP, FAHA

CONTENTS

SUMMARY

Over 100 years have passed since the discovery of renin as a "pressor substance" in 1898 by Robert Tigerstedt at Karolinska Institute. The 48-page publication "Niere und Kreislauf" in *Skandinävisches Archiev für Physiologie* in 1898 by Tiegerstedt and Bergman detailed their meticulous approaches, even including the design of a flow meter to measure blood pressure changes and documentation of long-lasting pressor effects of renin and tachyphylaxis *(1)*. The kidney became the target of studies again 30 some years later in independently conducted studies by Goldblatt, a pathologist who succeeded in making a dog model of renovascular hypertension by constricting the renal artery with silver clips. This work is based on Goldblatt's repeated observations that renal arterial stenosis frequently accompanies hypertension. He also found that venous plasma of ipsilateral kidney contains a vasopressor substance *(2)*.

Study of renin-angiotensin was given a solid base when renin was found to be a peptidase that produces the pressor peptide angiotensin (a hybrid of angiotonin and hypertensin), demonstrated by Page and Braun-Menendez and their associates in the late 1930s. Angiotensin I (ANG I) was

From: *Contemporary Endocrinology: Cardiovascular Endocrinology: Shared Pathways and Clinical Crossroads*
Edited by: V. A. Fonseca © Humana Press, New York, NY

isolated by Skeggs et al., and the structure of angiotensin II (ANG II) was determined by Lentz et al. Its synthesis was reported by Bumpus' and Schwyzer's groups in 1950. Skeggs et al. discovered two forms of angiotensin and two steps of Ang II formation from angiotensinogen by way of ANG I. Skeggs' group also discovered angiotensin-converting enzyme (ACE). Later, ACE was identified as kininase II by Erdös. This discovery by Erdös demonstrated an intimate relationship between angiotensin formation and bradykinin destruction *(3)*.

Key Words: Angiotensin, Angiotensinogen, Renin Inhibitors, ACE inhibitors, Angiotensin receptor blockers, Renin, Cardiovascular, Renin Angiotensin system, AT1 receptors, AT2 receptors

RENIN-ANGIOTENSIN SYSTEM

This system can be activated when there is a loss of blood volume or a drop in blood pressure. If the perfusion of the juxtaglomerular apparatus (JGA) in the kidneys decreases, then the juxtaglomerular (JG) cells release the enzyme renin. Renin cleaves an inactive liver-derived glycoprotein angiotensinogen, converting it into the decapeptide angiotensin I (ANG 1–10). Angiotensin I is then converted to angiotensin II (ANG 1–8) by angiotensin-converting enzyme (ACE), which is found in endothelial cells throughout the circulation especially the lung. The ANG II receptors exert its effects by acting through its receptors type 1 and 2 (AT1 and AT2). Ang I can be converted by endopeptidases to heptapeptide angiotensin 1–7 (ANG (1–7)). ANG (1–7) can also be produced from ANG II by ACE 2. ACE 2 is also capable of making ANG 1–9 from ANG I (1–10). ANG II is the major active product of the circulating renin angiotensin system (RAS) but it is not the only biologically active product. ANG II (1–8) can be converted to ANG III (1–8) by amino peptidase A. ANG III (2–8) can be converted to hexapeptide ANG IV (3–8) by aminopeptidases. In addition to ACE, chymases also can convert ANG I (1–10) to ANG II *(4)* (Fig. 1).

We will discuss about each of these components in detail in this chapter.

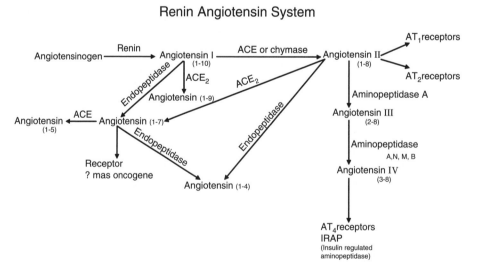

Fig. 1. Renin-angiotensin system.

THE CIRCULATING AND TISSUE RAS

In the past circulating RAS was reviewed as an endocrine system that mediated its effects through the production of angiotensin peptides by the effects of renin on angiotensinogen. A large number of studies have shown that the existence of a local RAS. Brain, heart, blood vessels, ovary, testes, adipose tissue, skin, adrenal gland, and lymphatic system are some of the tissues where this tissue RAS has been described. The local system seems to be operating in whole or in part independent of the circulating RAS. Major portion of the ANG I and ANG II seems to be produced in the tissues with the help of plasma-derived or locally formed renin and angiotensinogen. We will discuss this in detail later in this chapter.

RENIN

Renin is the rate-limiting enzyme in the formation of the vasoconstrictor ANG II. Renin is synthesized, stored, and secreted into the circulation by the JG cells that lie in the afferent arterioles of the kidney as they enter the glomeruli.

Genetics

The complete protein precursor of human kidney renin has been determined from the sequence of cloned genomic DNA. The gene spans 12 kilobases of DNA and is interrupted by eight intervening sequences *(5)*. The Ren 1-c gene is responsible for renin messenger RNA (mRNA) formation, which then initiates synthesis of an enzymatically inactive preprorenin (406 amino acids) by mRNA. This intermediate form is transported into the rough endoplasmic reticulum. The 23-amino-acid "pre" sequence is cleaved, leaving prorenin, which is also an inactive form of the enzyme (47,000 Da); in turn, prorenin is passed through the golgi apparatus, glycosylated, and deposited in the lysosomal granules. There the carboxy-terminal 43-amino-acid prosequence is cleaved to form the enzymatically active form of renin (40,000 Da). It is thought that cleavage and activation within the granules are initiated by the enzyme cathepsin B. Once the prosequence is removed, unmasking the active aspartyl residues of the molecule, secretion or release of active renin (340 amino acids) occurs in response to various regulatory stimuli *(6)*.

Pathophysiology of Renin Release

Physiological studies on the control of renin release from JG cells have revealed very intricate mechanisms.

REGULATION OF RELEASE OF ACTIVE RENIN

(a) *Macula densa pathway.* The macula densa lies adjacent to the JG cells and is composed of specialized columnar epithelial cells located in the wall of that portion of the cortical thick ascending limb that passes between the afferent and efferent arterioles of the glomerulus. A change in the NaCl reabsorption by the macula densa results in the transmission to nearby JG cells of chemical signals that modify renin release. Increase in NaCl flux across the macula densa inhibits renin release, and decrease in NaCl flux stimulates renin secretion. The chemical signals mediating macula densa pathway involves both adenosine and prostaglandins with the former being released when NaCl transport increases and the latter being released when NaCl transport decreases. In this regard adenosine acting via an A1 adenosine receptor inhibits renin release, and prostaglandins stimulate renin release *(7)*.

(b) *Renal baroreceptors.* The most powerful stimulus for renin secretion is a reduction in renal perfusion pressure. An intrarenal vascular stretch receptor in the afferent arteriole stimulates renin secretion in response to reduced renal perfusion pressure and attenuates it as renal perfusion pressure is increased. Obviously, a stretch receptor mechanism in JG cells is responsible for the decrease in renin secretion, most likely by increasing intracellular calcium in response to increased perfusion pressure. The chronic stimulation of renal baroreceptors contribute to the hyperreninemic phase of renovascular hypertension (HTN) *(6,8)*.

(c) *Sympathetic nerve activity.* Sympathetic nerve endings are found in close proximity to JG cells which express β_1-adrenergic receptors. Stimulation of these receptors by circulating or locally released catecholamine activates adenyl cyclase and increases intracellular cAMP, thereby stimulating renin synthesis and release *(9)*. This pathway is one of the best-documented mechanisms of renin regulation and may exert a tonic stimulatory influence on renin synthesis and secretion *(10)*. However, it affects renin-synthesizing cells only in the vicinity of the JG apparatus where nerve endings are localized, since these are the only cells that express β_1-adrenergic receptors*(11)*. Smooth muscle cells along other parts of the afferent arteriole are not responsive when they bear renin granules, and non expressing cells cannot be recruited for renin production by catecholamines *(9)*.

(d) Angiotensin-related short-loop and long-loop feedback mechanism. – Increase in renin secretion enhances the formation of ANG II that stimulates AT1 receptors on the JG cells to inhibit renin release. This is termed the short-loop negative-feedback mechanism. ANG II-mediated increase in blood pressure can inhibit renin release by *(1)* activation of high blood pressure baroreceptors, thereby reducing renal sympathetic tone, *(2)* increasing pressure in the pre-glomerular vessels, and *(3)* reducing NACL reabsorption in the proximal tubule (pressure natriuresis) which increases the tubular delivery of NaCl to the macula densa. This inhibition of renin release due to angiotensin II-induced increase in BP has been termed the long-loop negative-feedback mechanism *(7)*.

ANGIOTENSINOGEN

Angiotensinogen (AGT), the substrate for renin is the only precursor for the family of ANG peptides including ANG I, II, III, IV, Ang 1–7, Ang 1–9. AGT and renin are the rate-limiting steps in the formation of active Ang II in the circulation. Molecular cloning studies have shown that human AGT contains 452 amino acids and is synthesized as pre-AGT *(12)*

AGT Release

AGT is primarily synthesized in the liver although mRNA that codes the protein has been found in several other tissues *(13,14)*AGT is continuously synthesized and secreted by the liver, and its synthesis is stimulated by inflammation, insulin, estrogen, glucocorticoids, thyroid hormone, and angiotensin II *(15)*. During pregnancy plasma levels of AGT increases several fold under the influence of estrogen. Increase in AGT levels are associated with HTN. Oral contraceptive pills can increase the levels of circulating AGT and can induce HTN.

Role of AGT in HTN

Circulating levels of AGT are approximately equal to the K_m of renin for its substrate. Consequently, the rate of ANG II synthesis, and therefore blood pressure can be influenced by changes in AGT levels *(7)*. There is progressive relationship in genetically engineered mice in the number of copies of the AGT gene, plasma levels of AGT, and arterial blood pressure *(16)*. Mice with no AGT gene are hypotensive *(17)*.

ALLELIC ASSOCIATION

Linkage between *AGT* and essential HTN suggested that genetic variations in the *AGT* gene may affect individual predisposition to essential HTN. The *AGT* gene was scanned for the presence of such variation, and the frequencies of common genetic polymorphisms were compared between case and control subjects. Case subjects consisted of a proband randomly selected from each sibship with multiple hypertensive patients, whereas control subjects were selected from normotensive reference populations. The most significant observation was that at residue 235 of AGT, an allele encoding the presence of threonine (*T235*) instead of methionine (*M235*) was more frequent among case subjects than among control subjects. This association was significant for both the Salt Lake City and Paris samples. Plasma AGT levels were measured for study subjects, affording a test of association with the *T235/M235* polymorphism. Plasma AGT levels varied significantly with genotype, with *T235* homozygotes exhibiting approximately 20% higher levels than *M235* homozygotes *(18)* Statistical association indicates only correlation; therefore, those studies could not establish whether *T235* directly imparted disease predisposition or was only a marker for other, unidentified, variations in the gene *(19)*.

ASSOCIATION WITH ESSENTIAL HTN IN THE JAPANESE POPULATION

An AGT-mediated predisposition to essential HTN would be expected to affect sodium homeostasis and the regulation of fluid volume. Given the high prevalence of essential HTN in Japan and the likely significance of dietary sodium for this population, a study was undertaken to test the association between *T235* and essential HTN among Japanese subjects. An initial report revealed that *T235* occurred at high frequency among Japanese subjects and was indeed associated with essential HTN *(20)*.

ASSOCIATION WITH PREECLAMPSIA

Plasma AGT levels increase several fold in estrogenic states such as pregnancy or oral contraceptive use, and HTN may be induced by such states. Indeed, preeclampsia is a common form of pregnancy-induced HTN that has long been considered to involve a significant but unknown genetic component. *T235* occurred at higher frequency among Caucasian women with preeclampsia than among control subjects, a finding that was corroborated in a small Japanese sample *(21)*.

This information indicates that AGT is not just a precursor of the pathway but a major contributor and regulator of the actions of the RAS.

ENZYMES IN THE RAS

Angiotensin 1-Converting Enzyme

ANGIOTENSIN CONVERTING ENZYME (ACE; KININASE II; DIPEPTYDYL CARBOXYPEPTIDASE, CD 143, CARBOXY CATHEPSIN)

Angiotensin 1 converting enzyme (ACE) is a monomeric, membrane-bound, zinc- and chloride-dependent peptidyl dipeptidase that catalyzes the conversion of the decapeptide ANG

Action of Angiotensin Converting Enzyme (ACE)
on Angiotensin-Kininogen Pathways

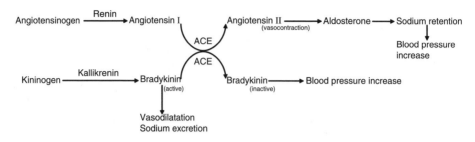

ACE increase blood pressure by activating vasocontractor, Angiotensin II, and inactivating vasodilator, Bradykinin.

Fig. 2.   Action of angiotensin converting enzyme (ACE) on angiotensin-kininogen pathways.

I to the octapeptide ANG II, by removing a carboxy-terminal dipeptide. ACE has long been known to be a key part of the RAS that regulates blood pressure, and ACE inhibitors are important for the treatment of HTN. In addition, ACE inactivates the vasodilator bradykinin by sequential removal of two carboxy-terminal dipeptides. Indeed, it is a broad-specificity dipeptidyl carboxypeptidase and may also act on nonvasoactive peptides *(22)*. Figure 2 shows how ACE contributes to elevated blood pressure by elevating vasoconstrictor angiotensin I and inactivating vasodilator bradykinin.

MOLECULAR ASPECTS

ACE is an ectoenzyme and a glycoprotein with an apparent MW of 170,000 Da. Human ACE contains 1277 amino acid residues and has two homologous domains, each with a catalytic site and a region for binding Zn. ACE has a large amino-terminal extracellular domain, and a 17-amino-acid hydrophobic stretch that anchors the ectoenzyme to the cell membrane. Circulating ACE represents membrane ACE that has undergone proteolysis at the cell surface by a secretase. Although slow conversion of angiotensin I to angiotensin II occurs in plasma, the very rapid metabolism that occurs is due largely to the activity of membrane-bound ACE present on the luminal aspect of the endothelial cells throughout the vascular system *(7)*.

The ACE gene encodes two isozymes. The somatic isozyme is expressed in many tissues, including vascular endothelial cells, epithelial kidney cells, and testicular Leydig cells, whereas the germinal is expressed only in sperm. Studies have shown that ACE plays an important functional role in fertilization because the absence of both ACE isozymes causes defects in sperm transport in the oviducts and in binding to zona pellucidae. However, because the absence of somatic ACE does not impair male fertility the conclusion is that it is the testis ACE isozyme that is important for reproductive function. These effects are not mediated by angiotensin I since the absence of angiotensin does not impair fertility *(23)*.

GENETIC VARIATION

The human *ACE* gene is found on chromosome 17 and contains a restriction fragment length polymorphism consisting of the presence (insertion, *I*) or absence (deletion, *D*) of a 287-bp repeat sequence in intron 16. The association of the *I* allele with lower ACE activity in both serum and tissues has ramifications throughout the RAS and the kallikrein-kinin system, and has stimulated much fascinating work with regard to various pathological and physiological states. Several cardiac and renal conditions appear to have a worse prognosis in subjects homozygous for the D allele (DD), whereas the I allele has been associated with enhanced endurance performance in elite distance runners, rowers, and mountaineers. The relationship between the *I* allele, low ACE activity, the increased half-life of bradykinin, and reduced production of Ang II might determine the physiological impact of the *ACE* genotype via enhanced endothelium-dependent vasodilatation and substrate delivery to the working muscles.

Neprilysin (Neutral Endopeptidase)

Neprilysin (NEP) was found first in the kidney proximal tubules as neutral endopeptidase 24.11, then as enkephalinase in brain, and subsequently as common acute lymphoblastic leukemia antigen (CALLA of CD10) in lymphocytes. NEP is constitutively expressed in all human endothelial cell types investigated, which suggests a systemic as well as a local regulatory role, for example, in the coronary circulation.

FUNCTION

Neutral endopeptidase 24.11, a membrane-bound metallopeptidase, cleaves and degrades vasoactive peptides such as atrial natriuretic peptide, endothelin, ANG I, substance P, and bradykinin. Therefore, the presence of this metallopeptidase may contribute to the regulation of vascular tone and local inflammatory responses in the vascular endothelium and elsewhere. It has been shown that endothelial NEP is mainly located on the membranes of human endothelial cells and contributes to the degradation of extracellular bradykinin, especially when ACE is inhibited. Since NEP is a potent inactivator of vasoactive and inflammatory peptides such as the chemotactic peptide *N*-formyl-L-methionyl-L-leucyl-L-phenylalanine, bradykinin, atrial natriuretic peptide, angiotensin I, endothelin, and tachykinins, its expression and upregulation might influence local vasomotor and inflammatory responses in the macrovasculature as well in the microvasculature *(24)*. In contrast to ACE, NEP does not release Ang II from Ang I, but cleaves it to a heptapeptide (ANG 1–7) and a tripeptide.

STRUCTURE

Human NEP is a type II integral membrane glycoprotein of 742 residues, inserted into the cell membrane near its N-terminus. It contains a short N-terminal cytoplasmic domain followed by a hydrophobic transmembrane sequence and a large extacellular domain. A single active center is present in the extracellular domain that contains the canonic HEXXH motif in which the glutamic acid serves as an important catalytic residue and the two histidines (and a glutamic acid 60 residues downstream) act as the zinc-coordinating ligands. The extracellular domain has two alpha helical lobes. The larger N-terminal region and the smaller C-terminal region *(25)*.

DISTRIBUTION

ACE and NEP are highly concentrated in the microvilli of the brush borders of the proximal tubules of the kidney and the male genital tract. Vascular endothelial cells express more ACE whereas epithelial cells and fibroblasts are richer in NEP.

Angiotensin Converting Enzyme 2

A new chapter in the story of the RAS began in 2000, with the discovery of ACE2 and its identification as an enzyme similar to ACE. ACE2 is expressed predominantly in vascular endothelial cells of the heart and kidney. ANG I is converted to angiotensin 1–9 (with nine amino acids) by ACE2 but is converted to ANG II, which has eight amino acids, by ACE. Whereas ANG II is a potent blood vessel constrictor, ANG 1–9 has no known effect on blood vessels but can be converted by ACE to a shorter peptide, ANG 1–7, which is a blood vessel dilator. Thus, it has been suggested that ACE2 prevents the formation of the vasopressor angiotensin II (Fig. 1).

Studies in mice have shown that loss of ACE 2 did not alter blood pressure homeostasis but did severely impair cardiac function. Mild thinning of the left ventricle and a severe reduction in contractility were observed. However, no interstitial cardiac fibrosis or myocyte hypertrophy was present. The constellation of findings (severe contractile dysfunction, mild dilatation, and no hypertrophy or cardiac fibrosis) was similar to that often observed in cardiac stunning, or hibernation (a reversible decline in cardiac contractility under ischemic conditions), in humans *(26)*. It has been found that loss of ACE2 was associated with upregulation of hypoxia-inducible genes, suggesting a role for ACE2 in mediating the response to cardiac ischemia *(27)*.

ACE2 can cleave ANG II and compete with ACE for the substrate ANG I. ACE and ACE2 have counterbalancing functions.

The final genetic approach used by Crackower et al. was to examine the expression pattern of heart-formation markers in *Drosophila*. In *Drosophila* lacking the fly homologue of ACE2, termed ACER, defective formation of the heart tube was observed. Loss of ACER led to a reduction in the number of cardiac progenitor cells and disorganization of the developing mesoderm. Thus, ACE2 also functions in cardiac morphogenesis. ACE2 is a critical regulator of cardiac function and may be an important therapeutic target. Modulation of the RAS by ACE inhibition and Ang II receptor blockade is a prime strategy for the treatment of cardiovascular diseases *(26)*. The work of Crackower and colleagues suggests that the new member of the RAS, ACE2, is a critical regulator of cardiac function and may be an important therapeutic target *(27)*. Drugs that specifically influence the production of ACE2, as well as dampen the activity of ANG II, may therefore have considerable clinical value *(26)*.

Aminopeptidases

Aminopeptidases catalyze the cleavage of amino acids from the amino-terminus of protein or peptide substrates. They are widely distributed throughout the animal and plant kingdoms and are found in many subcellular organelles, in cytoplasm, and as membrane components. Glutamyl aminopeptidase cleaves ANG II (1–8) to ANG III (2–8), and arginyl aminopeptidase cleaves ANG III (2–8) to ANG IV (3–8) *(28)*. Therefore, ANG III and IV are produced in tissues rich in aminopeptidases, such as brain.

Chymase

Some chymases are angiotensin forming while some other chymases are angiotensinases. The earliest physiologic evidence that non-ACE pathways contribute to ANG II formation showed incomplete suppression of plasma ANG II levels in patients undergoing ACE inhibitor therapy. ACE is a type I membrane protein located mainly on the luminal surface of endothelial cells. Chymase, the major Ang II-forming enzyme in the human heart, is located in the cardiac interstitium attached to the extracellular matrix through ionic interactions *(29)*.

ANGIOTENSIN PEPTIDES: THEIR ACTION, FORMATION, AND DEGRADATION (FIG. 1)

A family of angiotensins is derived from ANG I through the action of converting enzymes, chymases, aminopeptidases, and neuropeptidases. As we know, angitensinogen is converted to Ang I by renin. ANG I is a decapeptide. ANG I is converted to ANG II (1–8) which is an octapeptide by ACE and by chymase. ANG I per se is less than 1% as potent as ANG II on smooth muscle, heart, and the adrenal cortex. The conversion of Ang I to ANG II is done by removal of the two C-terminal amino acids (Table 1). ANG II is the major active product of the circulating RAS. Vasoconstriction and pressor response, aldosterone release, and vasopressin release are some of the functions of ANG II. Most of the cardiovascular effects of ANG II are exerted through angiotensin receptors type 1 and 2 (AT1 and AT2). Actions mediated through the receptors are listed under angiotensin receptors.

Physiologic Actions of Angiotensins

ANG II (1–8) can be converted to smaller peptides with biological activity by the action of aminopeptidases (glutamyl aminopeptidase). This removes a single amino acid from the N-terminus of ANG II to produce ANG III (ANG 2–8). ANG III seems to be very important because it shares many physiological functions with ANG II in the cardiovascular and central nervous system, including pressor response, vasopressin release, and water consumption. Some recent data suggest that ANG III could also be involved in some pathological processes. ANG III also presents proinflammatory properties *(30)*. ANG III also can bind to and signal through AT1 and AT2 receptors (has reduced affinity than angiotensin II).

Table 1
Angiotensin peptides

Angiotensin peptide	Receptor	No of amino acids	Amino acids
Angiotensin I		10	H- Asp- Arg- Val- Tyr-Ile-His-Pro-Phe-His-Leu-OH
Angiotensin 1–9		9	H-Asp-Arg-Val-Tyr-Lie-His-Pro-Phe-His-OH
Angiotensin II (1–8)	AT1, AT2	8	H-Asp-Arg-Val-Tyr-Ile-His-Pro-Phe-OH
Angiotensin 1–7	mass oncogene	7	H-Asp-Arg-Val-Tyr-Ile-His-Pro-OH
Angiotensin III (2–8)		7	H-Arg-Val-Tyr-Ile-His-Pro-Phe-OH
Angiotensin IV (3–8)	AT4	6	H-Val-Tyr-Ile-His-Pro-Phe-,OH

Further action of aminopeptidase (arginyl aminopeptidase) can generate the hexapeptide ANG IV (3–8) from angiotensin III. ANG IV binds to AT1 and AT2 receptors very poorly. ANG IV binds to a unique receptor that may have the ability to increase renal cortical blood flow and potentiate memory. This receptor may be the insulin-regulated aminopeptidase (IRAP) *(4)*. ANG IV (3–8) stimulates the expression of the plasminogen activator inhibitor I (PAI-I) in endothelial cells *(31)* and proximal tubular cells.

ANG 1 can be converted by prolyl endopeptidase (EC 3.4.21.6) and neural endopeptidase to heptapeptide ANG (1–7). Recently discovered ACE 2 enzyme is capable of removing a single amino acid from the C-terminus of either Ang1 or Ang II. Therefore it can make ANG (1–7) from ANG II. The ANG 1–7 produced by the action of the ACE 2 on Ang II has been reported to have a vasodilatory effect *(32)*. The effects of ANG (1–7) may be mediated by a specific ANG (1–7) receptor *(33)*. This receptor was previously misidentified as an ANG II receptor. This is the mas oncogene. ANG (1–7) releases vasopressin, stimulates prostaglandin synthesis, elicits depressor response when microinjected into certain brain muscle cells, and exerts natriuretic effect on the kidney. Ang (1–7) also inhibits proliferation of vascular smooth muscle cells *(7)*. There is a suggestion that ANG (1–7) may be counterbalancing the effects of ANG II. ACE inhibitors increase rather than decrease, tissue and plasma levels of ANG (1–7), because ANG I levels are increased and diverted away from ANG II formation and because ACE contributes importantly to the plasma clearance of ANG (1–7) *(34)* by converting ANG 1–7 to ang 1–5 (Fig. 1).

Angiotensin 1–4 is formed by the action of neutral endopeptidase on ANG II and ANG (1–7). ANG (1–9) is produced by the action of ACE 2 on ANG 1 (1–10). ANG (1–9) has no known function.

Since the relative importance of each of the biosynthetic pathways hinges on the abundance of catalyzing enzymes in any given tissue, the non ANG II peptide products of the RAS may have primarily autocrine or paracrine function.

The abundance of the peptides produced depends on the abundance of the substrate for the reaction. These non-ANG II peptides may become important when ACE inhibitors and angiotensin receptor blockers (ARBs) are used. ANG I may accumulate when ACE inhibitors are used and angiotensin II may accumulate when ARBs are used. Both of these can be converted to non-ANG II peptides. It is therefore possible to think that some of the physiological and pathological effects of the RAS are due to the action of non-ANG II peptides in certain situations *(4)*.

ANGIOTENSIN RECEPTORS

The actions of angiotensins are exerted through well-characterized receptors for ANG II known as AT1 and AT2 receptors. Both receptor subtypes have strong affinity for ANG II and virtually none for ANG I. AT2 receptor has a higher affinity for ANG III than AT1 receptor. The gene for AT1 is located on human chromosome 3 and the gene for AT2 is located on the X chromosome. They share only 34% of their amino acids *(35)*. Both AT1 and AT2 receptors are members of the G-protein-coupled receptor family with putative seven transmembrane regions. The AT1 receptor is 359-amino-acids long and the AT2 receptor is 363-amino-acids long. The AT1 and AT2 receptors have little sequence homology. Most of the biological effects of ANG II are mediated through the AT1 receptor. Evidence suggests that AT2 receptors may exert antiproliferative proapoptotic and vasodilator effects *(7)*.

Actions Mediated by Angiotensin Receptors (35,36)

Short-term actions mediated by AT1 receptors constitute a concerted response that supports the circulation when hemorrhage or dehydration depletes the plasma volume. These include vasoconstriction, aldosterone secretion, tubular sodium retention, and release of ADH. Most other rapid homeostatic actions of ANG II can be viewed as adjuncts to circulatory rescue: increased sympathetic nervous activity, increased thirst, intestinal fluid absorption, platelet agglutination, and increased cardiac contractility. These are short-term actions mediated by AT1 receptors. In addition to that there are long-term actions mediated by AT1 receptors.

The actions of angiotensin mediated through the AT1 receptors

1. *Vascular* This is important for cardiovascular homeostasis.

   (a) Vascular smooth muscle –vasoconstriction, hypertrophy, hyperplasia
   (b) Vascular endothelium – Prostaglandin, nitric oxide (NO), endothilin, and PAI production
   (c) Vascular connective tissue – Extracellular matrix synthesis
   (d) Myocardium – Strength of contraction, hypertrophy

2. *Blood and bone marrow*

   (a) Platelets – Aggregation by catecholamines
   (b) Monocytes – Adhesion to vessel wall
   (c) Bone marrow – Increases red cell production

3. *Adrenal gland*

   (a) Adrenal glomerulosa – Aldosterone secretion
   (b) Adrenal medulla – catecholamine secretion
   (c) Adrenal fasciculate – cortisol secretion

4. *Pituitary*

   (a) Posterior pituitary – Antidiuretic hormone release

5. *Kidney*

   (a) Kidney – embryogenesis
   (b) JG cells – inhibit renin release
   (c) Glomerulus – afferent and efferent vasoconstriction
   (d) Mesangial cells – Contraction
   (e) Proximal tubule – Sodium reabsorption

6. *Nervous System*

   (a) Sympathetic neurons – Norepinephrine release
   (b) Brain – Pressor center activation, baroreceptor blunting, antidiuretic hormone synthesis, thirst, prostaglandin release (angiotensin 1–7)

7. *Gastrointestinal tract*

   (a) Intestine – Salt and water absorption
   (b) Glycogenolysis – AGT synthesis

Long-term actions mediated by AT1 receptors include cell growth and organ hypertrophy, inflammation and remodeling, embryogenesis, and erythropoietic effects.

Actions Mediated by AT2 Receptors

The AT_2 receptor has several newly described functions related to cell growth, differentiation, and ultimate fate. In general, the AT_2 receptor inhibits cell growth and proliferation and promotes cell differentiation, counterbalancing the opposite effects of ANG II at the AT_1 receptor. Antiproliferative effects on ANG II by the AT_2 receptor have been identified in several different cell types including endothelial cells, neonatal cardiomyocytes, cardiac fibroblasts, and vascular smooth muscle cells. Recent studies also suggest that the AT_2 receptor inhibits angiogenesis. Although there is substantial evidence that the AT_2 receptor mediates apoptosis, the findings remain somewhat controversial *(36)*.

1. Regulation of blood pressure and kidney function – The AT_2 receptor mediates a vasodilator/natriuretic renal autacoids cascade that includes bradykinin, NO, and intracellular cyclic guanosine monophosphate (cGMP). This plays a protective role in renal vascular HTN. The AT_2 receptor also modulates renal prostaglandins, which play an important role in blood pressure regulation.
2. Jejuna sodium and water absorption inhibit sodium and water absorption through a prostaglandin E_2-dependent and cAMP-dependent mechanism *(37)*.
3. Nervous system – Neuronal cells inhibit norepinephrine release initiated by AT1 receptors, promotes neuronal differentiation and regeneration *(36)*.
4. Fetal development – There is a much higher concentration of AT2 receptors in the fetus than adults indicating its importance in the fetal development. AT2 receptors are important in the development of the fetal kidney.
5. Apoptosis and natriuresis

In general angiotensin II effects at the AT1 receptors are opposed by the actions of the AT2 receptor. This principle applies to neuronal effects, actions on cell proliferation and differentiation, angiogenesis, and chronotropic effects in the heart

TISSUE RAS

Renal JG cells are not the only source of renin in the body. Many tissues and organs can synthesize angitensin II independent of the classis blood – borne RAS. Angiotensin can be synthesized locally in many tissues, including the brain, pituitary, aorta, arteries, heart, ventricles, adrenal glands, kidneys, adipocytes, leukocytes, ovaries, testis, uterus, spleen, and skin. ANG II levels are much higher in tissue than in plasma so there must be local production of ANG II in tissue by intracellular or extracellular activity. These systems are known as the tissue RAS *(38)*.

The Heart and the Systemic Vasculature

Components of the RAS have been found in cardiomyocytes as well as in endothelial cells and vascular smooth muscle *(39)*.

The existence and relevance of cardiac renin expression has been a matter of debate. Although some investigators have found cardiac renin expression by detecting renin mRNA, these levels have been rather low. Less controversial is the evidence for the presence of renin protein in the heart attributed to uptake from the circulation *(40)*. AGT mRNA has been detected in humans *(41)*. Although cardiac mRNA levels of AGT are more readily detectable than those of renin they are low compared to those found in the liver. Therefore the major percentage of

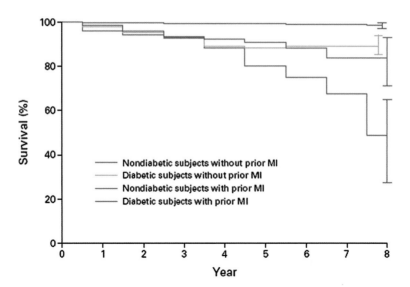

Color Plate 1. Kaplan-Meier estimates of the probability (with 95% confidence intervals) of death from coronary heart disease in 1059 subjects with type 2 diabetes and 1378 nondiabetic subjects with and without prior myocardial infarction (MI) in a Finnish population-based study (Chapter 2, Fig. 1; *see* discussion on p. 21).

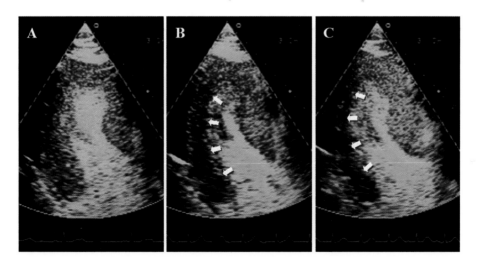

Color Plate 2. Example of myocardial perfusion performed by echocardiography after intravascular injection of echocontrast (microbubbles). The arrows point at an area of decreased perfusion of the inferior wall of the myocardium during dobutamine stress (panels B and C) (courtesy of Dr. Sanjiv Kaul, Oregon Health and Science University, Portland, OR) (Chapter 7, Fig. 3; *see* discussion on p. 101).

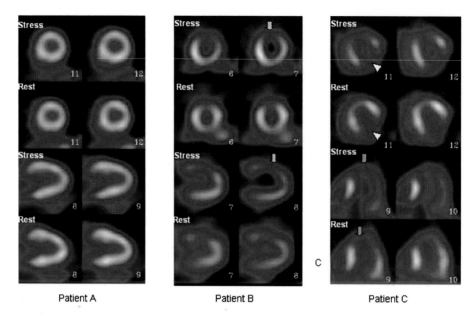

Patient A   Patient B   Patient C

Color Plate 3. Examples of nuclear myocardial perfusion imaging of the left ventricular myocardium. Patient A shows a homogeneous distribution of the radioactive tracer both at rest and during stress. Patient B shows a moderate size defect in the anterior wall of the left ventricle (yellow arrows) during stress (top row images). The defect disappears (i.e., is reversible) during rest (bottom row images). Patient C demonstrates a large and fixed perfusion defect of the infero-lateral wall (white arrow heads) and a partially reversible defect of the apex of the left ventricle (green arrows) (Chapter 7, Fig. 4; *see* discussion on p. 102).

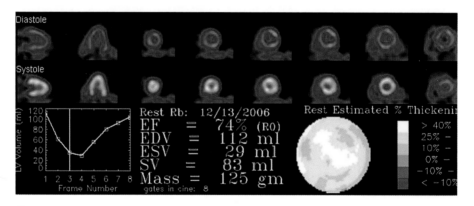

Color Plate 4. An example of assessment of left ventricular function on position emission tomography imaging. The calculated left ventricular ejection fraction is 74%. The top row shows diastolic images of the left ventricle (the chamber is larger and the walls are thinner) while the bottom row shows systolic frames (the chamber is almost virtual and the walls are thick) (Chapter 7, Fig. 5; *see* discussion on p. 102).

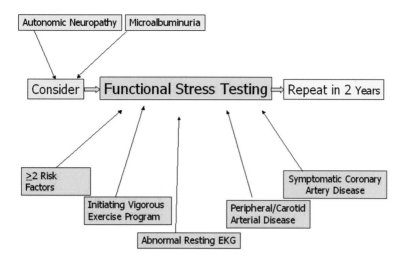

Color Plate 5. Guidelines proposed in 1998 by the American Diabetic Association on performance of exercise stress testing, with or without an imaging modality associated with it, in diabetic patients (modified from reference *(54)*) (Chapter 7, Fig. 10; *see* discussion on p. 112).

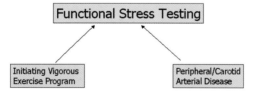

Color Plate 6. New standard of care from the American Diabetic Association on performance of exercise stress testing, with or without an imaging modality associated with it, in asymptomatic diabetic patients (modified from reference *(102)*) (Chapter 7, Fig. 11; *see* discussion on p. 112).

cardiac AGT may be due to plasma uptake *(42)*. Pig studies have shown that >90% of cardiac ANG I is synthesized locally in the heart and that >75% of cardiac ANG II is synthesized locally, most of it using local ANG I generation as a basis. ACE and ACE 2 expression has been demonstrated in the heart *(40)*. In the human heart chymase activates Ang I to Ang II but is not inhibited by ACE inhibitors and could act as an activator for alternative pathways of ANG II formation. It has been found that less than 20% of the angiotensin II is formed by ACE in the heart *(43)*. Both AT1 and AT2 receptors are expressed in the heart.

Cardiac RAS activity is increased by glucocorticoids, estrogen, thyroid hormone, and high-sodium diet all of which increase AGT mRNA. Pressure overload on the heart is associated with a rise in ACE content and AGT mRNA. Cardiac ACE and Ang II are generally considered to be major causative factors in left ventricular hypertrophy and cardiac fibrosis independent of the blood pressure *(38)*. In the heart the RAS is involved in positive inotropic effects, hypertrophic effects, remodeling, and apoptosis *(40)*.

Vasculature – Local synthesis of renin in the vasculature is controversial even though some renin mRNA has been detected in some blood vessels. ACE is localized in adventia of the blood vessels suggesting the importance of paracrine role of vascular RAS *(44)*. AGT mRNA has been detected in very small amounts in the rat adventitia. It was greatest in the periaortic adipose tissue *(45)*. Both AT1 and AT2 receptors have been identified in the vasculature. Vascular Ang II persists after bilateral nephrectomy (with dialysis) although plasma renin is undetectable proving local synthesis exists.

Endothelial ACE controls the activation of the ANG II and degradation of bradykinin. Therefore, synthesis of vascular ANG II probably is independent of the circulating RAS. Vascular ANG II plays a role in the development of atherosclerosis and inflammation. ACE accumulates in human plaque on inflammatory cells, leading to unstable plaque and myocardial infarction (MI) *(38)*. In the vasculature the RAS system maintains vascular tone and endothelial function *(40)*.

Central Nervous System (CNS)

The postulation of an independent brain RAS was one of the first indications of the presence of local ANG formation in the tissue. Renin mRNA has been found in brains of several animals. But the expression is low. Okamura et al. have screened several neuroblastoma cell lines of rat and mouse origin and found at least three cell lines that contain renin (EC 3.4.99.19), ACE (dipeptidyl carboxypeptidase; peptidyldipeptide hydrolase, EC 3.4.15.1), and angiotensins I and II. This finding was interpreted to indicate that in these cells angiotensin formation takes place by an intracellular mechanism, in contrast to the extracellular mechanism well known to occur in plasma. This study also demonstrates the existence of viable and cloned cell lines that produce renin *(46)*. With the use of double or triple immunogold labeling methods prorenin/renin and AGT have been identified in glandular cell types of the rat anterior pituitary. These were identified in lactotropes, gonadotropes, somatotropes, corticotropes, and thyrotropes. The simultaneous detection of the substrate (AGT) and both its specific cleavage enzyme and its proenzyme within the same granule suggest intragranular processing of this component. Moreover, the localization of these three constituents in the secretory granules also suggests that, in the rat anterior pituitary, they follow the regulated secretory pathway *(47)*. ACE mRNA has been localized in several parts of the brain. Other possible Ang II-forming enzymes in the brain are tonin, cathepsin, TPA, and chymase *(40)*. It has been shown that Ang-(1–7) is the major metabolite of dog brainstem homogenates both in the absence and in the presence of ACE inhibitors. Subsequent studies in the in vitro hypothalamoneurohypophysial system of the rat demonstrated that ANG-(1–7) is equipotent with Ang II in its activation of AVP release. Dr Ferrario's laboratory has also provided evidence for synthesis and storage of ANG-(1–7) in the brain *(48)*. AT1, AT2, and AT4 receptors have been described in different parts of brain in different animal studies. ANG IV receptors are found in the hippocampus, which is important in memory functions. ANG1–7 receptors are found on vasopressin forming neurons *(38)*. Studies indicate multiple functions of the brain RAS: central blood pressure regulation, water intake, maintenance of the blood-brain barrier, temperature regulation. Some central functions of the reproductive system, motor control, and functions associated with behavior and emotions are some of these.

Peripheral Nervous System

SYMPATHETIC NERVOUS SYSTEM

A direct relationship between the effect of ANG II and the sympathetic nervous system (SNS) is likely since sympathectomy or reserpine treatment attenuates the blood pressure response to ANG II. ANG II binding sites were localized and quantified in rat stellate and superior cervical ganglia by quantitative autoradiography. High concentrations of binding sites were localized in the areas rich in principal ganglion cells. These binding sites might mediate the facilitatory action of ANG II on the ganglionic transmission *(49)*. Upregulation of ANG II release and AGT mRNA expression can be induced by high-frequency preganglionic stimulation at the canine cardiac sympathetic ganglia. These results indicate that an intrinsic angiotensin I-dependent angiotensin system exists in the cardiac sympathetic ganglia *(50)*.

PARASYMPATHETIC NERVOUS SYSTEM

It has been shown that ANG II receptors are transported peripherally in the rat vagus nerve *(51)*. It has been demonstrated that there is a high density of AT_1 receptors in intracardiac ganglia and conduction systems of rat heart *(52)*.

Adrenal Glands

The adrenal gland contains the highest level of tissue ANG II that have been measured. The majority of the adrenal Ang II is localized within the zona glomerulosa and zona fasciculata of the cortex, where it stimulates aldosterone and corticosteroid synthesis. Cellular levels of renin in the rat adrenal cortex are independent of plasma renin levels. The adrenal medulla contains high levels of AT2 receptors and is a major source of epinephrine and norepinephrine, which increases vasoconstriction and cardiac output. Aldosterone also stimulates growth of fibrotic tissue of the heart *(38)*.

Reproductive Tract

Evidence has accumulated for the existence of local tissue RAS in the reproductive tissues. In the ovary the local RAS has been shown to influence ovulation and steroidogenesis.

In human ovaries renin-like immunoreactivity has been observed in theca, stromal, and luteal cells of the developing follicles. The heavily luteinized granulosa cells (GCs) of the preovulatory gonadotropin-stimulated follicles were strongly positive for immunoreactive renin and ANG II. These anatomic findings are consistent with gonadotropin-stimulated local production of both renin and angiotensin II in the human ovary and support the functional roles proposed for the ovarian RAS in follicle development, ovulation, and luteal function and during pregnancy *(53)*. A study done in women with a diagnosis of polycystic ovarian disease (PCOD) showed that large cystic follicles of polycystic ovaries (PCOs) presented intense immunostaining for renin and angiotensin in both theca and GCs. This study highlights the link between the ovarian RAS and those ovarian compartments known to be actively engaged in androgen secretion and/or luteinization and suggests that there may be an association between the ovarian RAS and PCOD. Luteal cells also consistently stained both in normal ovaries and in the occasional corpus luteum present in PCOs *(54)*. Renin-like activity has been found in the follicular fluid *(55)*.

The presence of renin mRNA in the endometrium, choriodecidua, and the fetal part of the placenta indicates local renin synthesis *(56)*. Renin has been demonstrated in the human endometrial glandular epithelium *(57)*. During late pregnancy the uterus is also a source of plasma prorenin *(58)*.

AGT mRNA has been shown to be expressed in ovaries of rat and mouse. AGT activity has been shown in rat ovary. AGT appears to be greater in preovulatory follicles than atretic follicles *(40)*. ANG II/III activity has been found in human follicular fluid *(55)*. It has been reported that ovary contained the fourth highest level of ANG II in 13 tissues examined *(59)*. AGT mRNA is expressed in spiral artery smooth muscle in the uterine deciduas *(60)*. Immunoreactive ANG II has been found in human uterus *(60)*. ANG II-like immunoreactivity was detected in human proliferate endometrium (glandular epithelium and stroma) with cyclic changes *(61)*.

ACE is abundant in rat ovary *(62)*. In the human ovary, ACE activity increases with age, which could be a result of the age-dependent reduction in the number of ovulating follicles rather than a direct regulatory effect *(63)*. ACE immunoreactivity showed a cyclic variation in the human endometrium with the highest expression in the late secretory phase at the menses *(64)*.

Angiotensin receptors have been demonstrated in high densities in the placenta and uterus, indicating an autocrine or paracrine action of ANG II *(57)*. Receptors for ANG II have been demonstrated to be present *(65)* in the human fallopian tube. Animal studies have demonstrated the presence of angiotensin receptors in the ovary *(40)*.

Function of RAS in the female reproductive tract has been proposed as a mediator of ovarian function and follicular maturation.

Several probable effects of the uteroplacental RAS can be defined. It is very likely that the uteroplacental RAS plays an important role during implantation and placentation by stimulation of decidualization and angiogenesis. Furthermore, ANG II may regulate synthesis and secretion of other hormones formed locally in the uteroplacental unit. During labor the action of ANG II may be important for contraction of the uterine musculature. ANG II is also involved in the complex regulation of the uteroplacental blood flow *(57)*.

Male Reproductive Tract

In the male reproductive system, local RAS function is thought to be relevant for fertility. This system is regulated independently from the plasma RAS, and the blood testicular barrier prevents ACE inhibitors and AT_1 blockers affecting fertility *(40)*.

Immunohistological studies have shown evidence of renin in human Leydig cells *(66)*. Animal studies have shown the same. Human prostate shows a positive signal after renin immnochemisstry *(67)*. The ACE gene encodes for two ACE proteins, the somatic ACE enzyme that has two identical lobes and the testicular ACE (tACE) molecule consisting of a single lobe. Molecular cloning of the human tACE cDNA indicates that the mRNA codes for 732 residues (vs. 1306 in endothelium) *(68)*. tACE is equally active despite the fact that it is translated from a shorter mRNA. tACE is highly tissue specific. tACE is expressed at high levels by male germ cells during spermatogenesis while somatic ACE is also expressed in other testicular cells. The regulation of tACE is tissue specific. The concentration of ACE in the testis is among the highest in all organs *(69)*. tACE was found in the seminiferous tubules of the testes in spermatocytes containing mature spermatids, and in spermatids within the epididymal tubular lumen in sexually mature, but not in immature, rabbits. Epididymal tubular cells contained pulmonary ACE *(70)*. High ACE activity has been determined in human seminal vesicles and seminal plasma *(71)*. Human benign hypertrophic prostate had significantly higher concentration of ACE than normal prostate *(72)*. Immunohistochemistry showed strong staining for somatic ACE in cells of the vas deferens in both young and adult rabbit *(71)*.

AGT mRNA has been detected in mouse testis and rat epididymal epithelium *(40)*. Existence of ANG II receptors has been demonstrated in rat and rhesus monkey testis *(73)*. AT1 and AT2 receptors have been detected in rat epididymis *(74)*. AT1 receptors have been found in human sperms *(75)*. Human prostate is found to have AT1 receptors *(76)*.

The high concentration of AT_1 receptors that has been found in the periurethral region of the prostate suggests a role for ANG II in modulating cell growth, smooth muscle tone, and possibly micturition. Furthermore, downregulation of AT_1 receptors in BPH may be due to receptor hyperstimulation by increased local levels of ANG II in BPH. Finally, Ang II may play a functional role in modulating sympathetic transmission in the prostate.

It has been shown that ACE is important for achieving in vivo fertilization and that sperm from mice lacking both ACE isozymes show defects in transport within the oviducts and in binding to zonae pellucidae. Male mice generated by gene targeting that lack somatic ACE but retain testis ACE are normally fertile, establishing that somatic ACE in males is not essential for their fertility but tACE is. tACE may play a role for the detachment of sperm from the oviduct epithelium and/or other structures in the female reproductive tract at capacitation. Furthermore, male and female mice lacking AGT have normal fertility, indicating that angiotensin I is not a necessary substrate for testis ACE *(77)*. There are suggestions for a function of AT_1 receptors as determinants of sperm motility, since ANG II increases both the percentage of motile sperm and their linear velocity and AT_1 receptor antagonists inhibit this action of ANG II *(76)*.

Adipose Tissue

Components of the RAS have been found in the white and brown adipose tissue (BAT). It is intriguing to assume that components of the RAS produced by adipocytes may play an autocrine, a paracrine, and/or an endocrine role in the pathophysiology of obesity and provide a potential pathway through which obesity leads to HTN and type 2 diabetes mellitus (DM) *(78)*.

Gene expression of AGT, renin, renin-binding protein, ACE and AT1 receptors have been demonstrated in human preadipocytes. ANG II was secreted both by undifferentiated preadipocytes and immature adipocytes, and its production was significantly elevated in differentiated cells. This concludes that preadipocytes from human adipose tissue express a functional RAS *(79)*. AGT and RAS and non-RAS enzymes required for the conversion of AGT to ANG II has been demonstrated in adipose tissue of obese subjects *(80)*. AGT, ACE, and type 1 angiotensin receptor genes are found to be widely expressed both in human adipose tissue and in cultured human adipocytes. Expression of the chymase and renin-binding protein genes also have been found in these samples *(81)*.

The receptor subtype that is present most abundantly in both white and BAT is the AT_1 receptor subtype *(40)*.

Cold exposure has shown to increase BAT ANG II content without detectable changes of the plasma components of the RAS. A role for ANG II in enhanced sympathetic activity of cold-induced thermogenesis in BAT has been demonstrated (82). It has been shown that ANG II significantly increased triglyceride content and the activities of two key lipogenic enzymes (fatty acid synthase (FAS) and glycerol-3-phosphate dehydrogenase (GPDH)) in 3T3-L1 adipocytes (83). AGT mRNA was expressed at variable levels in obese patients. It was significantly greater in visceral than in subcutaneous adipose tissue. Positive and significant correlation was found between the expression of AGT in visceral adipose tissue and BMI. These data suggest that AGT may be the determinant of fat distribution and may be involved in the metabolic syndrome of central obesity (84). Locally produced AngII directly increases leptin release from adipocytes (85).

A major source of AGT mRNA in blood vessels is the adipose tissue surrounding them. In obesity fatty tissue is more highly vascularized. Therefore it is possible that locally formed ANG II from adipocyte causes local and systemic vasoconstriction, altering local and systemic blood flow characteristics and perhaps increasing blood pressure (38).

Skin

Renin mRNA expression in subcutaneous tissue of mice has been shown (86). De novo production of ANG I and ANG II have been shown in the skin (87). ACE has been detected in subcutaneous tissue of rats (88). Mast cells are abundant in the skin. Mast cells have been shown to be an additional source of renin (89). Mast cell-derived chymases may act as a substitute for ACE at some tissues. Keratinocytes of the skin seem to express an angiotensin receptor different from AT1 and AT2 (90).

The local concentration of ANG II is greatly elevated after injury, although plasma levels are unchanged. For this reason it has been suggested that ANG II contributes to wound healing, perhaps by stimulating release of growth factors (38).

Gastrointestinal tract

The salivary gland of some mouse strains expresses significant amounts of renin (40). In humans the presence of (pro)renin both in the beta-cells of the islets of Langerhans, and in endothelial cells of the pancreatic vasculature has been demonstrated. Transcription of (pro)renin mRNA, however, was confined to connective tissue surrounding the blood vessels and in reticular fibers within the islets. Tissue RAS may directly affect beta-cell function as well as pancreatic blood flow (91). Renin gene expression has been found in humans (92). Presence of AGT messenger mRNA, AGT protein, Ang II has been demonstrated in canine pancreas (93). AGT mRNA has been identified in the stomach, large intestine, and mesentery but not in the small intestines (94). ACE is a prominent jejunal brush-border enzyme that behaves pharmacologically and kinetically like its peripheral circulation counterpart (95). AT receptors have been found in the rat submandibular region (96). Beta-cells of the human islets of Langerhans and endothelial cells of the pancreatic vasculature show AT2 receptors (92). A study has shown that there is predominant distribution of AT_1 and AT_2 receptor subtypes in the endothelia of the blood vessels and the epithelia of the pancreatic ductal system of rat and mouse (97). AT1 and AT2 receptors have been demonstrated in the small and large intestines (40).

Function The pancreatic RAS seems to regulate the secretion of pancreatic hormones. It has been shown that ANG II probably mediates pancreatic acinar cell apoptosis during the course of pancreatic fibrosis (98). ANG II and ANG III play a part in intestinal sodium and water absorption *(40)*. Intestinal brush-border membrane ACE functions as a digestive peptidase *(99)*. Jaszewski et al. have reported that mucosal levels of ANG I and II were elevated in patients with Crohn's colitis versus normal subjects and other forms of colitis and that mucosal levels of ANG I and ANG II correlated well with the degree of macroscopic inflammation in Crohn's disease *(100)*.

Sensory Organs

EYE

Renin mRNA, AGT mRNA, and ACE mRNA have been found in different parts of the eye *(40)*. It has been shown that ocular concentrations of ANG are too high to be caused by blood-borne peptides. This suggests local angiotensin production *(101)*.

Ocular RAS may be involved in the regulation of ocular vascular tone, regulation of aqueous fluid, and maintenance of normal secretory function in the epithelial cells of the ciliary body.

There is evidence for activation of local RAS in diabetes. This appears to be directly responsible, as well as indirectly through other mediators, for an increase in concentration of vascular endothelial growth factor (VEGF), a selective angiogenic and vasopermeability factor that is implicated in the pathogenesis of diabetic retinopathy *(102)*.

White Blood Cells

MONOCYTES

Renin mRNA has been detected in peritoneal macrophage monocyte cells *(103)*. Renin protein has been detected in rat and mice alveolar macrophages and monocytes *(104)*. ANG I and II has been found in rat and mouse macrophages and monocytes *(105)*. ANG II binding to human mononuclear cells is not easily reversible and poorly inhibited in a competitive manner suggesting that endocytosis occurs *(106)*.

It has been reported that ANG II increases monocyte binding to human as well as rabbit aortic endothelial cells, suggesting a role in arteriosclerosis *(107)*.

Granulocytes

In human neutrophils ANG I-to-ANG II conversion occur via cathepsin *(108)*. Cathepsin can also cleave AGT. Therefore human neutrophil angiotensin system may not require renin or ACE *(109)*.

Spleen

Renin mRNA *(110)* and AGT mRNA have been detected in rat spleen *(111)*. Mouse spleen lymphocytes seem to possess both types of Ang receptors *(112)*

PRENATAL DEVELOPMENT RAS

Local angiotensin formation and tissue-specific effects of angiotensin peptides on growth and differentiation are thought to be extremely important for embryonic and fetal development. There appears to be a close interaction between plasma and tissue RAS in this situation *(40)*.

ROLE OF RAS IN HTN AND CVD

We now know that the RAS which was once considered as an endocrine system has important paracrine and autocrine functions at tissue level. Therefore the RAS system is critical in both normal physiology and pathophysiological states such as HTN, congestive heart failure (CHF) and post infarction cardiac remodeling. Considerable evidence has recently accumulated suggesting that the RAS not only governs cellular function (e.g., sodium excretion, vasoconstriction, and ionotropic responses) but also contributes to tissue structure (e.g., inflammation, fibrosis, and hypertrophy). Indeed, the RAS stimulation, especially at the tissue level, seems to be an initiating event in several pathophysiological processes including diabetic nephropathy and cardiac remodeling in response to ischemia (113).

The actions of ANG II is mediated through AT1 and AT2 receptors. Even though ANG II has affinity to AT1 and AT2 receptors, vast majority of ANG II actions are mediated through AT1 receptors. As we know AT2 receptors are highly expressed in fetal tissue and the expression decreases after birth. But we know that AT2 receptors mediate effects that are opposed to the actions of AT1. The AT_2 receptor is often upregulated by tissue injury and/or disease processes, making it a likely candidate molecule in cardiovascular pathophysiology (114).

Modest changes in plasma concentrations of ANG II acutely increase BP. This is due to an increase in total peripheral resistance. This is a response that helps maintain arterial blood pressure in the face of an acute hypotensive challenge (e.g., blood loss, vasodilatation). Although ANG II directly increases the cardiac contractility and indirectly increases the heart rate (via facilitation of the sympathetic tone and enhanced noradrenergic neurotransmission and adrenal catecholamine release) the rapid increase in arterial blood pressure activates baroreceptor reflex that decreases the sympathetic tone and increases vagal tone. Therefore ANG II may increase, decrease, or not change cardiac contractility, heart rate, and cardiac output depending on the physiological state. Therefore, cardiac output contributes little if at all to the rapid pressor response induced by ANG II.

ANG II also causes a slow pressor response that helps stabilize the arterial BP over the long term. This is most likely mediated by a renal response, the mechanisms of which include a direct effect to increase sodium reabsorption in proximal tubule, release of aldosterone from adrenal cortex (increased Na reabsorption, and increased K excretion in the distal nephron) and altered renal hemodynamics (direct renal vasoconstriction, enhanced noradrenergic neurotransmission in the kidney, and increased renal sympathetic tone).

In addition to the effects on the BP, RAS has significant effects on the morphology of the cardiovascular system. These could be hemodynamically- or nonhemodynamically-mediated cardiovascular effects of ANG II. The nonhemodynamically-mediated effects are as follows. (1) ANG II stimulates migration, proliferation, hypertrophy, and or synthetic capacity of vascular smooth muscle cells, cardiac myocytes, and or fibroblasts in part by acting directly on the specific protooncogenes, (2) increased production of growth factors, and (3) increased production of extracellular matrix proteins such as collagen fibronectin and tenascin. The hemodynamically-mediated effects of ANG II are (1)increased preload and afterload (increased arterial BP) that contribute to cardiac hypertrophy and remodeling and (2) increased wall tension (vascular). The final effect of this is vascular and cardiac hypertrophy and remodeling (7).

The key to the pathogenesis of CV disease appears to be oxidative stress and consequent vicious actions of angiotensin. ANG II is a potent mediator of oxidative stress and stimulates the release of cytokines and the expression of leukocyte adhesion molecules that mediate vessel wall inflammation. Inflammatory cells release enzymes (including ACE) that generate angiotensin II. Thus, a local positive-feedback mechanism could be established in the vessel wall for oxidative stress, inflammation, and endothelial dysfunction. ANG II also acts as a direct growth factor for vascular smooth muscle cells and can stimulate the local production of metalloproteinases and PAI. Taken together, ANG II can promote vasoconstriction, inflammation, thrombosis, and vascular remodeling. ANG II also acts as a direct growth factor for vascular smooth muscle cells and can stimulate the local production of metalloproteinases and PAI-I. Taken together, ANG II can promote vasoconstriction, inflammation, thrombosis, and vascular remodeling *(115)*. Considering these effects the importance of the RAS blockage cannot be overemphasized. Results of trials with ACE inhibitors and ARBs have shown that blocking the RAS system has a positive impact on heart failure progression, post MI remodeling, diabetes, renal disease, and HTN. These drugs have shown to reduce cardiovascular mortality and morbidity.

DRUGS AFFECTING THE RAS

ACE Inhibitors

These inhibit the conversion of ANG I to ANG II, and therefore take part in inhibition of actions mediated by ANG II. ACE inhibitors also increase bradykinin levels (Fig. 2). Bradykinin stimulates prostaglandin synthesis. Therefore increased bradykinin and prostaglandin also may contribute to the pharmacological effects of ACE inhibition. ACE inhibitors interfere with both the short- and long-loop negative-feedback on renin release described early in this chapter. ACE inhibitors increase the release of renin and ANG I. This increases ANG 1–7 production. It is not known if some of the beneficial effects of ACE inhibitors are due to increased production of ANG1–7.

Therapeutic Effects of ACE Inhibitors

In HTN ACE inhibitors lower the systemic vascular resistance and mean diastolic and systolic BP. Systemic arteriolar dilatation and increased compliance of large arteries contribute to this. Studies have shown that ACE inhibitors are superior to other antihypertensives in patients with DM.

ACE inhibitors have been proven to be beneficial in patients with left ventricular systolic dysfunction. Studies have shown that ACE inhibitors decrease MI, stroke, progression of CHF, CVD death, and overall mortality. ACE inhibitors have shown to improve exercise tolerance and endothelial dysfunction *(7)*.

HOPE study showed that Ramipril significantly reduces the rates of death, MI, and stroke in a broad range of high-risk patients who are not known to have a low ejection fraction or heart failure. The study participant had vascular disease or diabetes plus one other cardiovascular risk factor *(116)*.

Angiotensin Receptor Blockers (ARBs)

It is now well established that ACE inhibitors can reduce CVD risk. Therefore attention is increasingly focused on the ARBs. Clinically available ARBs bind to AT1 receptors with high affinity and are generally 10,000-fold selective for AT1 versus AT2 receptors. Because ARBs block the AT1 receptor the actions of ANG II via AT1 receptor are blocked regardless of the biochemical pathway leading to ANG II production (ACE is not the only way to produce ANG II from ANG I; therefore, ACE inhibitors block only the ANG II produced by the action on

ACE on ANG I). For this reason ARBs are able to completely inhibit of the AT1 effects of the RAS. ARBs increase the levels of ANG II. Since AT1 receptor is blocked the peptide can stimulate the AT2 receptor. Therefore, activation of the AT2 receptor may mediate some of the antihypertensive effects of the ARBs *(36)*. Studies have shown that ARBs are useful in the treatment of HTN. In addition to that they reduce cardiovascular death in patients with CHF and reduce mortality in post MI patients. ARBs have also shown to have BP-independent benefits in patients with microalbuminuria and macroalbuminuria in addition to reducing progression to end-stage renal disease (ESRD).

If ACE Inhibitors and ARBs are Good What About the Combination of the Two?

Candesartan in Heart failure – Assessment and Reduction in Mortality and morbidity (CHARM) added study *(117)* showed that there was a 15% reduction in the risk of cardiovascular death or admission to hospital with heart failure and 4.6/3.00 mg reduction in systolic/diastolic BP in ACE inhibitor and ARB group compared to monotherapy. Patients with type 2 diabetes, HTN, and microalbuminuria recruited to the Candesartan And Lisinopril effect on Microalbuminuria (CALM) study achieved significantly greater reductions in blood pressure and albuminuria with combination therapy compared with monotherapy *(118)*. In the combination treatment of ANG II receptor blocker and ACE inhibitor in nondiabetic renal disease (COOPERATE) study, nondiabetic individuals receiving combination therapy for 3 years had a significantly reduced chance of doubling of serum creatinine or developing ESRD compared with those given monotherapy (11% compared with 23%, respectively; $P = 0.018$), despite similar changes in blood pressure *(123)*.

Renin Inhibitors

Renin catalyzes the first and rate-limiting step of the RAS. Renin inhibitors prevent the formation of Ang I and Ang II without affecting kinin metabolism, so may offer a therapeutic profile distinct from those of ACE inhibitors and ARBs. Aliskiren is an orally effective, nonpeptide, long-lasting renin inhibitor that in experimental models reduces blood pressure as effectively as valsartan or benazeprilat *(124)*. In hypertensive patients, once-daily oral doses of aliskiren (150-640 mg) decrease plasma Ang I and II levels for 48 h and its antihypertensive efficacy and tolerance is similar to enalapril *(125)*, losartan *(126)* and irbesartan *(127)*.

There are intriguing implications to the possibility that renin inhibitors may induce more complete blockade of the intrarenal RAS. While both diabetic and nondiabetic nephropathies are considerably retarded by ACE inhibition and AT_1 receptor blockade, it appears likely that ANG -II formation may still play an important role in those patients who show deterioration while on ACE inhibitors and ARB's. Hence, agents capable of inducing more complete blockade may further reduce progressive renal injury. Renin inhibitors could fulfill this role as a single agent or in combination with either an ACE inhibitor or a receptor blocker – this latter strategy could circumvent treatment resistance to these modes of RAS blockade by precluding the reactive rise in renin activity *(128)*.

Aliskiren is the first orally active renin inhibitor and provides a true alternative to ACE inhibitors and ARBs for HTN and other cardiovascular and renal disease.

As with ACE inhibitors and ARBs, the administration of a renin inhibitor increases circulating and intrarenal renin levels. In order to provide sustained inhibition of renin activity, a renin inhibitor should be potent and have a very high affinity to renin, its dissociation rate (k_{off})

should be slow, and its plasma and tissue concentrations should remain high long enough to inhibit each new renin molecule released into the bloodstream or kidney *(129)*.

Interruption of the generation of ANG-II by renin inhibitors at this highly specific initial step of the cascade would be expected to have similar but not identical effects to those of the already well-established RAS antagonists. Due to the lack of effective alternative enzyme pathways, blockade of ANG-II production may be more effective with renin inhibition than with ACE inhibition, and because of the high specificity of renin for only one substrate, namely AGT, adverse effects would be expected to be less frequent.

It appears likely that Aliskiren is the first of a new class of agents that may prove useful in the management of patients with nephropathy, heart failure, and atherosclerosis in addition to HTN *(130)*.

SUMMARY AND CONCLUSIONS

The RAS is a major hormonal system involved in the regulation of blood pressure, cardiovascular, and renal functions. This was initially considered as an endocrine system. Evidence from recent studies show that in addition to the circulating RAS there is a tissue RAS which functions as an autocrine/paracrine system. This local RAS system appears to be important in normal physiology and pathophysiology of disease states such as HTN, CHF, and post-infarction cardiac remodeling. There are several angiotensin peptides in the RAS. These act through different ANG receptors. The major peptide is ANG-I1 and the main receptors are AT1 and AT2 receptors. The main enzyme is ACE. Due to the several pathological conditions associated with the activation of the RAS system it appears that medications that block this system are beneficial in several medical conditions including HTN, CHF, diabetic nephropathy, and post MI. This has clearly been shown with ACE inhibitors and ARBs. The newest addition to this group is the renin blocker aliskiren.

Since the first discovery of renin as a "pressor substance" in 1898 by Robert Tiegerstedt there has been long and difficult but highly productive years of renin-angiotensin research. Considering the role of ANG II in CV disease, studies on RAS have occupied a central role in the cardiovascular research. Hopefully future research about the RAS system will enlighten us with more information on this fascinating endocrine , paracrine, and autocrine system.

REFERENCES

1. Tiegerstedt R, Bergman PG. Niere und Kreislauf. *Skandinävisches Archiev für Physiologie* 8: 223–271, 1898.
2. Tadashi Inagami A Memorial to Robert Tiegerstedt: The Centennial of Renin Discovery. *Hypertension* 32: 953–957, 1998
3. Robertson JIS. Renin and angiotensin: a historical review. In: Robertson JIS, Nicholls MG, eds. *The Renin-Angiotensin System*. Vol. 1. London, UK: Gower Medical Publishing; 1993: 1.1–1.18
4. Reudelhuber, TL. *Curr Opin Nephrol Hypertens* 14(2): 155–159, 2005
5. Hobart, PM, Fogliano, M, O'Connor, BA, Schaefer, IM, Chirgwin. JM: Human renin gene: structure and sequence analysis. *Proc Natl Acad Sci USA* 81(16): 5026–5030, 1984
6. William HB. Hypertension Primer. Third Edition Chapter A5. Renin synthesis and secretion. Pg 14–17
7. Edwin K Jackson Goodman and Gilman's The pharmacological basis of therapeutics. Chapter 31. Renin and angiotensin pg 809–841
8. Bader M, Ganten D. Regulation of rennin: new Evidence from cultured cells and genetically modified mice. *J Mol Med* 78: 130–139, 2000
9. Holmer SR, Kaissling B, Putnik K, Pfeifer M, Kramer BK, Riegger GA, Kurtz A. Beta-adrenergic stimulation of renin expression in vivo. *J Hypertens* 15: 1471–1479, 1997
10. Wagner C, Hinder M, Krämer BK, Kurtz A. Role of renal nerves in the stimulation of the renin system by reduced renal arterial pressure. *Hypertension* 34: 1101–1105,1999

11. Wagner C, Kurtz A.Regulation of renal renin release. *Curr Opin Nephrol Hypertens* 7: 437–441, 1998

12. Kageyama R, Ohkibo H, Nakanishi S. Primary structure of human preangiotensinogen deduced from the cloned cDNA sequence. *Biochemistry* 23: 3603–3609, 1984

13. Campbell DJ, Habener JF. Angiotensinogen gene is expressed differently and differentially regulated in multiple tissues of the rat. *J Clin Invest* 78: 31–39, 1986

14. Cassis lA, Saye J; Peach MJ. Location and regulation of rat angiotensinogen messenger RNA. *Hypertension* 11: 591–596, 1998

15. Ben – Ar ET, Garrison JC. Regulation of angiotensinogen mRNA accumulation in rat hepatocytes. *Am J Physiol* 255:E70–E79, 1988

16. Kim HS, Krege JH, Kluckman KD, Hagaman JR, et al. Genetic control of blood pressure and the angiotensinogen locus. *Proc Natl Acad Sci USA* 92: 2735–2739, 1995 (Mice with no angiotensinogen gene are hypotensive)

17. Tanimoto K, Sugiyama F, Goto Y Ishida J, et al. Angiotensinogen deficient mice with hypotension *J Biol Chem* 269: 31334–31337, 1994

18. Jeunemaitre X, Soubrier F, Kotelevtsev YV, Lifton RP, Williams CS, Charru A, Hunt SC, Hopkins PN, Williams RR, Lalouel JM, et al. Molecular basis of human hypertension: Role of angiotensinogen. *Cell*;71: 169–180, 1992

19. Lolauel JM, Rohrwasser A, Terreros D, Morgan K, et al. Angiotensinogen in essential HTN from genetics to nephrology. *J Am Soc Nephrolo* 12;606–615, 2001

20. Hata A, Namikawa C, Sasaki M, Sato K, Nakamura T, Tamura K, Lalouel JM. Angiotensinogen as a risk factor for essential hypertension in Japan. *J Clin Invest* 93: 1285–1287, 1994

21. Ward K, Hata A, Jeunemaitre X, Helin C, Nelson L, Namikawa C, Farrington PF, Ogasawara M, Suzumori K, Tomoda S, et al. A molecular variant of angiotensinogen associated with preeclampsia. *Nat Genet* 4: 59–61, 1993

22. James FR. Angiotensin converting enzymes and its relatives. *Genome Biol* 4(8): 225, 2003.

23. Hagaman JR, Moyer JS, Bachman ES, Sibony M. Angiotensin converting enzyme and male fertility. *Proc Natl Acad Sci USA* 95: 2552–2557, 1998

24. Erdös EG, Skidgel RA. Neutral endopeptidase 24.11 (enkephalinase) and related regulators of peptide hormones. *FASEB J* 3: 145–151, 1989.

25. Randal AS, Ervin GE. Angiotensin I converting enzyme and neprilysin (Neutral Endopeptidase). Hypertension Primer Third Edition Pg 16–19

26. Boehm M, Nabel EG, Angiotensin converting enzyme 2 – A new cardiac regulator *N Engl J Med* 347: 1795–1797, 2002

27. Crackower MA, Sarao R, Oudit GY, Yagil C, et al. Angiotensin-converting enzyme 2 is an essential regulator of heart function. *Nature* 417: 799–802, 2002

28. Carlos M Ferrario MD, Mark C, Chappell PhD Angiotensin formation and degradation Chapter 7 Hypertension Primer pg 19–21

29. Dell'Italia LJ, Husain A. Dissecting the role of chymase in angiotensin II formation and heart and blood vessel diseases [Hypertension]. *Curr Opin Cardiol* 17(4): 374–379, 2002

30. Ruiz-Ortega M, Lorenzo O, Rupérez M, Esteban V, et al. Egido role of the renin-angiotensin system in vascular diseases. *Hypertension* 38: 1382, 2001.

31. Kerins DM, Hao Q, Vaughan DE. Angiotensin Induction of PAI-I expression in endothelial cells is mediated by the hexapeptide angiotensin IV *J Clini Invest* 96: 2515-2520, 1995

32. Santos RA, Simoes e Silva AC, Maric C, et al. Angiotensin 1-7 is an endogenous ligand for the G protein coupled receptor Mas. *Proc Natl Acad Sci USA* 100;8258–8263, 2003

33. Tallant EA, Lu X, Weiss RB, Chappell MC, et al. Bovine aortic endothelial cell contains an angiotensin (1–7) receptor. *Hypertension* 29: 388–393, 1997

34. Yamada K, Iyer SN, Chappell MC, Ganten D et al. Converting enzyme determines the plasma clearance of angiotensin (1–7). *Hypertension* 32: 496–502, 1998

35. Theodore L, Good friend MD Angiotensins: Actions and Receptors Hypertension Primer. Third Edition 8–11

36. Carey RM, Wang ZQ, Siragy HM. Role of the angiotensin type 2 (AT2) receptor in the regulation of blood pressure and renal function. *Hypertension* 35: 155–16, 2000

37. Jin X-H, Wang Z-Q, Siragy HM, Guerrant RL, Carey RM. Regulation of jejunal sodium and water absorption by angiotensin subtype receptors. *Am J Physiol* 275:R515–R523, 1998

38. Phillips MI, Tissue renin angiotensin systems. Hypertension Primer Third edition Pg 21–23

39. Ingrid Fleming, Karin Kohlstedt, Rudy Busse The tissue rennin angiotensin system and intracellular signaling. *Curr Opin Nephrol Hypertens* 15: 8–13, 2006

40. Paul M, Mehr AP, Kreutz R. Physiology of local renin-angiotensin systems. *Physiol Rev* 86: 747–803, 2006

41. Paul M, Wagner J, Dzau VJ. Gene expression of the components of the renin-angiotensin system in human tissues: quantitative analysis by the polymerase chain reaction. *J Clin Invest* 91: 2058–2064, 1993

42. De Lannoy LM, Danser AH, van Kats JP, Schoemaker RG, Saxena PR, Schalekamp MA. Renin-angiotensin system components in the interstitial fluid of the isolated perfused rat heart: local production of angiotensin I. *Hypertension* 29: 1111–1117, 1997.

43. Urata H, Healy B, Stewart RW, Bumpus FM, Husain A. Angiotensin II-forming pathways in normal and failing human hearts. *Circ Res* 66: 883–890, 1990.

44. Zhuo J, Moeller I, Jenkins T, Chai SY, Allen AM, Ohishi M, Mendelsohn FA. Mapping tissue angiotensin-converting enzyme and angiotensin AT1, AT2 and AT4 receptors. *J Hypertens* 16;(12 Pt 2): 2027–2037, 1998.

45. Cassis LA, Lynch KR, Peach MJ. Localization of angiotensinogen messenger RNA in rat aorta. *Circulation Res* 62: 1259–1262, 1998

46. Okamura T, Clemens DL, Inagami T. Renin, angiotensins, and angiotensin-converting enzyme in neuroblastoma cells: evidence for intracellular formation of angiotensins. *Proc Natl Acad Sci USA* 78(11): 6940–6943, 1981

47. Vila-Porcile, E. Corvol, P. Angiotensinogen, prorenin, and renin are co-localized in the secretory granules of all glandular cells of the rat anterior pituitary: an immunoultrastructural study. *J Histochem Cytochem* 46(3): 301–311, 1998

48. Schiavone, MT. Khosla, MC. Ferrario, CM. Angiotensin-[1–7]: evidence for novel actions in the brain. [Review] *J Cardiovas Pharmacol* 16 Suppl 4:S19

49. Castren E, Kurihara M, Gutkind JS, Saavedra JM. Specific angiotensin II binding sites in the rat stellate and superior cervical ganglia. *Brain Res* 422: 347–351, 1987

50. Kushiku K, Yamada H, Shibata K, Tokunaga R, Katsuragi T, Furukawa T. Upregulation of immunoreactive angiotensin II release and angiotensinogen mRNA expression by high-frequency preganglionic stimulation at the canine cardiac sympathetic ganglia. *Circ Res* 88: 110–116, 2001

51. Allen AM, Lewis SJ, Verberne AJ, Mendelsohn FAO. Angiotensin receptors and the vagal system. *Clin Exp Hypertens* 10: 1239–1249, 1988.

52. Saito K, Gutkind JS, Saavedra JM. Angiotensin II binding sites in the conduction system of rat hearts. *Am J Physiol Heart Circ Physiol* 253:H1618–H1622, 1987

53. Palumbo A, Jones C, Lightman A, Carcangiu ML, DeCherney AH, Naftolin F. Immunohistochemical localizaton of renin and angiotensin II in human ovaries. *Am J Obstet Gynecol* 160: 8–14, 1989

54. Palumbo A, Pourmotabbed G, Carcangiu ML, Andrade-Gordon P, Roa L, DeCherney A, Naftolin F. Immuno-histochemical localization of renin and angiotensin in the ovary: comparison between normal women and patients with histologically proven polycystic ovarian disease. *Fertil Steril* 60: 280–284, 1993

55. Lightman A, Tarlatzis BC, Rzasa PJ, Culler MD, Caride VJ, Negro-Vilar AF, Lennard D, DeCherney AH, Naftolin F. The ovarian renin-angiotensin system: renin-like activity and angiotensin II/III immunoreactivity in gonadotropin-stimulated and unstimulated human follicular fluid. *Am J Obstet Gynecol* 156: 808–816, 1987

56. Hagemann A, Nielsen AH, Poulsen K. The uteroplacental renin-angiotensin system: a review. *Exp Clin Endocrinol* 102: 252–261, 1994

57. Raju GC, Lee YS. Immunohistochemical demonstration of renin in the endometrium. *Ann Acad Med Singapore* 18: 345–347, 1989.

58. Lee YA, Liang CS, Lee MA, Lindpaintner K. Local stress, not systemic factors, regulate gene expression of the cardiac renin-angiotensin system in vivo: a comprehensive study of all its components in the dog. *Proc Natl Acad Sci USA* 93: 11035–11040, 1996

59. Phillips MI, Speakman EA, Kimura B. Levels of angiotensin and molecular biology of the tissue renin angiotensin systems. *Regul Pept* 43: 1–20, 1993

60. Morgan T, Craven C, Nelson L, Lalouel JM, Ward K. Angiotensinogen T235 expression is elevated in decidual spiral arteries. *J Clin Invest* 100: 1406–1415, 1997

61. Ahmed A, Li XF, Shams M, Gregory J, Rollason T, Barnes NM, Newton JR. Localization of the angiotensin II and its receptor subtype expression in human endometrium and identification of a novel high-affinity angiotensin II binding site. *J Clin Invest* 96(2): 848–857, 1995

62. Cushman DW and Cheung HS. Concentrations of angiotensin-converting enzyme in tissues of the rat. *Biochim Biophys Acta* 250: 261–265, 1971

63. Erman A, Chen-Gal B, van Dijk DJ, Sulkes J, Kaplan B, Boner G, Neri A. Ovarian angiotensin-converting enzyme activity in humans: relationship to estradiol, age, and uterine pathology. *J Clin Endocrinol Metab* 81: 1104–1107, 1996

64. Li XF, Ahmed A. Compartmentalization and cyclic variation of immunoreactivity of renin and angiotensin converting enzyme in human endometrium throughout the menstrual cycle. *Hum Reprod* 12: 2804–2809, 1997

65. Saridogan E, Djahanbakhch O, Puddefoot JR, Demetroulis C, Collingwood K, Mehta JG, Vinson GP. Angiotensin II receptors and angiotensin II stimulation of ciliary activity in human fallopian tube. *J Clin Endocrinol Metab* 81: 2719–2725, 1996 (Angiotensin receptors have been demonstrated in ova)

66. Naruse K, Murakoshi M, Osamura RY, Naruse M, Toma H, Watanabe K, Demura H, Inagami T, Shizume K. Immunohistological evidence for renin in human endocrine tissues. *J Clin Endocrinol Metab* 61: 172–177, 1985.

67. Naruse K, Murakoshi M, Osamura RY, Naruse M, Toma H, Watanabe K, Demura H, Inagami T, Shizume K. Immunohistological evidence for renin in human endocrine tissues. *J Clin Endocrinol Metab* 61: 172–177, 1985

68. Lattion AL, Soubrier F, Allegrini J, Hubert C, Corvol P, and Alhenc-Gelas F. The testicular transcript of the angiotensin I-converting enzyme encodes for the ancestral, non-duplicated form of the enzyme. *FEBS Lett* 252: 99–104, 1989

69. Cushman DW, Cheung HS. Concentrations of angiotensin-converting enzyme in tissues of the rat. *Biochim Biophys Acta* 250: 261–265, 1971

70. Berg T, Sulner J, Lai CY, Soffer RL. Immunohistochemical localization of two angiotensin I-converting isoenzymes in the reproductive tract of the male rabbit. *J Histochem Cytochem* 34: 753–760, 1986

71. Van Sande M, Inokuchi J, Nagamatsu A, Scharpe S, Neels H, Van Camp K. Tripeptidyl carboxypeptidase activity of angiotensin-converting enzyme in human tissues of the urogenital tract. *Urol Int* 40: 100–102, 1985

72. Yokoyama M, Hiwada K, Kokubu T, Takaha M, Takeuchi M. Angiotensin-converting enzyme in human prostate. *Clin Chim Acta* 100: 253–258, 1980

73. Aguilera G, Millan MA, Harwood JP. Angiotensin II receptors in the gonads. *Am J Hypertens* 2: 395–402, 1989

74. Leung PS, Chan HC, Fu LX, Leung PY, Chew SB, Wong PY. Angiotensin II receptors: localization of type I and type II in rat epididymides of different developmental stages. *J Membr Biol* 157: 97–103, 1997.

75. Vinson GP, Puddefoot JR, Ho MM, Barker S, Mehta J, Saridogan E, Djahanbakhch O. Type 1 angiotensin II receptors in rat and human sperm. *J Endocrinol* 144(2): 369–378, 1995,

76. Dinh DT, Frauman AG, Sourial M, Casley DJ, Johnston CI, Fabiani ME. Identification, distribution, and expression of angiotensin II receptors in the normal human prostate and benign prostatic hyperplasia. *Endocrinology* 142: 1349–1356, 2001

77. Hagaman JR, Moyer JS, Bachman ES, Sibony M, Magyar PL, Welch JE, Smithies O, Krege JH, O'Brien DA. Angiotensin-converting enzyme and male fertility. *Proc Natl Acad Sci USA* 95: 2552–2557, 1998

78. Goossens GH. Blaak EE. van Baak MA. Possible involvement of the adipose tissue renin-angiotensin system in the pathophysiology of obesity and obesity-related disorders. [Review] [179 refs] *Obesity Rev* 4(1): 43–55, 2003 Feb

79. Schling P, Mallow H, Trindl A,, Loffler G. Evidence for a local renin angiotensin system in primary cultured human preadipocytes. *Int J Obes Relat Metab Disord* 23: 336–341, 1999.

80. Karlsson C, Lindell K, Ottosson M, Sjostrom L, Carlsson B, Carlsson LM. Human adipose tissue expresses angiotensinogen and enzymes required for its conversion to angiotensin II. *J Clin Endocrinol Metab* 83: 3925–3929, 1998

81. Engeli S, Gorzelniak K, Kreutz R, Runkel N, Distler A, Sharma AM. Co-expression of renin-angiotensin system genes in human adipose tissue. *J Hypertens* 17: 555–560, 1999.

82. Cassis LA. Role of angiotensin II in brown adipose thermogenesis during cold acclimation. *Am J Physiol Endocrinol Metab* 265: E860-E865, 1993

83. Jones BH, Standridge MK, Moustaid N. Angiotensin II increases lipogenesis in 3T3-L1 and human adipose cells. *Endocrinology* 138: 1512–1519, 1997

84. Giacchetti G, Faloia E, Sardu C, Camilloni MA, Mariniello B, Gatti C, Garrapa GG, Guerrieri M, and Mantero F. Gene expression of angiotensinogen in adipose tissue of obese patients. *Int J Obes Relat Metab Disord* 24 Suppl 2: S142–S143, 2000

85. Cassis LA, English VL, Bharadwaj K, Boustany CM. Differential effects of local versus systemic angiotensin II in the regulation of leptin release from adipocytes. *Endocrinology* 145: 169–174, 2004

86. Sigmund CD, Jones CA, Mullins JJ, Kim U, Gross KW. Expression of murine renin genes in subcutaneous connective tissue. *Proc Natl Acad Sci USA* 87: 7993–7997, 1990

87. Danser AH, Koning MM, Admiraal PJ, Sassen LM, Derkx FH, Verdouw PD, and Schalekamp MA. Production of angiotensins I and II at tissue sites in intact pigs. *Am J Physiol Heart Circ Physiol* 263: H429–H437, 1992

88. Sun Y, Diaz-Arias AA, Weber KT. Angiotensin-converting enzyme, bradykinin, and angiotensin II receptor binding in rat skin, tendon, and heart valves: an in vitro, quantitative autoradiographic study. *J Lab Clin Med* 123: 372–377, 1994

89. Silver RB, Reid AC, Mackins CJ, Askwith T, Schaefer U, Herzlinger D, Levi R. Mast cells: a unique source of renin. *Proc Natl Acad Sci USA* 101: 13607–13612, 2004

90. Steckelings UM, Artuc M, Paul M, Stoll M, Henz BM. Angiotensin II stimulates proliferation of primary human keratinocytes via a non-AT_1, non-AT_2 angiotensin receptor. *Biochem Biophys Res Commun* 229: 329–333, 1996.

91. Tahmasebi M, Puddefoot JR, Inwang ER, Vinson GP. The tissue renin-angiotensin system in human pancreas. *J Endocrinol* 161: 317–322, 1999

92. Seo MS, Fukamizu A, Saito T, Murakami K. Identification of a previously unrecognized production site of human renin. *Biochim Biophys Acta* 1129: 87–89, 1991

93. Chappell MC, Milsted A, Diz DI, Brosnihan KB, Ferrario CM. Evidence for an intrinsic angiotensin system in the canine pancreas. *J Hypertens* 9: 751–759, 1991

94. Campbell DJ, Habener JF. Angiotensinogen gene is expressed and differentially regulated in multiple tissues of the rat. *J Clin Invest* 78: 31–39, 1986

95. Stevens BR, Fernandez A, Kneer C, Cerda JJ, Phillips MI,, Woodward ER. Human intestinal brush border angiotensin-converting enzyme activity and its inhibition by antihypertensive ramipril. *Gastroenterology* 94: 942–947, 1988

96. Matsubara S, Saito K, Kizawa Y, Sano M, Osawa M, Iwamoto K, Murakami H. Evidence for the AT_1 subtype of the angiotensin II receptor in the rat submandibular gland. *Biol Pharm Bull* 23: 1185–1188, 2000

97. Leung PS, Chan HC, Fu LX, Wong PY. Localization of angiotensin II receptor subtypes AT_1 and AT_2 in the pancreas of rodents. *J Endocrinol* 153: 269–274, 1997

98. Wang XP, Zhang R, Wu K, Wu L, Dong Y. Angiotensin II mediates acinar cell apoptosis during the development of rat pancreatic fibrosis by $AT_1 R$. *Pancreas* 29: 264–270, 2004.

99. Yoshioka M, Erickson RH, Woodley JF, Gulli R, Guan D, Kim YS. Role of rat intestinal brush-border membrane angiotensin-converting enzyme in dietary protein digestion. *Am J Physiol Gastrointest Liver Physiol* 253: G781–G786, 1987

100. Jaszewski R, Tolia V, Ehrinpreis MN, Bodzin JH, Peleman RR, Korlipara R, Weinstock JV. Increased colonic mucosal angiotensin I and II concentrations in Crohn's colitis. *Gastroenterology* 98: 1543–1548, 1990

101. Danser AH, van den Dorpel MA, Deinum J, Derkx FH, Peperkamp E, de Jong PT, Schalekamp MA. Prorenin in vitreous and subretinal fluid of the human eye. *Clin Exp Hypertens* 10: 1297–1299, 1988

102. Strain WD, Chaturvedi N. The renin-angiotensin-aldosterone system and the eye in diabetes. *J Renin Angiotensin Aldosterone Syst* 3: 243–246, 2002.

103. Iwai N, Inagami T, Ohmichi N, Kinoshita M. Renin is expressed in rat macrophage/monocyte cells. *Hypertension* 27: 399–403, 1996

104. Dezso B, Nielsen AH, and Poulsen K. Identification of renin in resident alveolar macrophages and monocytes: HPLC and immunohistochemical study. *J Cell Sci* 91: 155–159, 1988

105. Dezso B, Jacobsen J, Poulsen K. Evidence for the presence of angiotensins in normal, unstimulated alveolar macrophages and monocytes. *J Hypertens* 7: 5–11, 1989

106. Simon MR, Kamlay MT, Khan M, Melmon K. Angiotensin II binding to human mononuclear cells. *Immunopharmacol Immunotoxicol* 11: 63–80, 1989.

107. Kim JA, Berliner JA, Nadler JL. Angiotensin II increases monocyte binding to endothelial cells. *Biochem Biophys Res Commun* 226: 862–868, 1996.

108. Klickstein LB, Kaempfer CE, Wintroub BU. The granulocyte-angiotensin system. Angiotensin I-converting activity of cathepsin G. *J Biol Chem* 257: 15042–15046, 1982.

109. Wintroub BU, Klickstein LB, Dzau VJ, Watt KW. Granulocyte-angiotensin system. Identification of angiotensinogen as the plasma protein substrate of leukocyte cathepsin G. *Biochemistry* 23: 227–232, 1984

110. Ekker M, Tronik D, Rougeon F. Extra-renal transcription of the renin genes in multiple tissues of mice and rats. *Proc Natl Acad Sci USA* 86: 5155–5158, 19

111. Campbell DJ, Habener JF. Angiotensinogen gene is expressed and differentially regulated in multiple tissues of the rat. *J Clin Invest* 78: 31–39, 1986

112. Kunert-Radek J, Stepien H, Komorowski J, Pawlikowski M. Stimulatory effect of angiotensin II on the proliferation of mouse spleen lymphocytes in vitro is mediated via both types of angiotensin II receptors. *Biochem Biophys Res Commun* 198: 1034–1039, 1994

113. Carey Robert Angiotensin type-2 receptors and cardiovascular function: are angiotensin type-2 receptors protective?. *Curr Opin Cardiol* 20(4): 264–269, 2005 Jul

114. de Gasparo M, Catt KJ, Inagami T, et al. International union of pharmacology. XXIII. The angiotensin II receptors. *Pharmacol Rev* 52: 415–472, 2000

115. Victor J. Dzau Tissue angiotensin and pathobiology of vascular disease a unifying hypothesis. *Hypertension* 37: 1047, 2001

116. The heart Outcomes Prevention Evaluation Study investigators. Effect of and Angiotensin Converting Enzyme Inhibitor, ramipril on the Cadiovascular events in high risk patients. *New Eng J Med* 342: 145–153 2000

117. McMurray JJ, Ostergren J, Swedberg K, Granger CB, Held P, Michelson EL, et al. Effects of candesartan in patients with chronic heart failure and reduced left-ventricular systolic function taking angiotensin-converting-enzyme inhibitors: the CHARM-Added trial. *Lancet* 362: 767–771, 2003.

118. Mogensen CE, Neldam S, Tikkanen I, Oren S, Viskoper R, Watts RW, et al. Randomised controlled trial of dual blockade of renin-angiotensin system in patients with hypertension, microalbuminuria, and non-insulin dependent diabetes: the candesartan and lisinopril microalbuminuria (CALM) study. *BMJ* 321: 1440–1444, 2000

119. Nakao N, Yoshimura A, Morita H, Takada M, Kayano T, Ideura T. Combination treatment of angiotensin-II receptor blocker and angiotensin-converting-enzyme inhibitor in non-diabetic renal disease (COOPERATE). A randomized controlled trial. *Lancet* 361: 117–124, 2003

120. Wood JM, Schnell CR, Cumin F et al. Aliskiren, a novel, orally effective renin inhibitor, lowers blood pressure in marmosets and spontaneously hypertensive rats. *J Hypertens* 2005; 23:417–426

121. Nussberger J, Wuerzner G, Jensen C, Brunner HR. Angiotensin II suppression in humans by the orally active renin inhibitor Aliskiren (SPP100): comparison with enalapril. *Hypertension* 39:E1–E8, 2002

122. Stanton A, Jensen C, Nussberger J, et al. Blood pressure lowering in essential hypertension with an oral renin inhibitor, aliskiren. *Hypertension* 42: 1137–1143, 2003.

123. Gradman AH, Schmieder RE, Lins RL, et al. Aliskiren, a novel orally effective renin inhibitor, provides dose-dependent antihypertensive efficacy and placebo-like tolerability in hypertensive patients. *Circulation* 111: 1012–1018, 2005.

124. Wood JM, Schnell CR, Cumin F, et al. Aliskiren, a novel, orally effective renin inhibitor, lowers blood pressure in marmosets and spontaneously hypertensive rats. *J Hypertens* 23: 417–426, 2005

125. Nussberger J, Wuerzner G, Jensen C, Brunner HR. Angiotensin II suppression in humans by the orally active renin inhibitor Aliskiren (SPP100): comparison with enalapril. Hypertension 2002; 39:E1–E8

126. Stanton A, Jensen C, Nussberger J, et al. Blood pressure lowering in essential hypertension with an oral renin inhibitor, aliskiren. *Hypertension* 42: 1137–1143, 2003.

127. Gradman AH, Schmieder RE, Lins RL, et al. Aliskiren, a novel orally effective renin inhibitor, provides dose-dependent antihypertensive efficacy and placebo-like tolerability in hypertensive patients. *Circulation* 111: 1012–1018, 2005.

128. Stanton A. Therapeutic potential of renin inhibitors in the management of cardiovascular disorders. [Review] [57 refs] [Journal Article. Review] *Am J Cardiovas Drugs* 3(6): 389–94, 2003. UI: 14728059

129. Azizi M. Webb R. Nussberger J. Hollenberg NK. Renin inhibition with aliskiren: where are we now, and where are we going?. [Review] [75 refs] [Journal Article. Research Support, Non-U.S. Gov't. Review] *J Hypertens* 24(2): 243–256, 2006 Feb.

130. Stanton A. Therapeutic potential of renin inhibitors in the management of cardiovascular disorders. [Review] [57 refs] [Journal Article. Review] *Am J Cardiovas Drugs* 3(6): 389–394, 2003.

9 Microalbuminuria and Chronic Kidney Disease as Cardiovascular Risk Factors

Pantelis A. Sarafidis, MD, PhD
and George L. Bakris, MD

Contents

Summary

Retrospective analyses of data from outcome trial and large databases demonstrate that presence of either microalbuminuria (MA) or a glomerular filtration rate (GFR) below 60 ml per min is associated with an increased risk for cardiovascular (CV) events such as stroke or myocardial infarction. Presence of microalbuminuria does not imply presence of kidney disease although a GFR below 60 ml per min generally has some degree of albuminuria associated with its presence. The mechanisms proposed for the increased CV risk associated with MA are numerous. They range from increases in vascular oxidant stress associated with underlying causes of inflammation such as atherosclerosis to increases in advanced glycation products as seen in diabetes. Monitoring for MA is useful as it may uncover an inflammatory condition not otherwise appreciated as it has been shown to be better than c-reactive protein as a prediction of CV mortality in many studies. Reduced kidney function is a risk factor for higher CV event rates. The mechanisms posited for this interaction are far less clear and range from reductions in nitric oxide production secondary to an enzyme deficiency to increases in factors associated with atherosclerosis such as homocysteine. None of the factors proposed alone explains the risk, thus it is unclear. However, aggressive daily dialysis and transplantation markedly lower CV risk in those individuals. We conclude that aggressive screening for both MA and CKD be undertaken in clinical practice and that physicians aggressively seek to achieve recommended CV risk reduction guideline goals to reduce the risk of nephropathy progression.

From: *Contemporary Endocrinology: Cardiovascular Endocrinology: Shared Pathways and Clinical Crossroads*
Edited by: V. A. Fonseca © Humana Press, New York, NY

Key Words: ACE inhibitors, Angiotensin II receptor blockers, CV disease, Diabetes mellitus, Hypertension, Microalbuminuria, Nephropathy

INTRODUCTION

The first observations on the association between renal failure and increased rates for cardiovascular complications and death date back several decades ago *(1,2)*. Similarly, it has long been noted that subclinical elevations of urinary albumin excretion (UAE) are related to higher risk of subsequent development of clinical nephropathy in patients with diabetes mellitus *(3,4)*, as well as that increased UAE was associated with higher risk for cardiovascular events and cardiovascular or overall mortality in both diabetic and nondiabetic individuals *(4–7)*. Since then, a substantial amount of data have accumulated, providing solid evidence that both the decline in renal function and the elevation in UAE are independently associated with increased risk for cardiovascular disease (CVD). Moreover, current knowledge suggests that elevated UAE and decreased renal function are related to the development of CVD through quite different background mechanisms. This chapter reviews the roles of microalbuminuria (MA) and chronic kidney disease (CKD) as risk factors of CVD, discussing the progress of the epidemiologic and clinical evidence on the field.

DEFINITIONS AND MEASUREMENT OF MA AND CKD

In the first description of MA as a predictor of nephropathy in patients with type 1 diabetes in 1982, Viberti et al. defined MA as overnight UAE rate between 30 mg/min and 140 mg/min, and clinical nephropathy as an "Albustix" stick positive for proteinuria *(3)*. Since then, the definition of MA has been refined to include all the possible methods of UAE measurement. Currently, MA is defined as UAE between 30 mg/day and 300 mg/day, if measured in a 24-h urine collection, and 20–200 ţg/min, if measured in a timed urine collection, or 30–300 mg/g, if measured with the use of urinary albumin to creatinine ratio (UACR) in a spot urine collection, as shown in Table 1. Any urine albumin value below these limits is considered as normal UAE, whereas any value above them reflects the presence of macroalbuminuria or clinical proteinuria *(8,9)*.

While 24-h or other timed collections were the traditional way to measure UAE, measuring UACR in a spot collection of morning urine in the fasting state arose as a simple, quick, and comparably accurate way of determining albuminuria *(10)*. The use of this approach, however, requires knowledge of the factors that can affect spot UACR measurement (Table 2). It is important to note that the range of UAE excretion is about 25% lower during sleep than during the hours of being awake. Furthermore, MA can exhibit a daily intraindividual variation between 40% and 100% *(11–14)*. This can be largely attributed to biological variations due to inflammation associated with small injury, toothaches, etc., as well as changes in dietary sodium and protein intake *(15)*. Caution is also required when interpreting the UACR in patients with higher muscle mass (i.e. males, African Americans), as these populations have higher levels of creatinine excretion *(16)*: that is why the Kidney Disease Outcomes Quality Initiative (K/DOQI) proposed different levels for MA in males and females (Table 1) *(9)*. After taking all of these factors into account, the use of the UACR in place of timed urine collections is currently recommended *(8,17,18)*. However, the imprecise nature of MA and creatinine measurement requires at least three measures to be made over a period of 2–3 months before determining the actual UACR for a particular individual *(10)*. Ideally, these measurements should be obtained in the fasting state and collected from the first morning void, to avoid the effect of physical activity

Table 1
Definitions of microalbuminuria and proteinuria. Adapted from KDOQI guidelines 2004 *(9)*

	Urine Collection Method	Normal	Microalbuminuria	Albuminuria or Clinical Proteinuria
Total Protein	24-h excretion	<300 mg/d	NA	>300 mg/d
	Spot urine dipstick	<30 mg/dl	NA	>30 mg/dl
	Spot urine protein-to-creatinine ratio	<200 mg/g	NA	>200 mg/g
Albumin	24-h excretion	<30 mg/d	30–300 mg/d	>300 mg/d
	Spot urine albumin-specific dipstick	<3 mg/dl	>3 mg/dl	NA
	Spot urine albumin-to-creatinine ratio	<30 mg/g	30–300 mg/g	>300 mg/g
	Spot urine albumin-to-creatinine ratio (gender-specific definition)	<17 mg/g (men)<25 mg/g (women)	17–250 mg/g (men)25–355 mg/g (women)	>250 mg/g (men)>355 mg/g (women)

Table 2
Factors that can affect measurement of urine albumin to creatinine in a spot specimen

Albumin Excretion
1. Blood pressure
2. Time of day
3. Fasting versus nonfasting sample
4. Salt intake
5. Volume status

Creatinine excretion
1. Gender
2. Race
3. Muscle mass

during the day *(19)*. Repeat specimens should follow the same protocol since, as noted above, dietary intake of sodium and protein can modify albuminuria.

According to the National Kidney Foundation (NKF) CKD is defined either as kidney damage, as confirmed by kidney biopsy (structural abnormalities) or markers of damage (abnormalities in blood, urine, or imaging tests indicating functional abnormalities), or as the presence of glomerular filtration rate (GFR) under the level of 60 ml/min/1.73 m^2, each for a period greater than 3 months *(17)*. The clinical syndrome of CKD is divided in terms of severity into five stages, which are based on the level of GFR, irrespective of the cause of kidney damage (Table 3). Decreased kidney function starts at a GFR below 89 ml/min/1.73 m^2, and is considered to be pronounced if GFR is less than 60 ml/min/1.73 m^2 for more than 3 months *(17)*. In

Table 3
Stages and estimated prevalence of chronic kidney disease in the United States. Adapted
from KDOQI guidelines 2002 *(17)*

Stage	Description	GFR (mL/min/1.73 m²)	Prevalence	
			N (1000's)	(%)
1	Kidney damage with normal or ↑ GFR	≥90	5900	3.3
2	Kidney damage with mild ↓ GFR	60–89	5300	3.0
3	Moderate ↓ GFR	30–59	7600	4.3
4	Severe ↓ GFR	15–29	400	0.2
5	Kidney failure	<15 of dialysis	300	0.1

clinical terms, the latter is reflected in an elevation of serum creatinine levels above the normal range (=1.5 mg/dl (133 ţmol/l) in men and =1.3 mg/dl (115 ţmol/l) in women). This decrease in renal function along with an increase in the level of MA or development of albuminuria is usually a clear indication of the presence of renal dysfunction. A definitive diagnosis could be assigned after biopsy or imaging studies, but in most patients, well-defined clinical presentations and causal factors provide sufficient basis for CKD diagnosis without these procedures. Diagnosis of the type of CKD based on aetiology is also very important, but in a considerable amount of cases CKD cannot be attributed to a single factor, since it is diagnosed in a late stage, when multiple aetiologic factors coexist in the patient.

Of particular importance is the establishment of the stage of CKD, as the level of kidney dysfunction determines the rate of kidney disease progression but also the risk of CVD *(17)*. Serum creatinine has been long considered as an imprecise index of renal function, since the levels of serum creatinine are affected from various factors, apart from creatinine filtration and, thus, patients with mild renal impairment can have normal, or near-normal, serum creatinine levels *(20,21)*. This is why stages of CKD are defined with the use of GFR levels, which is considered the best index of renal function in both health and disease *(17)*. Most accurate estimations of GFR require the measurement of renal clearance of inulin which is cumbersome and time-consuming, whereas the use of various radioactive substances, which also gives accurate results *(22)*, seems again difficult for everyday clinical practice. To overcome these limitations, a number of equations using serum creatinine and demographic variables have been developed to estimate GFR through creatinine clearance, such as the Cockcroft–Gault formula, the Modification of Diet in Renal Disease (MDRD) study formula and others *(23,24)*. The MDRD study formula seems to provide a much more accurate estimate of GFR than other commonly used equations *(24)* and thus the NKF recommends this formula to be used for GFR estimation *(17,18)*

PREVALENCE AND NATURAL COURSE OF MA AND CKD

Early observations suggested a high prevalence of MA in patients with diabetes, but later and larger studies failed to confirm these results *(25–30)*. These variations in prevalence can be attributed to differences in the populations studied in terms of age, race, blood pressure, or

Table 4
Factors known to influence the development of
microalbuminuria in subjects without diabetes

1. Elevated blood pressure (systolic, diastolic, mean)
2. Increased body mass index
3. Endothelial dysfunction
4. Decrease in high-density lipoprotein levels
5. Insulin resistance (hyperinsulinemia)
6. Smoking
7. Salt sensitivity
8. Increased age
9. DD ACE-genotype

renal function levels, as well as the techniques used for detection of MA. The prevalence of MA in patients with type 2 diabetes is estimated at about 20% and about 30% in type 2 diabetic subjects older than 55 years of age *(25,31,32)*. Without specific intervention the rate of progression to diabetic nephropathy (i.e., development of macroalbuminuria) in patients with type 2 diabetes with MA would be 5% per year, whereas in patients with type 1 diabetes and MA would be 7.5% per year *(3,4)*. Subsequent end-stage renal disease (ESRD) occurs at a rate of 1% annually in type 2 diabetes patients while the risk for those with type 1 diabetes approaches 75% after 20 years *(8,33,34)*. It should be noted, however, that the rate of nephropathy progression, as well as cardiovascular risk, is far lower in diabetic patients who have tight control of the glucose and blood pressure early in the course of their disease {Nathan, 2005 NATHAN2005 /id;Adler, 2003 245 /id}. Among nondiabetic individuals with essential hypertension the prevalence of MA varies widely from 5% to 40% *(35–37)* The reason for this high variability lies again in differences among the populations studies in the actual blood pressure levels, and other factors known to influence MA levels (Table 4).

In regard to the prevalence of CKD, it is needless to say that during the past decades CKD has grown to a worldwide public health problem. Data from National Health and Nutrition Examination Survey (NHANES) III (1988–1994) suggest that the prevalence of CKD in the adult population of the United States was roughly 11%; thus, about 20 million adult individuals were estimated to suffer from CKD, among which more than 8 million have CKD of at least stage 3 and 300,000 require dialysis treatment (Table 3) *(17,38)*. The incidence and prevalence of kidney failure treated by dialysis and transplantation is continuously increasing, as shown in Fig. 1. In 2002 the number of patients with kidney failure rose up to more than 430,000 and the incident rate of kidney failure has increased to 333 new cases per million people, a number almost four times higher than that in 1980 *(39)*. The number one cause for ESRD is diabetic nephropathy, with the prevalence rising to 35–40% of patients with ESRD, and the second is hypertensive nephrosclerosis, accounting roughly around 20% of ESRD cases *(8,17,39)*.The United States Renal Data System, taking into consideration the enormous growth of both the elderly and type 2 diabetic populations, estimates that by the year 2030 more than 2.2 million people in the United States will require treatment for ESRD *(39)*. Of note, among patients on dialysis 5-year survival rates are extremely low, about 32%, a fact mostly due to the parallel high prevalence of CVD.

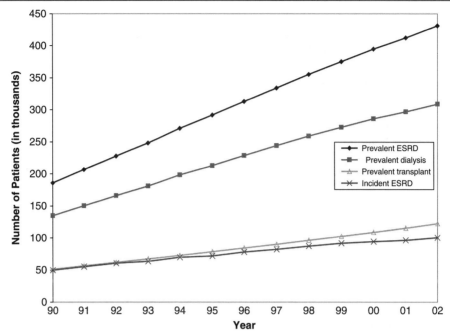

Fig. 1. Incident and prevalent end-stage renal disease patient counts, by modality. Adapted from USRDS 2004 *(39)*.

PATHOGENESIS OF MA

The pathophysiological role of MA as a participant in or accelerant to the atherosclerotic process is uncertain, but current available evidence suggests it is more a marker than a pathogenic factor. All patients with MA have an elevated transcapillary escape rate of albumin and share a higher prevalence of the risk factors included in the metabolic syndrome (insulin resistance, hypertension, hyperlipidemia, obesity, and elevated procoagulant factors) *(26,28,30)* However, the current paradigm suggests that the mechanism of vascular injury leading to MA is somehow different in the nondiabetic and diabetic populations *(34,40,41)*.

In nondiabetic patients with MA, generalized vascular leakiness is caused by alterations in the extracellular matrix. These alterations are largely triggered by increases in microvascular pressure which lead to injury to the endothelium and generalized endothelial dysfunction. In response to this injury, excess protein is deposited in the extracellular matrix and, as a result, the capillary basement membrane becomes sclerosed.*(34,42)* The resultant defect in endothelial permeability permits lipid influx into the vessel wall causing atherosclerotic changes. This response is the final common pathway of many acute and chronic illnesses and is mediated through various stimuli including complement activation, macrophages, neutrophils, and endothelial stimulation from diverse inflammatory insults *(40)*.

The presence of diabetes accelerates this process in a manner similar to adding "gasoline to an already burning fire". The glycated state under which albumin exists in diabetics transforms it into an antigenic-like molecule that is associated with generation of reactive oxygen species *(42,43)*. These free radicals cause direct injury to the epithelial cells of the glomerular membrane, vascular smooth muscle cells, and mesangial cells, and they chelate the proteins on the glomerular membrane. This impairs the ability of the glomerulus to filter proteins and thus albumin excretion is increased *(44)*. Further evidence from animal studies supports the notion that albumin must be glycated to be pathogenic. An interesting finding from these animal models is that intermittent elevation of serum glucose induces similar changes in cell membranes to that seen in people with diabetes.*(42)* Thus, the link between diabetic and nondiabetic MA may be the pre-diabetic state associated with insulin resistance leading to an increased amount of glycated albumin.

The presence of diabetes also increases MA by other mechanisms. Direct injury to the glomerular membrane by advanced glycosylation end products results in a loss of glomerular membrane size selectivity *(45)*. This has a direct effect of increasing albuminuria, but also allows for passage of more lipids into the vessel wall. The cycle is worsened by the body's increased production of albumin in response to renal losses *(34,46)*. It should be noted, however, it is difficult to predict what form of dysfunction a particular diabetic patient will exhibit. This may explain the different course of diabetic renal diseases between different types of diabetes and between patients with the same type of disease.

MA AND CARDIOVASCULAR DISEASE

MA and the Risk for Cardiovascular Outcomes

Yudkin et al. were the first to report cross-sectional associations between MA and the prevalence of coronary artery disease (CAD) and peripheral vascular disease (PVD) in a selected sample of 187 nondiabetic subjects *(47)*. Since then, several studies, either in the general population or in high-risk individuals, have examined the relationship of MA with an adverse cardiovascular risk profile or the occurrence of CVD. Both descriptive and observational studies reported associations of MA with established cardiovascular risk factors (age, elevated blood pressure, hyperglycemia, obesity, high total and LDL-cholesterol, high triglycerides, low HDL-cholesterol, smoking) as well as emerging cardiovascular risk factors and other unfavorable conditions (high C-reactive protein, insulin resistance, hyperinsulinemia, endothelial dysfunction, hyperhomocysteinemia, high fibrinogen levels, high tissue-type plasminogen activator antigen, and others) *(28,30,31,48–70)*. Furthermore, MA has long been suggested to be an independent risk factor for cardiovascular morbidity and mortality in various populations either with or without diabetes mellitus *(71–75)*.

In patients with type 1 or type 2 diabetes early observations in small cohorts of subjects followed for periods up to many years linked the presence of MA with increased risk of cardiovascular morbidity and total or cardiovascular mortality, in parallel to an enormous elevation of the risk for future development of clinical proteinuria *(4,6,7)*. A subsequent prospective cohort study examined the impact of MA and macroalbuminuria on about 440 hypertensive men with and without type 2 diabetes. In the diabetic patients there was a lower cardiovascular mortality in the normoalbuminuric group compared with both the microalbuminuric and the macroalbuminuric group and the logarithm of UAE was an independent predictor of both total and cardiovascular mortality during the 6.3 years of follow-up *(76)*. In another prospective cohort study in 840 patients with type 2 diabetes, MA was associated with 1.84 times and MA with a 2.61 times higher risk of cardiovascular mortality, after adjustment for multiple confounders *(77)*. Further, a previous meta-analysis including more than 2000 type 2 diabetes patients from 11 cohort studies showed that the overall odds ratio in patients with MA was 2.4 for total mortality and 2.0 for cardiovascular morbidity and mortality *(25)*.

Similar to patients with diabetes, early observations in nondiabetic individuals reported significant associations between elevated UAE and overall mortality *(5)*. Subsequently, a cross-sectional study including 11,343 nondiabetic hypertensive patients showed that subjects with

MA had significantly higher prevalence of CHD, stroke, PVD, and left ventricular hypertrophy in relation to those without MA (31%, 6%, 7%, and 24% in patients with MA compared to 22%, 4%, 5%, and 14% in those without MA) *(54)*. In a cohort of more than 1000 elderly non-diabetic Finnish subjects, after adjustment for all classic cardiovascular risk factors, MA was associated with elevated risk of cardiovascular morbidity and mortality during the 3.5 years of follow-up, whereas the simultaneous presence of both MA and hyperinsulinemia further increased this risk *(78)*. Furthermore, in a cohort of more than 2000 subjects free of diabetes aged 30–60 years MA was the strongest predictor of development of CHD during follow-up, with a relative risk adjusted for all major cardiovascular risk factors of 3.5 *(79)* In contrast to these data, there are some observations that did not confirm the association of MA with increased cardiovascular risk in nondiabetic patients. For example, in the above-mentioned cohort study of Agewall et al. *(76)*, no significant difference in cardiovascular mortality between the normo- and MA groups of nondiabetics was observed and only macroalbuminuria, but not MA, predicted cardiovascular mortality.

In addition to the above, more recent cross-sectional studies indicated significant associations between MA and prevalent CVD (angina, previous myocardial infarction, previous stroke, etc.) in the general population *(62,64,67)*. However, the best evidence of the association between MA and the risk for CVD comes from post-hoc analyses of long-term, multicenter, randomized clinical trials studying the effect of various interventions on hard cardiovascular outcomes, as well as from recent large prospective cohort studies. In about 9000 individuals with a history of CVD or diabetes included in the Heart Outcomes Prevention Evaluation (HOPE) trial, the presence of MA was associated with an adjusted relative risk of 1.83 for major cardiovascular events (myocardial infarction, stroke, or cardiovascular death), 2.09 for all-cause mortality, and 3.23 for hospitalization for congestive heart failure *(80)*. The relative risks seen for participants with or without diabetes was quite similar (e.g., the adjusted relative risk for major cardiovascular events was 1.97 and 1.61 in those with and without diabetes, respectively). Of note, the risk for the primary endpoint started from UACR levels well below the cut-off for MA and increased continuously. For every 0.4-mg/mmol increase in the UACR level, the adjusted hazard of major cardiovascular events increased by 5.9%.

A post-hoc analysis of the Losartan Intervention For Endpoint reduction in hypertension (LIFE) study examined the relationship between UAE and cardiovascular risk in a population of the original randomized clinical trial consisting of 8206 hypertensive patients with left ventricular hypertrophy *(81)*. In patients without diabetes the risk for the primary composite endpoint (CV death, fatal and nonfatal stroke, and fatal and nonfatal myocardial infarction) increased continuously as albumin excretion increased and from much lower values of UAE than previously reported for diabetic patients. For every 10-fold increase in UACR, hazard ratios for the composite endpoint increased by 57%, for cardiovascular mortality by 97.7%, for all-cause mortality by 75.2%, for stroke by 51.0%, and for myocardial infarction by 45%. Similar were the results for diabetic patients, with the exception of myocardial infarction where the elevation in risk was not significant.

The association between MA and cardiovascular risk was also examined in recently published large prospective cohort studies. In a subpopulation of the NHANES II study, examined between 1976 and 1980 and followed for 16 years, after adjustment for potential confounders, the relative hazards for cardiovascular and all-cause mortality were 1.57 and 1.64 for subjects with urinary protein levels of 30–299 mg/dl, and 1.77 and 2.00, respectively, in subjects with urinary protein levels ≥300 mg/dl, compared with individuals having levels of <30 mg/dl *(82)*. A series of studies on subpopulations of 20,000–23,600 individuals from the population-based European Prospective Investigation into Cancer and Nutrition study at the city of Norfolk,

United Kingdom (the EPIC-Norfolk Study) further supports the above. In these studies after mean follow-up of 6.2–7.2 years, the presence of MA at baseline was independently associated with a significantly greater risk of 36% for incident coronary heart disease (83), 49% for stroke (84), 103% for cardiovascular mortality, and 48% for all-cause mortality (85). Of note, the risk for cardiovascular events associated with the presence of macroalbuminuria was again even higher (83,84). In another recent prospective observational study more than 3500 nondiabetic hypertensive patients were evaluated for MA and tubular proteinuria and were openly treated with the angiotensin-converting enzyme inhibitor ramipril. The presence of MA at baseline was also independently associated with future cardiovascular events after an average follow-up of 42.5 months (86).

In contrast to the above findings, the evidence linking reduction of MA with reduction in cardiovascular endpoints is not as strong. However, based on the existing data this case should be considered possible. Another analysis of the LIFE trial demonstrated that the group with the lowest cardiovascular event rate had also the greatest reduction in UAE from baseline and that the cardiovascular benefits in favor of losartan versus atenolol treatment tended to be more pronounced in patients with higher baseline levels of UAE. It was also estimated that one-fifth of the difference in favor of losartan on the primary composite endpoint was explained by the greater reduction in albuminuria on losartan (87). In the above-mentioned study from Schrader et al. (86), a change of UAE either from pathologic to normal showed a clear trend to correlate with cerebrovascular endpoints. In the Prevention of Renal and Vascular Endstage Disease Intervention Trial (PREVEND IT), 864 inhabitants of the city of Groningen in the Netherlands with MA (UAE between 15 mg/day and 300 mg/day) were randomized to fosinopril 20 mg/day or matching placebo and pravastatin 40 mg/day or matching placebo. During a mean follow-up of 46 months, fosinopril reduced UAE by 26%, but the reduction in cardiovascular mortality or cardiovascular hospitalization in patients treated with this agent showed only a trend toward statistical significance (88). This study, however, was limited by the low overall number of cardiovascular events, as well as submaximal doses of fosinopril.

MA as a Marker of Target Organ Damage

It has been hypothesized that MA can also serve as a market for subclinical cardiovascular organ damage. In various previous studies MA has been associated with larger left ventricular mass and higher degrees of left ventricular hypertrophy, documented by both electrocardiogram and echocardiogram criteria (28,89–93). Even among hypertensive patients who are normoalbuminuric, those with higher absolute levels of UAE have greater left ventricular wall thickness and more frequent concentric left ventricular hypertrophy than those with lower levels (94). The relationship between MA and left ventricular mass was not apparent in populations who were relatively young (aged between 18 and 45 years) and had mild hypertension (53), and the possibility that this association is due to higher blood pressure loads leading to both MA and left ventricular hypertrophy could not be excluded. However, in the population of the LIFE study not only UAE was correlated with left ventricular hypertrophy, at baseline and after 1 year of treatment, independently of systolic blood pressure, plasma glucose, and age, but also the changes in these parameters during the 1-year period were also correlated independently of systolic blood pressure and plasma glucose changes (95). Such observations stress the need for further evaluation of the associations of these parameters and the acute prognostic importance of MA for left ventricular hypertrophy.

The presence of MA has been also associated with the degree of atherosclerotic disease, evaluated with the use of ultrasound imaging of the intima-media thickness in the carotid artery. This relation was noted in both nondiabetic and diabetic MA subjects *(28,92,93,96,97)*. In another study including both diabetic and nondiabetic subjects, MA was associated with increased prevalence of CHD documented by angiography *(98)*. Vascular retinal changes are also more common in hypertensive patients with MA than those with normal UAE *(28,99)*.Interestingly, the incidence of hypertensive retinopathy is lower if MA is reversible with treatment than if it is not.

Overall, a large number of patients with diabetes, hypertension, or other risk factors for CVD progress to major cardiovascular events through an asymptomatic phase that is characterized by the presence of subclinical organ damage (left ventricular hypertrophy, peripheral atherosclerosis, etc.) and this asymptomatic phase not only precedes but also predicts the occurrence of major events *(100)*. Thus, screening for MA can be an invaluable tool for identifying patients with subclinical damage in order to prevent the occurrence of major events, as well as reverse subclinical changes, through a multifactorial intervention.

Disease Severity Assessment

Measurement of UAE has been considered a very sensitive tool for assessment of the severity of any inflammatory condition, including CVD. The level of UAE is proportional to the severity of many acute inflammatory processes, such as trauma, sepsis, and surgery *(41)*. The severity of conditions like ischemic and reperfusion injuries is also associated with the level of UAE. For example, MA was found to be an early response in patients with acute myocardial infarction and to be proportional to the severity of the infarct *(101)*. In patients with peripheral vascular disease and claudication, the level of UACR after exercise was related to the severity of muscle ischemia during it *(102)*. Another study sought to evaluate the predictive value of MA for conditions like acute respiratory failure and multiple organ failure in intensive care unit patients. Increasing of MA had high negative but low positive predictive value and this concept should be examined further *(103)*.

Clinical Utility of Monitoring MA

The presence of MA alone may have limited diagnostic value since it represents a very sensitive but disease-nonspecific marker of increased vascular permeability and inflammation *(41)*. However, in patients at increased risk for CVD or CKD, measurement of UAE can be a very useful guide for CVD risk assessment, disease severity evaluation, and as a marker of target organ damage. The benefit of using MA in lieu of other markers to evaluate the CVD risk, or screen for target organ injury, is that it is inexpensive, easy to obtain in the clinical setting, and the results are rapidly available *(45,104,105)*.

The utility of assessment of MA in patients with increased risk for CVD and CKD, like patients with diabetes or hypertension, seems clear. These patients should be screened annually for MA. Documented persistent elevations of UAE (2 out of 3 measurements above reference range) in individuals undergoing treatment for these disorders should be retested within 6 months. After complete diagnosis and evaluation, continued surveillance is recommended to assess response to therapy *(106)*. The routine determination of MA in the general population is debatable, in part due to the relatively low prevalence of MA in the general population and uncertainty of the significance of its modification in individuals free of major risk factors for CVD and CKD *(71,105)* However, targeting high-risk patients may be of greater value. A recent cost-effectiveness analysis of screening for proteinuria to slow progression of CKD and decrease mortality reported that it is not cost-effective, unless selectively directed toward high-risk groups (older persons and persons with hypertension) or conducted at an infrequent interval of 10 years *(107)*. However the authors took into account only the utility of protein-uria to assess risk for renal outcomes. Future research is needed to assess the cost-effectiveness of MA screening in various groups, taking also into account its possible use as a marker of increased CVD risk.

CKD AS CARDIOVASCULAR RISK FACTOR

Historically, the first observations that patients with ESRD had elevated rates for cardiovas-cular complications and death were made more than 30 years ago *(1,2)*, as mentioned above. Recent data suggest that among patients in the Medicare database in the United States, 80% of those with CKD submitted CVD claims over a 2-year period compared with only 45% of those without CKD, and the prevalence of heart failure was four times higher in CKD patients compared to those without CKD *(39)*. In ESRD patients treated by dialysis, the risk of CVD is enormously elevated, with cardiovascular mortality rates in various studies being approximately 15 times higher than age- and sex-matched controls in the general population *(108)*.

As evident from several of the above studies linking MA with CVD risk, there is a continuous association between the level of UAE and the risk for cardiovascular morbidity and mortal-ity and, thus, the presence of macroalbuminuria or clinical proteinuria was associated with a higher risk for cardiovascular events than MA *(76,80–84)*. Since the presence of macroalbu-minuria or clinical proteinuria is a clear manifestation of overt nephropathy and is associated with faster deterioration of kidney function *(9,17,109)*, the underlying mechanisms for the increase in cardiovascular risk in macroalbuminiric patients is somehow different from those in patients with MA; that is, the excess cardiovascular risk in patients with macroalbumin-uria could be attributed not only to the presence of a generalized vascular injury, as in the case of MA, but also to the appearance of a number of uremia-related factors which can also promote CVD.

In parallel to the common presence of many of the traditional (hypertension, diabetes, obesity etc.) or nontraditional (i.e., hyperhomocysteinemia) cardiovascular risk factors in patients with CKD *(9)*, as GFR falls below 60 ml/min/1.73 m^2 and most physiological functions of the kidney start to wane, a number of factors that are related to impaired renal function and can further con-tribute to CVD also appear *(110,111)*, providing explanations for the independent connection between renal function loss and cardiovascular risk. These factors become obvious clinically when the GFR falls below 45 ml/min/1.73 m^2 and blatant at a GFR of 30 ml/min/1.73 m^2. The most important of these uremia-related factors seem to be changes in calcium/phosphorus and related hormones homeostasis and anemia resulting from reduced production of erythropoietin. In particular, changes in calcium, phosphorus, and parathyroid hormone (PTH) metabolism have been associated with increased vascular calcification, arteriosclerosis, and cardiovascu-lar risk, while recent evidence suggests that reduced levels of vitamin D also contribute in increased cardiovascular mortality in CKD patients *(112)*. On the other hand, the decrease in erythropoietin production results in anemia which through various effects on the cardiovascu-lar system, mainly left ventricular hypertrophy, is also associated with adverse cardiovascular outcomes in CKD patients *(113)*. Moreover, preliminary evidence suggests that both vitamin D supplementation and partial correction of hemoglobin levels are associated with reduction of cardiovascular events *(112,113)*.

Since the very first observations in ESRD patients *(1,2)*, a considerable amount of studies tried to investigate the association between renal function and cardiovascular outcomes or over-all mortality either in populations with or without CVD. Most of these studies suggested that mild-to-moderate elevations in serum creatinine levels were associated with increased risk of cardiovascular events or cardiovascular death *(114–118)*, as well as of death from any cause *(5,114,115,117–122)*, whereas a few did not confirm these results *(123)*. A major limitation of these studies was the use of only serum creatinine levels to assess the level of renal function *(5,114–117,119–123)* with different cut-off values to define the presence or the stages of CKD *(5,114–116,119–123)*, as well as the use of dichotomous groups of estimated kidney function *(5,114,115,118–121,123)*. Several were also characterized by relatively small numbers of individuals with CKD *(5,114,115,117–121,123)* and others were restricted to study of selected populations (elderly subjects, patients with CVD, etc.) *(116–119,122)*.

Thus, it is only very recently that studies performed either on the general population *(82,124,125)* or in patients with pre-existing CVD *(126,127)* evaluated the association between the continuum of kidney function loss and cardiovascular risk using the level of GFR and gave more precise information. In the above-mentioned study in the subcohort of the NHANES II population, the investigators also examined the associations of the level of GFR estimated with the MDRD formula with cardiovascular and overall mortality *(82)*. Cardiovascular disease-related mortality rates were 4.1, 8.6, and 20.5 deaths/1000 person-years of follow-up among participants with estimated GFR of $\geq$90 ml/min, 70–89 ml/min, and <70 ml/min, respectively. In addition, after adjustment for multiple related confounders, individuals with estimated GFR of <70 ml/min had a 68% higher risk of death from CVD, 51% higher risk of death from all causes compared with subjects with estimated GFR of $\geq$90 ml/min during the 16 years of follow-up. Similarly, Manjunath et al. examined the association between GFR levels and cardiovascular events in 15,350 subjects from the population-based Atherosclerosis Risk in Communities (ARIC) study that were followed up for a mean of 6.2 years *(124)*. Subjects with GFR of 15–59 ml/min/1.73 m^2 had a 38% higher risk for cardiovascular events and subjects with GFR of 60–89 ml/min/1.73 m^2 had a 16% higher risk compared with subjects with GFR of 90–150 ml/min/1.73 m^2, after adjustment for multiple CVD risk factors. Moreover, each 10 ml/min/1.73 m^2 lower GFR was associated with a significant adjusted hazard ratio of 1.05, 1.07, and 1.06 for CVD, de novo CVD, and recurrent CVD, respectively. Comparable were the findings in a cohort of almost 5000 subjects over 65 years of age that were followed for 5 years. In this study, after adjustment for multiple confounders each 10 ml/min/1.73 m^2 lower GFR was associated with a significantly elevated hazard ratio of 1.05 for CVD, 1.07 for de novo CVD, 1.04 for recurrent CVD, and 1.06 for all-cause mortality *(128)*.

In addition to the above, a recently published prospective cohort study on a sample of more than 1.1 million individuals participating in a large, integrated system of healthcare delivery in the area of San Francisco in the United States, which used again the MDRD formula for GFR to estimate the level of kidney function, seem to provide the best evidence on the field *(125)*. After a median follow-up of 2.84 years, which amounts for over 3 million person-years of follow-up, the adjusted hazard ratio for cardiovascular events was 1.4 for individuals with a GFR 45–59 ml/min/1.73 m^2, 2.0 for those with GFR 30–44 ml/min/1.73 m^2, 2.8 for those with GFR 15–29 ml/min/1.73 m^2, and 3.4 for individuals with GFR <15 ml/min/1.73 m^2, respectively, compared to subjects with GFR $\geq$60 ml/min/1.73 m^2, which were used as the reference group. The adjusted risk of death from all causes also increased inversely with the estimated GFR, being 1.2, 1.8, 3.2, and 5.9 for individuals with a GFR 45–59 ml/min/1.73 m^2, 30–44 ml/min/1.73 m^2, 15–29 ml/min/1.73 m^2, and <15 ml/min/1.73 m^2, respectively, compared to those with GFR $\geq$60 ml/min/1.73 m^2, while the adjusted risk of hospitalization followed the same pattern. Of note, the confidence intervals for the calculated adjusted risks were very small, obviously due to the enormous sample size; thus, the results provide very accurate estimates of the actual risks. In spite of some limitations (e.g., lack of information for some confounders and concerns about the generalizability of the findings), this study seems to provide the definite evidence on the association between the continuum of renal function and the risk of CVD in the general population.

In regards to patients that already had suffered a cardiovascular event, a recent study also reported an independent association between declining GFR estimated with the MDRD formula and increasing cardiovascular risk *(126)*. This study included 14,527 patients with acute myocardial infarction complicated by clinical or radiologic signs of heart failure, left ventricular dysfunction, or both, that had a serum creatinine measurement from the original population of the prospective Valsartan in Acute Myocardial Infarction Trial (VALIANT). After a median follow-up of 24.7 months, the adjusted hazard ratio for the composite endpoint (death from cardiovascular causes, congestive heart failure, recurrent myocardial infarction, resuscitation after cardiac arrest and stroke) was 1.10 for individuals with a GFR 60–74.9 ml/min/1.73 m^2, 1.26 for those with GFR 45–59.9 ml/min/1.73 m^2, and 1.49 for those with GFR <45 ml/min/1.73 m^2, respectively, compared to subjects of the reference group with GFR ≥75 ml/min/1.73 m^2. The adjusted risk from overall death was 1.14, 1.38, and 1.70 for individuals with GFR 60–74.9 ml/min/1.73 m^2, 45–59.9 ml/min/1.73 m^2, and <45 ml/min/1.73 m^2, respectively, compared to the subjects with GFR ≥75 ml/min/1.73 m^2. Furthermore, for baseline estimated GFR values below a considerably high renal function level, that of 81.0 ml/min/1.73 m^2, each 10-unit decrease in GFR was associated with an adjusted hazard ratio of 1.10 for death and nonfatal cardiovascular outcomes.

Similarly, based on previous observations linking decreased renal function with increased risk for cardiovascular outcomes in patients with chronic heart failure (CHF) and reduced left ventricular ejection fraction, a recent study examined this association in patients with various levels of left ventricular function, with the use of GFR derived from the MDRD formula *(127)*. The analysis included 2680 patients from the population of The Candesartan in Heart Failure: Assessment of Reduction in Mortality and Morbidity (CHARM) programme of clinical trials. After a median follow-up of 34.4 months, the adjusted hazard ratio for the primary outcome of cardiovascular death or hospitalization for worsening CHF was 1.54 for patients with GFR 45–60 ml/min/1.73 m^2 and 1.86 for those with GFR <45 ml/min/1.73 m^2 compared to patients with GFR >60 ml/min/1.73 m^2. Further, the adjusted hazard ratio for all-cause mortality was 1.50 for patients with GFR 45–60 ml/min/1.73 m^2 and 1.91 for those with GFR <45 ml/min/1.73 m^2. This effect of GFR was not related to the level of left ventricular ejection fraction, which was also found to be an independent predictor of worse outcomes.

Studies that examined the prognostic importance of renal dysfunction after coronary artery bypass graft (CABG) surgery in patients with CAD yielded comparable results. Previous studies on the field have showed that both ESRD *(129,130)* and severe renal dysfunction not requiring renal replacement therapy *(131–133)* are associated with increased morbidity and mortality after CABG. However, the latter studies also identified patients with renal dysfunction by splitting the examined populations into dichotomized groups on the basis of serum creatinine level and not measuring renal function as a continuous variable *(111)*. Again, recent studies that used GFR as a measure of renal function, estimated either with the Cockcroft–Gault *(134)* or the MDRD formula *(135,136)*, have clearly showed that reduced GFR was independently associated with elevated operative morbidity and mortality as well as postoperative mortality. Of note, as in the general population, in the latter studies the relation between renal dysfunction and mortality risk was not linear but presented a steep increase when GFR fell below a threshold of about 60 ml/min/1.73 m^2 *(135,136)*.

CONCLUSION

Recently accumulated data have allowed a better understanding of the pathophysiology, epidemiology, and clinical significance of the relationships between MA or CKD and the risk of CVD. Both MA and CKD are clearly associated with a higher risk for cardiovascular events, as well as cardiovascular and overall mortality in the general population and in patients with other cardiovascular risk factors or prevalent CVD. Therefore, the routine assessments of MA with the use of UACR, and level of the renal function with estimation of GFR, can be a very useful guide for overall CVD risk evaluation and should be both implemented in clinical practice, at least for individuals with high cardiovascular risk. Further research should define in detail the populations that would benefit from these routine measurements and future guidelines should provide clear recommendations for their clinical use.

REFERENCES

1. Ma KW, Masler DS, Brown DC. Hemodialysis in diabetic patients with chronic renal failure. *Ann Intern Med* 1975; **83**(2):215–217.
2. Maher JF, Bryan CW, Ahearn DJ. Prognosis of chronic renal failure. II. Factors affecting survival. *Arch Intern Med* 1975; **135**(2):273–278.
3. Viberti GC, Hill RD, Jarrett RJ, Argyropoulos A, Mahmud U, Keen H. Microalbuminuria as a predictor of clinical nephropathy in insulin-dependent diabetes mellitus. *Lancet* 1982; **1**(8287):1430–1432.
4. Mogensen CE. Microalbuminuria predicts clinical proteinuria and early mortality in maturity-onset diabetes. *N Eng J Med* 1984; **310**(6):356–360.
5. Damsgaard EM, Froland A, Jorgensen OD, Mogensen CE. Microalbuminuria as predictor of increased mortality in elderly people. *Br Med J* 1990; **300**(6720):297–300.
6. Messent JW, Elliott TG, Hill RD, Jarrett RJ, Keen H, Viberti GC. Prognostic significance of microalbuminuria in insulin-dependent diabetes mellitus: a twenty-three year follow-up study. *Kidney Int* 1992; **41**(4):836–839.
7. Stehouwer CD, Nauta JJ, Zeldenrust GC, Hackeng WH, Donker AJ, den Ottolander GJ. Urinary albumin excretion, cardiovascular disease, and endothelial dysfunction in non-insulin-dependent diabetes mellitus. *Lancet* 1992; **340**(8815):319–323.
8. American Diabetes Association. Nephropathy in diabetes. *Diabetes Care* 2004; **27**(Suppl 1):S79-S83.
9. Kidney Disease Outcomes Quality Initiative (K/DOQI). K/DOQI clinical practice guidelines on hypertension and antihypertensive agents in chronic kidney disease. *Am J Kidney Dis* 2004; **43**(5 Suppl 1):S1–290.
10. Busby DE, Bakris GL. Comparison of commonly used assays for the detection of microalbuminuria. *J Clin Hypertens (Greenwich)* 2004; **6**(11 Suppl 3):8–12.
11. Rowe DJ, Bagga H, Betts PB. Normal variations in rate of albumin excretion and albumin to creatinine ratios in overnight and daytime urine collections in non-diabetic children. *Br Med J (Clin Res Ed)* 1985; **291**(6497):693–694.
12. Metcalf PA, Baker JR, Scragg RK, Dryson E, Scott AJ, Wild CJ. Microalbuminuria in a middle-aged workforce. Effect of hyperglycemia and ethnicity. *Diabetes Care* 1993; **16**(11):1485–1493.
13. James MA, Fotherby MD, Potter JF. Microalbuminuria in elderly hypertensives: reproducibility and relation to clinic and ambulatory blood pressure. *J Hypertens* 1994; **12**(3):309–314.
14. Metcalf PA, Scragg RK. Epidemiology of microalbuminuria in the general population. *J Diabetes Complications* 1994; **8**(3):157–163.
15. Bakris GL, Smith A. Effects of sodium intake on albumin excretion in patients with diabetic nephropathy treated with long-acting calcium antagonists. *Ann Intern Med* 1996; **125**(3):201–204.
16. Mattix HJ, Hsu CY, Shaykevich S, Curhan G. Use of the albumin/creatinine ratio to detect microalbuminuria: implications of sex and race. *J Am Soc Nephrol* 2002; **13**(4):1034–1039.
17. National Kidney Foundation. K/DOQI clinical practice guidelines for chronic kidney disease: evaluation, classification, and stratification. Kidney Disease Outcome Quality Initiative. *Am J Kidney Dis* 2002; **39**(2 Suppl 1):S1–266.
18. Levey AS, Coresh J, Balk E, Kausz AT, Levin A, Steffes MW, et al. National Kidney Foundation practice guidelines for chronic kidney disease: evaluation, classification, and stratification. *Ann Intern Med* 2003; **139**(2):137–147.
19. Howey JE, Browning MC, Fraser CG. Biologic variation of urinary albumin: consequences for analysis, specimen collection, interpretation of results, and screening programs. *Am J Kidney Dis* 1989; **13**(1):35–37.

20. Levey AS. Measurement of renal function in chronic renal disease. *Kidney Int* 1990; **38**(1):167–184.
21. Perrone RD, Madias NE, Levey AS. Serum creatinine as an index of renal function: new insights into old concepts. *Clin Chem* 1992; **38**(10):1933–1953.
22. Perrone RD, Steinman TI, Beck GJ, Skibinski CI, Royal HD, Lawlor M, et al. Utility of radioisotopic filtration markers in chronic renal insufficiency: simultaneous comparison of 125I-iothalamate, 169Yb-DTPA, 99mTc-DTPA, and inulin. The Modification of Diet in Renal Disease Study. *Am J Kidney Dis* 1990; **16**(3): 224–235.
23. Cockcroft DW, Gault MH. Prediction of creatinine clearance from serum creatinine. *Nephron* 1976; **16**(1): 31–41.
24. Levey AS, Bosch JP, Lewis JB, Greene T, Rogers N, Roth D. A more accurate method to estimate glomerular filtration rate from serum creatinine: a new prediction equation. Modification of Diet in Renal Disease Study Group. *Ann Intern Med* 1999; **130**(6):461–470.
25. Dinneen SF, Gerstein HC. The association of microalbuminuria and mortality in non-insulin-dependent diabetes mellitus. A systematic overview of the literature. *Arch Intern Med* 1997; **157**(13):1413–1418.
26. Bennett PH, Haffner S, Kasiske BL, Keane WF, Mogensen CE, Parving HH, et al. Screening and management of microalbuminuria in patients with diabetes mellitus: recommendations to the Scientific Advisory Board of the National Kidney Foundation from an ad hoc committee of the Council on Diabetes Mellitus of the National Kidney Foundation. *Am J Kidney Dis* 1995; **25**(1):107–112.
27. Mogensen CE, Poulsen PL. Epidemiology of microalbuminuria in diabetes and in the background population. *Curr Opin Nephrol Hypertens* 1994; **3**(3):248–256.
28. Pontremoli R, Viazzi F, Sofia A, Tomolillo C, Ruello N, Bezante GP, et al. Microalbuminuria: a marker of cardiovascular risk and organ damage in essential hypertension. *Kidney Int Suppl* 1997; **63**:S163–S165.
29. Jensen JS, Clausen P, Borch-Johnsen K, Jensen G, Feldt-Rasmussen B. Detecting microalbuminuria by urinary albumin/creatinine concentration ratio. *Nephrol Dial Transplant* 1997; **12**(Suppl 2):6–9.
30. Cirillo M, Senigalliesi L, Laurenzi M, Alfieri R, Stamler J, Stamler R, et al. Microalbuminuria in nondiabetic adults: relation of blood pressure, body mass index, plasma cholesterol levels, and smoking: The Gubbio Population Study. *Arch Intern Med* 1998; **158**(17):1933–1939.
31. Mimran A, Ribstein J, DuCailar G, Halimi JM. Albuminuria in normals and essential hypertension. *J Diabetes Complications* 1994; **8**(3):150–156.
32. Effects of ramipril on cardiovascular and microvascular outcomes in people with diabetes mellitus: results of the HOPE study and MICRO-HOPE substudy. Heart outcomes prevention evaluation study investigators. *Lancet* 2000; **355**(9200):253–259.
33. Mathiesen ER, Ronn B, Storm B, Foght H, Deckert T. The natural course of microalbuminuria in insulin-dependent diabetes: a 10-year prospective study. *Diabet Med* 1995; **12**(6):482–487.
34. Schmitz A. Microalbuminuria, blood pressure, metabolic control, and renal involvement: longitudinal studies in white non-insulin-dependent diabetic patients. *Am J Hypertens* 1997; **10**(9 Pt 2):189S-197S.
35. Gerber LM, Shmukler C, Alderman MH. Differences in urinary albumin excretion rate between normotensive and hypertensive, white and nonwhite subjects. *Arch Intern Med* 1992; **152**(2):373–377.
36. Parving HH, Mogensen CE, Jensen HA, Evrin PE. Increased urinary albumin-excretion rate in benign essential hypertension. *Lancet* 1974; **1**(7868):1190–1192.
37. Bigazzi R, Bianchi S, Campese VM, Baldari G. Prevalence of microalbuminuria in a large population of patients with mild to moderate essential hypertension. *Nephron* 1992; **61**(1):94–97.
38. Coresh J, Astor BC, Greene T, Eknoyan G, Levey AS. Prevalence of chronic kidney disease and decreased kidney function in the adult US population: Third National Health and Nutrition Examination Survey. *Am J Kidney Dis* 2003; **41**(1):1–12.
39. U.S. Renal Data System: USRDS 2004 Annual Data Report: Atlas of End-Stage Renal Disease in the United States. Bethesda, MD: National Institutes of Health, National Institute of Diabetes and Digestive and Kidney Diseases. 2004. Ref Type: Serial (Book,Monograph)
40. Gosling P. Microalbuminuria: a marker of systemic disease. *Br J Hosp Med* 1995; **54**(6):285–290.
41. Jensen JS. Renal and systemic transvascular albumin leakage in severe atherosclerosis. *Arterioscler Thromb Vasc Biol* 1995; **15**(9):1324–1329.
42. Deckert T, Kofoed-Enevoldsen A, Norgaard K, Borch-Johnsen K, Feldt-Rasmussen B, Jensen T. Microalbuminuria. Implications for micro- and macrovascular disease. *Diabetes Care* 1992; **15**(9):1181–1191.
43. Stehouwer CD, Lambert J, Donker AJ, van H, V. Endothelial dysfunction and pathogenesis of diabetic angiopathy. *Cardiovasc Res* 1997; **34**(1):55–68.
44. Yaqoob M, McClelland P, Patrick AW, Stevenson A, Mason H, White MC, et al. Evidence of oxidant injury and tubular damage in early diabetic nephropathy. *QJM* 1994; **87**(10):601–607.
45. Bakris GL. Microalbuminuria: prognostic implications. *Curr Opin Nephrol Hypertens* 1996; **5**(3):219–223.

46. Mogyorosi A, Ziyadeh FN. Update on pathogenesis, markers and management of diabetic nephropathy. *Curr Opin Nephrol Hypertens* 1996; **5**(3):243–253.
47. Yudkin JS, Forrest RD, Jackson CA. Microalbuminuria as predictor of vascular disease in non-diabetic subjects. Islington Diabetes Survey. *Lancet* 1988; **2**(8610):530–533.
48. Haffner SM, Stern MP, Gruber MK, Hazuda HP, Mitchell BD, Patterson JK. Microalbuminuria. Potential marker for increased cardiovascular risk factors in nondiabetic subjects? *Arteriosclerosis* 1990; **10**(5):727–731.
49. Winocour PH, Harland JO, Millar JP, Laker MF, Alberti KG. Microalbuminuria and associated cardiovascular risk factors in the community. *Atherosclerosis* 1992; **93**(1–2):71–81.
50. Woo J, Cockram CS, Swaminathan R, Lau E, Chan A, Cheung R. Microalbuminuria and other cardiovascular risk factors in nondiabetic subjects. *Int J Cardiol* 1992; **37**(3):345–350.
51. Haffner SM, Morales PA, Gruber MK, Hazuda HP, Stern MP. Cardiovascular risk factors in non-insulin-dependent diabetic subjects with microalbuminuria. *Arterioscler Thromb* 1993; **13**(2):205–210.
52. Groop PH, Viberti GC, Elliott TG, Friedman R, Mackie A, Ehnholm C, et al. Lipoprotein(a) in type 1 diabetic patients with renal disease. *Diabet Med* 1994; **11**(10):961–967.
53. Palatini P, Graniero GR, Mormino P, Mattarei M, Sanzuol F, Cignacco GB, et al. Prevalence and clinical correlates of microalbuminuria in stage I hypertension. Results from the Hypertension and Ambulatory Recording Venetia Study (HARVEST Study). *Am J Hypertens* 1996; **9**(4 Pt 1):334–341.
54. Agrawal B, Berger A, Wolf K, Luft FC. Microalbuminuria screening by reagent strip predicts cardiovascular risk in hypertension. *J Hypertens* 1996; **14**(2):223–228.
55. Hodge AM, Dowse GK, Zimmet PZ. Microalbuminuria, cardiovascular risk factors, and insulin resistance in two populations with a high risk of type 2 diabetes mellitus. *Diabet Med* 1996; **13**(5):441–449.
56. Jensen JS, Feldt-Rasmussen B, Borch-Johnsen K, Clausen P, Appleyard M, Jensen G. Microalbuminuria and its relation to cardiovascular disease and risk factors. A population-based study of 1254 hypertensive individuals [see comments]. *J Hum Hypertens* 1997; **11**(11):727–732.
57. Mykkanen L, Zaccaro DJ, Wagenknecht LE, Robbins DC, Gabriel M, Haffner SM. Microalbuminuria is associated with insulin resistance in nondiabetic subjects: the insulin resistance atherosclerosis study. *Diabetes* 1998; **47**(5):793–800.
58. Kim CH, Kim HK, Park JY, Park HS, Hong SK, Park SW, et al. Association of microalbuminuria and atherosclerotic risk factors in non-diabetic subjects in Korea. *Diabetes Res Clin Pract* 1998; **40**(3):191–199.
59. Hoogeveen EK, Kostense PJ, Jager A, Heine RJ, Jakobs C, Bouter LM, et al. Serum homocysteine level and protein intake are related to risk of microalbuminuria: the Hoorn Study. *Kidney Int* 1998; **54**(1):203–209.
60. Tomura S, Kawada K, Saito K, Lin YL, Endou K, Hirano C, et al. Prevalence of microalbuminuria and relationship to the risk of cardiovascular disease in the Japanese population. *Am J Nephrol* 1999; **19**(1):13–20.
61. Halimi JM, Forhan A, Balkau B, Novak M, Wilpart E, Tichet J, et al. Is microalbuminuria an integrated risk marker for cardiovascular disease and insulin resistance in both men and women? *J Cardiovasc Risk* 2001; **8**(3):139–146.
62. Hillege HL, Janssen WM, Bak AA, Diercks GF, Grobbee DE, Crijns HJ, et al. Microalbuminuria is common, also in a nondiabetic, nonhypertensive population, and an independent indicator of cardiovascular risk factors and cardiovascular morbidity. *J Intern Med* 2001; **249**(6):519–526.
63. Kim YI, Kim CH, Choi CS, Chung YE, Lee MS, Lee SI, et al. Microalbuminuria is associated with the insulin resistance syndrome independent of hypertension and type 2 diabetes in the Korean population. *Diabetes Res Clin Pract* 2001; **52**(2):145–152.
64. Romundstad S, Holmen J, Hallan H, Kvenild K, Kruger O, Midthjell K. Microalbuminuria, cardiovascular disease and risk factors in a nondiabetic/nonhypertensive population. The Nord-Trondelag Health Study (HUNT, 1995–1997), Norway. *J Intern Med* 2002; **252**(2):164–172.
65. Nakamura M, Onoda T, Itai K, Ohsawa M, Satou K, Sakai T, et al. Association between serum C-reactive protein levels and microalbuminuria: a population-based cross-sectional study in northern Iwate, Japan. *Intern Med* 2004; **43**(10):919–925.
66. Barzilay JI, Peterson D, Cushman M, Heckbert SR, Cao JJ, Blaum C, et al. The relationship of cardiovascular risk factors to microalbuminuria in older adults with or without diabetes mellitus or hypertension: the cardiovascular health study. *Am J Kidney Dis* 2004; **44**(1):25–34.
67. Yuyun MF, Khaw KT, Luben R, Welch A, Bingham S, Day NE, et al. Microalbuminuria, cardiovascular risk factors and cardiovascular morbidity in a British population: the EPIC-Norfolk population-based study. *Eur J Cardiovasc Prev Rehabil* 2004; **11**(3):207–213.
68. Tsioufis C, Dimitriadis K, Chatzis D, Vasiliadou C, Tousoulis D, Papademetriou V, et al. Relation of microalbuminuria to adiponectin and augmented C-reactive protein levels in men with essential hypertension. *Am J Cardiol* 2005; **96**(7):946–951.

69. Kistorp C, Raymond I, Pedersen F, Gustafsson F, Faber J, Hildebrandt P. N-terminal pro-brain natriuretic peptide, C-reactive protein, and urinary albumin levels as predictors of mortality and cardiovascular events in older adults. *JAMA* 2005; **293**(13):1609–1616.

70. De Cosmo S, Minenna A, Ludovico O, Mastroianno S, Di Giorgio A, Pirro L, et al. Increased urinary albumin excretion, insulin resistance, and related cardiovascular risk factors in patients with type 2 diabetes: evidence of a sex-specific association. *Diabetes Care* 2005; **28**(4):910–915.

71. Alzaid AA. Microalbuminuria in patients with NIDDM: an overview. *Diabetes Care* 1996; **19**(1):79–89.

72. Bakris GL, Sowers JR. Microalbuminuria in diabetes: focus on cardiovascular and renal risk reduction. *Curr Diab Rep* 2002; **2**(3):258–262.

73. Karalliedde J, Viberti G. Microalbuminuria and cardiovascular risk. *Am J Hypertens* 2004; **17**(10):986–993.

74. Weir MR. Microalbuminuria in type 2 diabetics: an important, overlooked cardiovascular risk factor. *J Clin Hypertens (Greenwich)* 2004; **6**(3):134–141.

75. Pontremoli R, Leoncini G, Viazzi F, Parodi D, Vaccaro V, Falqui V, et al. Role of microalbuminuria in the assessment of cardiovascular risk in essential hypertension. *J Am Soc Nephrol* 2005; **16 Suppl 1**:S39-S41.

76. Agewall S, Wikstrand J, Ljungman S, Fagerberg B. Usefulness of microalbuminuria in predicting cardiovascular mortality in treated hypertensive men with and without diabetes mellitus. Risk Factor Intervention Study Group. *Am J Cardiol* 1997; **80**(2):164–169.

77. Valmadrid CT, Klein R, Moss SE, Klein BE. The risk of cardiovascular disease mortality associated with microalbuminuria and gross proteinuria in persons with older-onset diabetes mellitus. *Arch Intern Med* 2000; **160**(8):1093–1100.

78. Kuusisto J, Mykkanen L, Pyorala K, Laakso M. Hyperinsulinemic microalbuminuria. A new risk indicator for coronary heart disease. *Circulation* 1995; **91**(3):831–837.

79. Jensen JS, Feldt-Rasmussen B, Strandgaard S, Schroll M, Borch-Johnsen K. Arterial hypertension, microalbuminuria, and risk of ischemic heart disease. *Hypertension* 2000; **35**(4):898–903.

80. Gerstein HC, Mann JF, Yi Q, Zinman B, Dinneen SF, Hoogwerf B, et al. Albuminuria and risk of cardiovascular events, death, and heart failure in diabetic and nondiabetic individuals. *JAMA* 2001; **286**(4):421–426.

81. Wachtell K, Ibsen H, Olsen MH, Borch-Johnsen K, Lindholm LH, Mogensen CE, et al. Albuminuria and cardiovascular risk in hypertensive patients with left ventricular hypertrophy: the LIFE study. *Ann Intern Med* 2003; **139**(11):901–906.

82. Muntner P, He J, Hamm L, Loria C, Whelton PK. Renal insufficiency and subsequent death resulting from cardiovascular disease in the United States. *J Am Soc Nephrol* 2002; **13**(3):745–753.

83. Yuyun MF, Khaw KT, Luben R, Welch A, Bingham S, Day NE, et al. A prospective study of microalbuminuria and incident coronary heart disease and its prognostic significance in a British population: the EPIC-Norfolk study. *Am J Epidemiol* 2004; **159**(3):284–293.

84. Yuyun MF, Khaw KT, Luben R, Welch A, Bingham S, Day NE, et al. Microalbuminuria and stroke in a British population: the European Prospective Investigation into Cancer in Norfolk (EPIC-Norfolk) population study. *J Intern Med* 2004; **255**(2):247–256.

85. Yuyun MF, Khaw KT, Luben R, Welch A, Bingham S, Day NE, et al. Microalbuminuria independently predicts all-cause and cardiovascular mortality in a British population: The European Prospective Investigation into Cancer in Norfolk (EPIC-Norfolk) population study. *Int J Epidemiol* 2004; **33**(1):189–198.

86. Schrader J, Luders S, Kulschewski A, Hammersen F, Zuchner C, Venneklaas U, et al. Microalbuminuria and tubular proteinuria as risk predictors of cardiovascular morbidity and mortality in essential hypertension: final results of a prospective long-term study (MARPLE Study)*. *J Hypertens* 2006; **24**(3):541–548.

87. Ibsen H, Wachtell K, Olsen MH, Borch-Johnsen K, Lindholm LH, Mogensen CE, et al. Does albuminuria predict cardiovascular outcome on treatment with losartan versus atenolol in hypertension with left ventricular hypertrophy? A LIFE substudy. *J Hypertens* 2004; **22**(9):1805–1811.

88. Asselbergs FW, Diercks GF, Hillege HL, van Boven AJ, Janssen WM, Voors AA, et al. Effects of fosinopril and pravastatin on cardiovascular events in subjects with microalbuminuria. *Circulation* 2004; **110**(18):2809–2816.

89. Cerasola G, Cottone S, D'Ignoto G, Grasso L, Mangano MT, Carapelle E, et al. Micro-albuminuria as a predictor of cardiovascular damage in essential hypertension. *J Hypertens Suppl* 1989; **7**(6):S332-S333.

90. Pedrinelli R, Bello VD, Catapano G, Talarico L, Materazzi F, Santoro G, et al. Microalbuminuria is a marker of left ventricular hypertrophy but not hyperinsulinemia in nondiabetic atherosclerotic patients. *Arterioscler Thromb* 1993; **13**(6):900–906.

91. Redon J, Liao Y, Lozano JV, Miralles A, Baldo E, Cooper RS. Factors related to the presence of microalbuminuria in essential hypertension. *Am J Hypertens* 1994; **7**(9 Pt 1):801–807.

92. Pontremoli R, Nicolella C, Viazzi F, Ravera M, Sofia A, Berruti V, et al. Microalbuminuria is an early marker of target organ damage in essential hypertension. *Am J Hypertens* 1998; **11**(4 Pt 1):430–438.

93. Leoncini G, Sacchi G, Ravera M, Viazzi F, Ratto E, Vettoretti S, et al. Microalbuminuria is an integrated marker of subclinical organ damage in primary hypertension. *J Hum Hypertens* 2002; **16**(6):399–404.

94. Dell'Omo G, Penno G, Giorgi D, Di B, V, Mariani M, Pedrinelli R. Association between high-normal albuminuria and risk factors for cardiovascular and renal disease in essential hypertensive men. *Am J Kidney Dis* 2002; **40**(1):1–8.

95. Olsen MH, Wachtell K, Borch-Johnsen K, Okin PM, Kjeldsen SE, Dahlof B, et al. A blood pressure independent association between glomerular albumin leakage and electrocardiographic left ventricular hypertrophy. The LIFE Study. Losartan Intervention For Endpoint reduction. *J Hum Hypertens* 2002; **16**(8):591–595.

96. Bigazzi R, Bianchi S, Nenci R, Baldari D, Baldari G, Campese VM. Increased thickness of the carotid artery in patients with essential hypertension and microalbuminuria. *J Hum Hypertens* 1995; **9**(10):827–833.

97. Mykkanen L, Zaccaro DJ, O'Leary DH, Howard G, Robbins DC, Haffner SM. Microalbuminuria and carotid artery intima-media thickness in nondiabetic and NIDDM subjects. The Insulin Resistance Atherosclerosis Study (IRAS). *Stroke* 1997; **28**(9):1710–1716.

98. Tuttle KR, Puhlman ME, Cooney SK, Short R. Urinary albumin and insulin as predictors of coronary artery disease: An angiographic study. *Am J Kidney Dis* 1999; **34**(5):918–925.

99. Biesenbach G, Zazgornik J. High prevalence of hypertensive retinopathy and coronary heart disease in hypertensive patients with persistent microalbuminuria under short intensive antihypertensive therapy. *Clin Nephrol* 1994; **41**(4):211–218.

100. Devereux RB, Alderman MH. Role of preclinical cardiovascular disease in the evolution from risk factor exposure to development of morbid events. *Circulation* 1993; **88**(4 Pt 1):1444–1455.

101. Gosling P, Hughes EA, Reynolds TM, Fox JP. Microalbuminuria is an early response following acute myocardial infarction. *Eur Heart J* 1991; **12**(4):508–513.

102. Hickey NC, Shearman CP, Gosling P, Simms MH. Assessment of intermittent claudication by quantitation of exercise-induced microalbuminuria. *Eur J Vasc Surg* 1990; **4**(6):603–606.

103. Abid O, Sun Q, Sugimoto K, Mercan D, Vincent JL. Predictive value of microalbuminuria in medical ICU patients: results of a pilot study. *Chest* 2001; **120**(6):1984–1988.

104. Gosling P. Microalbuminuria and cardiovascular risk: a word of caution. *J Hum Hypertens* 1998; **12**(4):211–213.

105. Lydakis C, Efstratopoulos A, Lip GY. Microalbuminuria in hypertension: is it up to measure? *J Hum Hypertens* 1997; **11**(11):695–697.

106. Bakris GL. Clinical importance of microalbuminuria in diabetes and hypertension. *Curr Hypertens Rep* 2004; **6**(5):352–356.

107. Boulware LE, Jaar BG, Tarver-Carr ME, Brancati FL, Powe NR. Screening for proteinuria in US adults: a cost-effectiveness analysis. *JAMA* 2003; **290**(23):3101–3114.

108. Sarnak MJ, Levey AS. Cardiovascular disease and chronic renal disease: a new paradigm. *Am J Kidney Dis* 2000; **35**(4 Suppl 1):S117-S131.

109. Lasaridis AN, Sarafidis PA. Diabetic nephropathy and antihypertensive treatment: what are the lessons from clinical trials? *Am J Hypertens* 2003; **16**(8):689–697.

110. Sarnak MJ. Cardiovascular complications in chronic kidney disease. *Am J Kidney Dis* 2003; **41**(5 Suppl):11–17.

111. Sarafidis PA, Bakris GL. Level of kidney function determines cardiovascular fate after coronary bypass graft surgery. *Circulation* 2006; **113**(8):1046–1047.

112. Levin A, Li YC. Vitamin D and its analogues: do they protect against cardiovascular disease in patients with kidney disease? *Kidney Int* 2005; **68**(5):1973–1981.

113. Locatelli F, Pozzoni P, Del VL. Anemia and heart failure in chronic kidney disease. *Semin Nephrol* 2005; **25**(6):392–396.

114. Wannamethee SG, Shaper AG, Perry IJ. Serum creatinine concentration and risk of cardiovascular disease: a possible marker for increased risk of stroke. *Stroke* 1997; **28**(3):557–563.

115. Mann JF, Gerstein HC, Pogue J, Bosch J, Yusuf S. Renal insufficiency as a predictor of cardiovascular outcomes and the impact of ramipril: the HOPE randomized trial. *Ann Intern Med* 2001; **134**(8):629–636.

116. Shlipak MG, Simon JA, Grady D, Lin F, Wenger NK, Furberg CD. Renal insufficiency and cardiovascular events in postmenopausal women with coronary heart disease. *J Am Coll Cardiol* 2001; **38**(3):705–711.

117. Wang JG, Staessen JA, Fagard RH, Birkenhager WH, Gong L, Liu L. Prognostic significance of serum creatinine and uric acid in older Chinese patients with isolated systolic hypertension. *Hypertension* 2001; **37**(4):1069–1074.

118. Ruilope LM, Salvetti A, Jamerson K, Hansson L, Warnold I, Wedel H, et al. Renal function and intensive lowering of blood pressure in hypertensive participants of the hypertension optimal treatment (HOT) study. *J Am Soc Nephrol* 2001; **12**(2):218–225.

119. Langford HG, Stamler J, Wassertheil-Smoller S, Prineas RJ. All-cause mortality in the Hypertension Detection and Follow-up Program: findings for the whole cohort and for persons with less severe hypertension, with and without other traits related to risk of mortality. *Prog Cardiovasc Dis* 1986; **29**(3 Suppl 1):29–54.

120. Shulman NB, Ford CE, Hall WD, Blaufox MD, Simon D, Langford HG, et al. Prognostic value of serum creatinine and effect of treatment of hypertension on renal function. Results from the hypertension detection and follow-up program. The Hypertension Detection and Follow-up Program Cooperative Group. *Hypertension* 1989; **13**(5 Suppl):I80-I93.

121. Culleton BF, Larson MG, Wilson PW, Evans JC, Parfrey PS, Levy D. Cardiovascular disease and mortality in a community-based cohort with mild renal insufficiency. *Kidney Int* 1999; **56**(6):2214–2219.

122. Shlipak MG, Heidenreich PA, Noguchi H, Chertow GM, Browner WS, McClellan MB. Association of renal insufficiency with treatment and outcomes after myocardial infarction in elderly patients. *Ann Intern Med* 2002; **137**(7):555–562.

123. Garg AX, Clark WF, Haynes RB, House AA. Moderate renal insufficiency and the risk of cardiovascular mortality: results from the NHANES I. *Kidney Int* 2002; **61**(4):1486–1494.

124. Manjunath G, Tighiouart H, Ibrahim H, Macleod B, Salem DN, Griffith JL, et al. Level of kidney function as a risk factor for atherosclerotic cardiovascular outcomes in the community. *J Am Coll Cardiol* 2003; **41**(1):47–55.

125. Go AS, Chertow GM, Fan D, McCulloch CE, Hsu CY. Chronic kidney disease and the risks of death, cardiovascular events, and hospitalization. *N Eng J Med* 2004; **351**(13):1296–1305.

126. Anavekar NS, McMurray JJ, Velazquez EJ, Solomon SD, Kober L, Rouleau JL, et al. Relation between renal dysfunction and cardiovascular outcomes after myocardial infarction. *N Eng J Med* 2004; **351**(13):1285–1295.

127. Hillege HL, Nitsch D, Pfeffer MA, Swedberg K, McMurray JJ, Yusuf S, et al. Renal function as a predictor of outcome in a broad spectrum of patients with heart failure. *Circulation* 2006; **113**(5):671–678.

128. Manjunath G, Tighiouart H, Coresh J, Macleod B, Salem DN, Griffith JL, et al. Level of kidney function as a risk factor for cardiovascular outcomes in the elderly. *Kidney Int* 2003; **63**(3):1121–1129.

129. Rinehart AL, Herzog CA, Collins AJ, Flack JM, Ma JZ, Opsahl JA. A comparison of coronary angioplasty and coronary artery bypass grafting outcomes in chronic dialysis patients. *Am J Kidney Dis* 1995; **25**(2):281–290.

130. Liu JY, Birkmeyer NJ, Sanders JH, Morton JR, Henriques HF, Lahey SJ, et al. Risks of morbidity and mortality in dialysis patients undergoing coronary artery bypass surgery. Northern New England Cardiovascular Disease Study Group. *Circulation* 2000; **102**(24):2973–2977.

131. Anderson RJ, O'brien M, MaWhinney S, VillaNueva CB, Moritz TE, Sethi GK, et al. Renal failure predisposes patients to adverse outcome after coronary artery bypass surgery. VA Cooperative Study #5. *Kidney Int* 1999; **55**(3):1057–1062.

132. Hirose H, Amano A, Takahashi A, Nagano N. Coronary artery bypass grafting for patients with non-dialysis-dependent renal dysfunction (serum creatinine > or =2.0 mg/dl). *Eur J Cardiothorac Surg* 2001; **20**(3): 565–572.

133. Szczech LA, Best PJ, Crowley E, Brooks MM, Berger PB, Bittner V, et al. Outcomes of patients with chronic renal insufficiency in the bypass angioplasty revascularization investigation. *Circulation* 2002; **105**(19): 2253–2258.

134. Reddan DN, Szczech LA, Tuttle RH, Shaw LK, Jones RH, Schwab SJ, et al. Chronic kidney disease, mortality, and treatment strategies among patients with clinically significant coronary artery disease. *J Am Soc Nephrol* 2003; **14**(9):2373–2380.

135. Hillis GS, Croal BL, Buchan KG, El-Shafei H, Gibson G, Jeffrey RR, et al. Renal function and outcome from coronary artery bypass grafting: impact on mortality after 2.3 year follow-up. *Circulation* 2006; **113**:1056–1062.

136. Cooper WA, O'Brien SM, Thourani VH, Guyton RA, Bridges CR, Szczech LA, et al. The impact of renal dysfunction on outcomes of coronary artery bypass surgery: results from the Society of Thoracic Surgeon's National Cardiac Database. *Circulation* 2006; **113**:1063–1070.

III OBESITY IN CARDIOVASCULAR DISEASE

10 Adiponectin and Cardiovascular Disease

Medhavi Jogi, MD and Mandeep Bajaj, MD

CONTENTS

ADIPONECTIN: STRUCTURE AND FUNCTION
ADIPONECTIN AND CVD
HYPOADIPONECTINEMIA: TREATMENT STRATEGIES
REFERENCES

SUMMARY

Adiponectin, an adipocytokine secreted by adipose tissue, enhances insulin sensitivity and inhibits vascular inflammation. Hypoadiponectinemia is associated with endothelial dysfunction, hypertension, coronary heart disease, and other cardiovascular complications. Furthermore, enhancing adiponectin concentrations by lifestyle changes or pharmacological therapy can have cardiovascular-protective effects. In this chapter, we review the association between adiponectin and cardiovascular disease and discuss treatment strategies to ameliorate hypoadiponectinemia.

Key Words: Adipokine, Adiponectin, Atherosclerosis, Cardiovascular disease, Endothelial dysfunction

Obesity is a major health problem worldwide and is characterized by generalized expansion of all adipose tissue depots. The adipocyte functions not only as a storage depot for fat, but also as an endocrine organ that releases hormones in response to specific extracellular stimuli or changes in metabolic status. These secreted hormones, referred to collectively as adipokines, carry out a variety of diverse functions and include among them TNF-α, leptin, resistin, adiponectin, and others. The adipokines have been postulated to play an important role in the pathogenesis of hypertension, disorders of coagulation, dyslipidemia, glucose intolerance, and abnormalities associated with the insulin resistance syndrome (1,2). The WHO has recognized the key components of the metabolic syndrome to be insulin resistance, impaired glucose tolerance, hypertension, dyslipidemia, hyperuricemia, central obesity, microalbuminuria, and a hypercoagulable state (3). These are recognized risk factors for cardiovascular disease (CVD) and explain the increased prevalence of CVD in patients with type 2 diabetes mellitus (T2DM) (4).

From: *Contemporary Endocrinology: Cardiovascular Endocrinology: Shared Pathways and Clinical Crossroads*
Edited by: V. A. Fonseca © Humana Press, New York, NY

ADIPONECTIN: STRUCTURE AND FUNCTION

The adipokine, adiponectin, was originally identified independently by four different groups in the 1990s. It is also termed Acrp30 *(5)*, apM1 *(6)*, or GBP28 *(7)*. Adiponectin is a secreted protein that has a carboxyl-terminal globular domain and an amino-terminal collagen domain. It is structurally similar to complement 1q, which belongs to a family of proteins that form characteristic multimers *(8,9)*. This adipose tissue-specific 30-kDa protein is synthesized by adipocytes. Circulating adiponectin exists as complexes in plasma and combines via its collagen domain to create three major oligomeric forms: a low-molecular-weight (LMW) trimer, a middle-molecular-weight (MMW) hexamer, and a high-molecular-weight (HMW) 12–18-multimer adiponectin *(5)*. Plasma levels of the HMW isoform have stronger correlations with glucose tolerance than total adiponectin, suggesting that the HMW isoform of adiponectin is the active form *(10)*. A strong relationship has been demonstrated between total plasma adiponectin levels and both hepatic and peripheral tissue insulin sensitivity in patients with type 2 diabetes *(11)*. One of the primary effects of adiponectin is to increase fatty acid oxidation in muscle, leading to a decrease in intracellular fatty acid metabolites, that is, fatty acyl coenzyme A, diacylglycerol, ceramides, and enhanced insulin signal transduction *(12)* (Fig. 1).

Two adiponectin receptors have been cloned. The identification of adiponectin receptors in mice by Yamauchi et al. represents a significant breakthrough in our understanding of the mechanism of adiponectin action. Yamauchi et al. identified two adiponectin receptors – AdipoR1 and AdipoR2. In mice, AdipoR1 is abundantly expressed in skeletal muscle, whereas AdipoR2 is mainly expressed in the liver. AdipoR1 and AdipoR2 serve as receptors for globular and

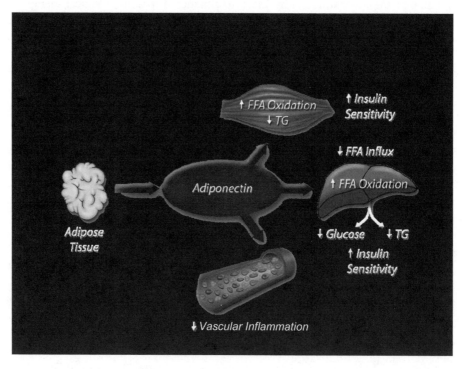

Fig. 1. Adiponectin modulates insulin sensitivity and vascular inflammation. [Reproduced with permission from the American Diabetes Association © 2003. From Chandran M, et al. Diabetes Care 26: 2442–2450, 2003.]

full-length adiponectin, and they mediate adiponectin stimulation of 5′-AMP-activated protein kinase (AMPK), fatty acid oxidation, and glucose uptake *(13)*. More recently, the expression of AdipoR1 and AdipoR2 has also been demonstrated in human monocytes and macrophages *(14)*. Skeletal muscle adiponectin receptors AdipoR1 and AdipoR2 expression levels are strongly related to peripheral (muscle) insulin sensitivity in humans in vivo *(15)*.

ADIPONECTIN AND CVD

Adiponectin and the Metabolic Syndrome

Excessive storage of fat in both adipocytes and ectopic locations plays an important role in the development of insulin resistance *(16,17)*. In addition, adipocyte size is strongly correlated with insulin resistance *(18)*. Specifically, large adipocytes are severely resistant to the antilipolytic effects of insulin. As a result, there is an increase in circulating plasma free fatty acids (FFAs), peripheral (muscle) insulin resistance *(19,20)*, impaired suppression of hepatic glucose production *(19,21)*, and impairment in insulin secretion *(22)*. Thus, elevated plasma FFA levels contribute to the early metabolic defects in patients with type 2 diabetes.

Adiponectin levels are inversely associated with several parameters of the metabolic syndrome. Although adiponectin is secreted by adipose tissue, plasma levels of this adipokine are significantly lower in obese subjects than in nonobese subjects. Human cross-sectional studies have shown that plasma adiponectin levels are negatively correlated with obesity *(23)*, waist–hip ratio, insulin resistance *(18)*, and diabetic dyslipidemia *(24)*. Studies in humans have shown that low plasma adiponectin levels are associated with peripheral insulin resistance and the individual components of the metabolic syndrome i.e. elevated plasma triglyceride and glucose levels, and decreased HDL cholesterol *(18,25)* (Fig. 2).

Studies in rodents have confirmed the negative associations of adiponectin and the metabolic syndrome. Adiponectin expression is reduced in obese, insulin-resistant rodent models *(26)*. Yamauchi et al. showed a reduction in fat cell mRNA and circulating adiponectin levels in high-fat-feeding mice and clear reversal of insulin resistance after administration of adiponectin *(27)*. Transgenic mice also show correlations between adiponectin and the metabolic syndrome. Adiponectin-deficient mice develop features of metabolic syndrome with insulin resistance, hyperlipidemia, and hypertension *(28)*. Mice that overexpress adiponectin show partial improvements in insulin resistance, diabetes, and insulin-mediated glucose production. These studies strongly suggest that increasing endogenous adiponectin levels has direct effects on insulin sensitivity *(29)*. Adiponectin enhances AMPK activity and fat oxidation in the muscle and liver. The reduction in hepatic and intramyocellular triglyceride content is associated with enhanced hepatic and peripheral (muscle) insulin sensitivity *(27)*.

Adiponectin and Vascular Biology

Vascular inflammatory and fibroproliferative responses, as well as endothelial dysfunction play an important role in the development of atherosclerosis *(30)*. Endothelial dysfunction is considered to represent the initial step in atherogenesis and precedes any morphologic changes in the arterial vessel wall. There are multiple mechanisms that can initiate vascular inflammation. Abnormal nitric oxide (NO) metabolism is an important contributor to endothelial dysfunction. Nuclear factorκB (NFκB) is an important component to the inflammatory response *(31)*. The elevated FFAs associated with obesity/insulin resistance/metabolic syndrome also play an important role in endothelial dysfunction by activating inflammatory

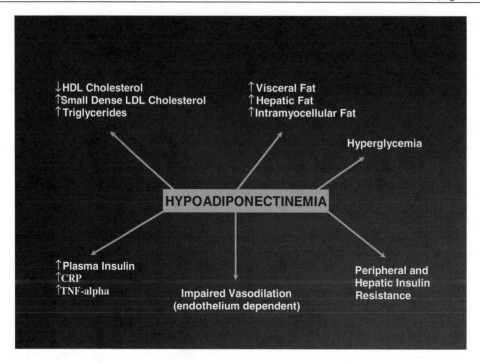

Fig. 2. Adiponectin: metabolic correlates.

pathways *(32)*. Thus, inflammation contributes to endothelial dysfunction, and the markers of acute inflammation reflect increased cardiovascular risk *(33)*.

There is considerable in vivo evidence in rodents that adiponectin is an important regulator of NO synthesis and could explain some of the observed vasoprotective properties of adiponectin, as well as its beneficial effects on the cardiovascular system. Many studies have provided evidence for a link between hypoadiponectinemia and impaired NO generation *(34,35)*. Diminished brachial arterial endothelium-dependent vasodilatation has been associated with reduced adiponectin levels in subjects with type 2 diabetes and with hypertension *(36,37)*. Animal models of adiponectin deficiency are characterized by severe neointimal hyperplasia that can be reversed with adiponectin repletion *(28)*. Recent in vitro studies *(38,39)* using bovine aortic endothelial cells have shown that adiponectin stimulates NO production by increasing eNOS enzyme activity and eNOS expression via a phophatidylinositol 3-kinase-dependent pathway that causes phosphorylation/activation of eNOS at Ser1179 by AMP-activated protein kinase (AMPK). Conversely, transfection of bovine aortic endothelial cells with dominant-inhibitory mutants of AMP-activated protein kinase (AMPKK45R) inhibited NO production in response to adiponectin. In a rat model of NO synthesis deficiency produced by L-NAME, plasma adiponectin concentration and adiponectin mRNA levels in the aorta were noted to be reduced. Treatment with pioglitazone increased fat adiponectin mRNA levels and normalized the plasma adiponectin concentration in association with an increase in NO synthesis in arterial tissue *(40)*.

Plasma adiponectin rapidly accumulates in the subendothelial space of the injured human artery and seems to have antiatherogenic effects. Adiponectin inhibits TNF-α-induced activation of NFκB-dependent proinflammatory pathways, expression of endothelial adhesion molecules, macrophage-to-foam cell transformation, lipid accumulation in macrophages, and

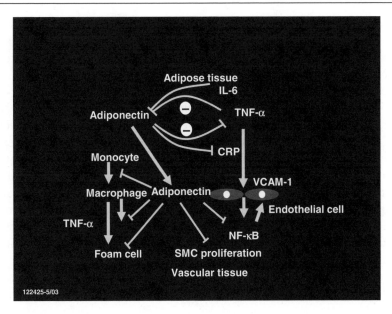

Fig. 3. Adiponectin and vascular inflammation. [Reproduced with permission from the Lippincott Williams & Wilkins, Inc. © 2003. From Ouchi N, et al. Curr Opin Lipidol. 14:561–566, 2003.]

smooth muscle cell proliferation *(41–43)* (Fig. 3). Hypoadiponectinemia is also closely associated with increased levels of the inflammatory markers *(44)* and is known to induce the expression of anti-inflammatory cytokines such as IL-10 and IL-1RA in macrophages *(45)*. Adiponectin inhibits growth factor-induced proliferation and migration of vascular smooth muscle cells *(46)*. There is an inverse correlation between adiponectin and IL-6 concentrations *(44,47)*. Plasma CRP levels are negatively correlated with plasma adiponectin levels in male patients with coronary artery disease (CAD). There is a significant inverse correlation between CRP and adiponectin gene expression in human adipose tissues *(48)*.

Adiponectin and Coronary Artery Disease

There are several in vitro and animal studies that suggest a protective role for adiponectin against coronary disease. In rodents, the role of adiponectin in myocardial remodeling in response to acute injury has been examined. Ischemia-reperfusion in adiponectin-deficient mice resulted in increased myocardial infarct size, myocardial apoptosis, and TNF-α expression compared with wild-type mice *(49)*. Administration of adiponectin reversed these abnormalities in both adiponectin-deficient and wild-type mice. In cultured cardiac cells, adiponectin inhibited apoptosis and TNF-α production. Dominant-negative AMP-activated protein kinase (AMPK) reversed the inhibitory effects of adiponectin on cell apoptosis. Adiponectin-induced cyclooxygenase (COX)-2-dependent synthesis of prostaglandin E2 in cardiac cells, and COX-2 inhibition reversed the inhibitory effects of adiponectin on TNF-α production and infarct size. These data suggest that adiponectin protects the heart from ischemia-reperfusion injury through both AMPK- and COX-2-dependent mechanisms *(49)*. Furthermore, the expression levels (and protein) of the adiponectin receptor, AdipoR1, have been shown to be decreased both in the infarcted and remote area after myocardial infarction in rodent hearts *(50)*.

Adiponectin levels are strongly correlated with the degree of CAD in patients without diabetes. Several cross-sectional studies have shown low circulating adiponectin to be linked to the presence of CAD *(51–53)*. Kumada et al. demonstrated a twofold increased risk for CHD in patients with less than 4 μg/ml circulating adiponectin levels *(51)*. An inverse association between circulating adiponectin concentrations and risk of CHD has been shown in patients with angiographically defined CHD and this association was significantly reduced after adjustment for HDL cholesterol reflecting a close relationship between adiponectin and HDL cholesterol *(52)*. In the Health Professionals' Follow-Up Study, the risk of recurrent myocardial infarction was reduced in association with higher circulating adiponectin concentrations.

The relationship between adiponectin and CAD is less apparent in the presence of type 2 diabetes, and the association is likely to be dependent on the prevalence of obesity and associated metabolic disorders. Although a relationship between adiponectin and CHD events in T2DM patients has been demonstrated, the strength of this association was reduced when HDL-C was included into the model. Thus, the effects of adiponectin on CHD in type 2 diabetics may be mediated largely by its effect on HDL cholesterol *(54,55)*.

Low adiponectin levels are also independently associated with the progression of coronary artery calcification, a marker of subclinical CAD and a strong predictor of future CHD events *(56)*.

Adiponectin and Acute Coronary Syndrome

Hypoadiponectinemia may contribute to coronary plaque vulnerability. Otsuka et al. have demonstrated that low plasma adiponectin levels are associated with angiographic coronary lesion complexity in men with CAD. In addition, they demonstrate that patients with acute coronary syndrome (ACS) have lower plasma adiponectin concentration than patients with stable CAD *(57)*. These findings are important given the higher prevalence of diabetes and impaired glucose tolerance in patients with ACS and suggest that hypoadiponectinemia may be the link between type 2 diabetes, CAD, enhanced plaque vulnerability, and ACS *(58–60)*. Understanding the clinical significance of plasma adiponectin may be helpful in preventing the development of atherosclerotic vascular disease.

Adiponectin may be a useful predictor of clinical events after percutaneous coronary intervention (PCI). Pre-procedural hypoadiponectinemia may be an independent predictor of major adverse cardiac and cerebrovascular (MACCE) after PCI. MACCE includes death from any cause, re-infarction, repeat coronary revascularization, hospitalization due to CHF, and cerebral infarction. Those patients with the lowest circulating adiponectin concentrations had a high rate of MACCE compared to the upper three quartiles of serum adiponectin levels *(61)*.

Some, but not all studies, have demonstrated the protective association of adiponectin with ACS. In a prospective study (that excluded diabetics) higher plasma adiponectin levels were associated with a lower risk of ACS, independent of other traditional metabolic and cardiovascular risk factors. The authors found the greatest increase in risk for ACS was seen at adiponectin levels less than 5.5 μg/ml, suggesting a potential clinically useful cut-off value *(62)*. Similarly, Pischon et al. found low levels of adiponectin to be an independent predictor of adverse cardiovascular events in a population of healthy male patients that were free of diagnosed CVD *(63)*. On the other hand, Cavusoglu et al. found that high baseline plasma adiponectin levels are independently associated with an increased risk of both death and MI (as individual endpoints) at 2-year follow-up in a cohort of men with stable angina, unstable angina, and NSTEMI referred for coronary angiography *(64)*. Along similar lines, Pilz et al.

showed that among the patients with angiographic CAD, higher adiponectin levels were a predictor of all-cause, cardiovascular and noncardiovascular mortality, respectively, independent from established and emerging risk factors *(65)*.

Adiponectin and Heart Failure

Insulin resistance and obesity is associated with chronic heart failure. Pathological cardiac remodeling characterized by myocardial hypertrophy occurs with many obesity-related conditions, and diastolic dysfunction is one of the earliest manifestations of insulin resistance *(66,67)*. In addition, cardiac steatosis and lipoapoptosis has been shown in an animal model of obesity *(68)*. In adiponectin-deficient rodents, pressure overload has been shown to enhance concentric cardiac hypertrophy and increase mortality and was associated with increased extracellular signal-regulated kinase (ERK) and diminished AMPK signaling in the myocardium *(69)*. Cardiac hypertrophy, in response to pressure overload, was attenuated by adenovirus-mediated supplementation of adiponectin. In cultures of cardiac myocytes, adiponectin activates AMPK, inhibits hypertrophy, and inhibits ERK activation. Transduction with a dominant-negative form of AMPK has been shown to reverse these effects, suggesting that adiponectin inhibits hypertrophic signaling in the myocardium through activation of AMPK signaling *(69)*. Recently, adiponectin receptors AdipoR1 and AdipoR2 have been shown to mediate the suppressive effects of full-length and globular adiponectin on endothelin-1-induced hypertrophy in cultured cardiac myocytes *(50)*.

Adiponectin may influence the development of chronic heart failure, but at this time, only a few studies have been done to elucidate the effects of this adipokine on left ventricular remodeling. These studies have shown that concentrations of adiponectin are surprisingly high in patients with CHF. Elevated plasma adiponectin levels have been shown to be associated with increased mortality in patients with congestive heart failure; however, causality could not be proven. Furthermore, obesity was also related to a reduced mortality risk in this study, although this association was not independent of baseline levels of adiponectin *(70)*. Other studies have shown similar associations between elevated plasma adiponectin levels and increasing severity of CHF as well as BNP levels *(71,72)*. Further studies are needed to understand if the augmentation in circulating adiponectin levels is a physiological response to enhanced neurohumoral and inflammatory activation.

Genetics

The adiponectin protein encoding gene ADIPOQ is located on chromosome 3q27. The gene is encoded by three exons which span approximately 16 kb. The *Adiponectin* gene appears to be a candidate susceptibility gene for type 2 diabetes, the metabolic syndrome, and CVD. There are a number of single-nucleotide polymorphisms (SNPs) that have been studied in relation to CVD.

There have been several studies done that show an association of adiponectin SNPs with CAD. Ohashi et al. examined these associations in 383 Japanese patients with confirmed CAD by angiogram and matched healthy controls. They demonstrated an increased frequency of I164T with CAD patients. Similar results were reported by Jung et al. *(73,74)*. In 162 Caucasian patients with type 2 diabetes, SNP+45 also was associated with CAD *(75)*. The G allele of the −11377 C>G proximal promoter polymorphism has been shown to be associated with coronary atherosclerosis and predictive of vascular events among men undergoing coronary angiography

(76). SNP+276 in intron 2 is associated with type 2 diabetes and obesity but there are conflicting studies on whether SNP 276 is truly associated with CAD *(74,75,77–79)*.

HYPOADIPONECTINEMIA: TREATMENT STRATEGIES

The effects of lifestyle modifications and drugs on hypoadiponectinemia and insulin resistance are briefly reviewed. A major future advancement in the field is likely to be the development of drugs that enhance the gene expression of adiponectin and/or its receptors.

Dietary Factors

Some dietary factors, such as soy protein *(80)*, fish oils *(81)*, and linoleic acid have been shown to increase plasma adiponectin levels. The effect of fish oil on adiponectin secretion in mice has been examined. Feeding mice fish oil raised plasma adiponectin concentrations twofold to threefold in a dose-dependent manner within 15 days of initiating feeding. Within 24 h, fish oil markedly induced transcription of the adiponectin gene in epididymal adipose tissue but not in subcutaneous fat. The increase of plasma adiponectin by fish oil was blocked by administration of the peroxisome proliferator-activated receptor (PPAR) inhibitor bisphenol-A-diglycidyl ether. There was no effect of fish oil feeding on adiponectin secretion in PPAR-alpha-null mice *(82)*.

Lifestyle changes

There are a number of lifestyle changes that are associated with increased adiponectin levels. Prolonged weight loss increases plasma adiponectin levels in both diabetic and nondiabetic patients *(83)*. The HMW isoform of adiponectin is significantly increased, and levels of trimer and hexamer adiponectin decline during weight loss *(84)* In premenopausal obese women without diabetes, hypertension, or hyperlipidemia, 2 years of weight loss and lifestyle changes led to significantly increased adiponectin levels *(47)* . Obese patients who underwent gastric partition surgery had a significant increase in adiponectin levels *(85)*. Plasma adiponectin levels are significantly lower in smokers and a negative association between adiponectin and smoking status has been shown in patients with CAD. The combination of low serum adiponectin levels and smoking predisposes to a significantly high risk for coronary stenosis. This risk is likely to be a synergistic rather than an additive effect *(86–88)*.

Drug Therapy

THIAZOLIDINEDIONES

Treatment with a thiazolidinedione increases circulating adiponectin concentrations by almost threefold in patients with type 2 diabetes. The increase in plasma adiponectin levels following thiazolidinedione treatment correlates with the improvement in glycemic control and hepatic and peripheral (muscle) insulin sensitivity *(11)*. Adiponectin expression is influenced by the stimulation of PPAR-γ. Specific activation of PPAR-γ induces the differentiation of preadipocytes into mature insulin-sensitive adipocytes *(89,90)* as well as the intracellular fatty acid transport, activation of fatty acids, and fatty acid esterification in adipocytes *(91,92)*. PPAR-γ stimulation also results in an increase in circulating adiponectin levels and the subsequent enhancement of fat oxidation in the liver and skeletal muscle*(93)*. More recently, adiponectin has also been shown to enhance mitochondrial biogenesis *(94)*. These effects may explain the reduction in hepatic and intramyocellular fat and the increment in hepatic and peripheral insulin sensitivity observed following thiazolidinedione (PPAR-γ agonists) treatment. Furthermore, the increase in plasma adiponectin concentrations may be playing an important role in inhibiting vascular inflammation observed following thiazolidinedione treatment.

ACE INHIBITORS/ARBS

A modest but significant increase in plasma adiponectin levels has been observed after treatment with ACE inhibitors and ARBs in patients with hypertension *(95,96)*. Japanese adults with essential hypertension had significant increases in plasma adiponectin concentrations following 3 months of losartan treatment *(97)*. Blocking the renin-angiotensin system (RAS) is associated with an increase in plasma adiponectin levels. Furthermore, angiotensin II (Ang II) infusion decreases plasma adiponectin concentrations and adipose tissue adiponectin expression *(98)*. *Olmesartan*, an Ang II type-1 (AT$_1$) receptor blocker (ARB), reverses obesity-induced hypoadiponectinemia *(99)*. The precise molecular mechanisms by which renin-angiotensin-system inhibition stimulates adiponectin production remain unclear.

RIMONABANT

The endocannabinoid system is an intercellular signaling system that plays an important role in regulating cardiovascular risk factors associated with excess body weight and obesity. Adipose tissue also expresses CB$_1$ receptors, and the level is increased in obese animals. Rimonabant increased the expression of adiponectin in cultured mouse 3T3 F442A preadipocytes but had no effect on adiponectin expression in adipose tissue of CB$_1$ receptor knockout mice, suggesting a CB$_1$ receptor-mediated effect *(100)*. In the RIO-Lipids study, rimonabant treatment (20 mg/day) was associated with an increase in plasma adiponectin levels by 57% ($P<0.001$). This increase in plasma adiponectin correlated with weight loss in both the placebo and rimonabant groups, but more than half of the rimonabant-induced increase in plasma adiponectin levels observed in those receiving 20 mg rimonabant could not be attributed to weight loss alone. This suggested a direct enhancement of adiponectin expression by rimonabant in adipose tissue *(101)*. These results suggest a primary effect of rimonabant on circulating adiponectin concentrations and further studies are needed to evaluate the benefits of such an effect on liver and intramyocellular fat and vascular inflammation.

REFERENCES

1. Kahn BB, Flier JS: Obesity and insulin resistance. J Clin Invest 106: 473–481, 2000.
2. Bajaj M, Ben-Yehuda O: A big fat wedding: association of adiponectin with coronary vascular lesions: J Am Coll Cardiol 48: 1163–1165, 2006.
3. Alberti KG, Zimmet PZ: Definition, diagnosis and classification of diabetes mellitus and its complications. Diabetes Med 15: 539–553, 1998.
4. Reaven GM: Banting Lecture 1988. Role of insulin resistance in human disease. Diabetes 37: 1595–1607, 1988.
5. Scherer PE, Williams S, Fogliano M, Baldini G, Lodish HF: A novel serum protein similar to C1q, produced exclusively in adipocytes. J Biol Chem 270: 26746–26749, 1995.
6. Maeda K, Okubo K, Shimomura I, Funahashi T, Matsuzawa Y, Matsubara K: cDNA cloning and expression of a novel adipose specific collagen-like factor, apM1 (AdiPose Most abundant Gene transcript). Biochem Biophys Res Commun 221: 286–289, 1996.
7. Nakano Y, Tobe T, Choi-Miura NH, Mazda T, Tomita M: Isolation and characterization of GBP28, a novel gelatin-binding protein purified from human plasma. J Biochem (Tokyo) 120: 803–812, 1996.

8. Shapiro L, Scherer PE: The crystal structure of a complement-1q family protein suggests an evolutionary link to tumor necrosis factor. Curr Biol 8: 335–338, 1998.

9. Crouch E, Persson A, Chang D, Heuser J: Molecular structure of pulmonary surfactant protein D (SP-D). J Biol Chem 269:17311–17319, 1994.

10. Lara-Castro C, Luo N, Wallace P, Klein RL, Garvey WT: Adiponectin multimeric complexes and the metabolic syndrome trait cluster. Diabetes 55: 249–259, 2006.

11. Bajaj M, Suraamornkul S, Piper P, Hardies LJ, Glass L, Cersosimo E, Pratipanawatr T, Miyazaki Y, DeFronzo RA: Decreased plasma adiponectin concentrations are closely related to hepatic fat content and hepatic insulin resistance in pioglitazone-treated type 2 diabetic patients. J Clin Endocrinol Metab 89: 200–206, 2004.

12. Yamauchi T, Kamon J, Waki H, Terauchi Y, Kubota N, Hara K, Mori Y, Ide T, Murakami K, Tsuboyama-Kasaoka N, Ezaki O, Akanuma Y, Gavrilova O, Vinson C, Reitman ML, Kagechika H, Shudo K, Yoda M, Nakano Y, Tobe K, Nagai R, Kimura S, Tomita M, Froguel P, Kadowaki T: The fat-derived hormone adiponectin reverses insulin resistance associated with both lipoatrophy and obesity. Nat Med 7: 941–946, 2001.

13. Yamauchi T, Kamon J, Ito Y, Tsuchida A, Yokomizo T, Kita S, Sugiyama T, Miyagishi M, Hara K, Tsunoda M, Murakami K, Ohteki T, Uchida S, Takekawa S, Waki H, Tsuno NH, Shibata Y, Terauchi Y, Froguel P, Tobe K, Koyasu S, Taira K, Kitamura T, Shimizu T, Nagai R, Kadowaki T: Cloning of adiponectin receptors that mediate antidiabetic metabolic effects. Nature 423: 762–769, 2003.

14. Chinetti G, Zawadski C, Fruchart JC, Staels B: Expression of adiponectin receptors in human macrophages and regulation by agonists of the nuclear receptors PPARalpha, PPARgamma, and LXR. Biochem Biophys Res Commun 14: 151–158, 2004.

15. Civitarese AE, Jenkinson CP, Richardson D, Bajaj M, Cusi K, Kashyap S, Berria R, Belfort R, DeFronzo RA, Mandarino LJ, Ravussin E: Adiponectin receptor gene expression and insulin sensitivity in non-diabetic Mexican Americans with or without a family history of diabetes. Diabetologia 47: 816–820, 2004.

16. Bajaj M, Suraamornkul S, Romanelli A, Cline GW, Mandarino LJ, Shulman GI, DeFronzo RA: Effect of a sustained reduction in plasma free fatty acid concentration on intramuscular long-chain fatty acyl-CoAs and insulin action in type 2 diabetic patients. Diabetes 54: 3148–3153, 2005.

17. Danforth E: Failure of adipocyte differentiation causes type II diabetes mellitus? Nat Genet 26: 1, 2000.

18. Weyer C, Funahashi T, Tanaka S, Hotta K, Matsuzawa Y, Pratley RE, Tataranni PA: Hypoadiponectinemia in obesity and type 2 diabetes: close association with insulin resistance and hyperinsulinemia. J Clin Endocrinol Metab 86: 1930–1935, 2001.

19. Boden G, Jadali F, White J, Liang Y, Mozzoli M, Chen X, Coleman E, Smith C: Effects of fat on insulin-stimulated carbohydrate metabolism in normal men. J Clin Invest 88: 960–966, 1991.

20. Thiebaud D, DeFronzo RA, Jacot E, Golay A, Acheson K, Maeder E, Jequier E, Felber JP: Effect of long chain triglyceride infusion on glucose metabolism in man. Metabolism 31: 1128–1236, 1982.

21. Chen X, Iqbal N, Boden G: The effects of free fatty acids on gluconeogenesis and glycogenolysis in normal subjects. J Clin Invest 103: 365–372, 1999.

22. Kashyap S, Belfort R, Gastaldelli A, Pratipanawatr T, Berria R, Pratipanawatr W, Bajaj M, Mandarino L, DeFronzo R, Cusi K: A sustained increase in plasma free fatty acids impairs insulin secretion in nondiabetic subjects genetically predisposed to develop type 2 diabetes. Diabetes 52: 2461–2474, 2003.

23. Arita Y, Kihara S, Ouchi N, Takahashi M, Maeda K, Miyagawa J, Hotta K, Shimomura I, Nakamura T, Miyaoka K, Kuriyama H, Nishida M, Yamashita S, Okubo K, Matsubara K, Muraguchi M, Ohmoto Y, Funahashi T, Matsuzawa Y: Paradoxical decrease of an adipose-specific protein, adiponectin, in obesity. Biochem Biophys Res Commun 257: 79–83, 1999.

24. Matsubara M, Maruoka S, Katayose S: Decreased plasma adiponectin concentrations in women with dyslipidemia. J Clin Endocrinol Metab 87: 2764–2769, 2002.

25. Yu JG, Javorschi S, Hevener AL, Kruszynska YT, Norman RA, Sinha M, Olefsky JM: The effect of thiazolidinediones on plasma adiponectin levels in normal, obese, and type 2 diabetic subjects. Diabetes 51: 2968–2974, 2002.

26. Hu E, Liang P, Spiegelman BM: AdipoQ is a novel adipose-specific gene dysregulated in obesity. J Biol Chem 271: 10697–10703, 1996.

27. Yamauchi T, Kamon J, Minokoshi Y, Ito Y, Waki H, Uchida S, Yamashita S, Noda M, Kita S, Ueki K, Eto K, Akanuma Y, Froguel P, Foufelle F, Ferre P, Carling D, Kimura S, Nagai R, Kahn BB, Kadowaki T: Adiponectin stimulates glucose utilization and fatty-acid oxidation by activating AMP-activated protein kinase. Nat Med 8: 1288–1295, 2002.

28. Kubota N, Terauchi Y, Yamauchi T, Kubota T, Moroi M, Matsui J, Eto K, Yamashita T, Kamon J, Satoh H, Yano W, Froguel P, Nagai R, Kimura S, Kadowaki T, Noda T: Disruption of adiponectin causes insulin resistance and neointimal formation. J Biol Chem 277: 25863–25866, 2002.

29. Combs TP, Pajvani UB, Berg AH, Lin Y, Jelicks LA, Laplante M, Nawrocki AR, Rajala MW, Parlow AF, Cheeseboro L, Ding YY, Russell RG, Lindemann D, Hartley A, Baker GR, Obici S, Deshaies Y, Ludgate M, Rossetti L, Scherer PE: A transgenic mouse with a deletion in the collagenous domain of adiponectin displays elevated circulating adiponectin and improved insulin sensitivity. Endocrinology 145: 367–383, 2004.

30. Kim J, Montagnani M, Koh KK, Quon MJ: Reciprocal relationships between insulin resistance and endothelial dysfunction. Circulation113: 1888–1904, 2006.

31. de Winther MP, Kanters E, Kraal G, Hofker MH: Nuclear factor kappaB signaling in atherogenesis. Arterioscler Thromb Vasc Biol 25: 904–914, 2005.

32. Vincent MA, Montagnani M, Quon MJ: Molecular and physiologic actions of insulin related to production of nitric oxide in vascular endothelium, Curr Diab Rep 3: 279–288, 2003.

33. Rutter MK, Meigs JB, Sullivan LM, D'Agostino RB, Wilson PWF: C-reactive protein, the metabolic syndrome, and prediction of cardiovascular events in the Framingham Offspring Study, Circulation 110: 380–385, 2004.

34. Quyyumi AA, Dakak N, Andrews NP, Husain S, Arora S, Gilligan DM, Panza JA, Cannon RO: Nitric oxide activity in the human coronary circulation. Impact of risk factors for coronary atherosclerosis. J Clin Invest 95: 1747–1755, 1995.

35. Boger RH, Bode-Boger SM, Thiele W, Junker W, Alexander K, Frolich JC: Biochemical evidence for impaired nitric oxide synthesis in patients with peripheral arterial occlusive disease. Circulation 95: 2068–2074, 1997.

36. Ouchi N, Ohishi M, Kihara S, Funahashi T, Nakamura T, Nagarentani H, Kumada M, Ohashi K, Okamoto Y, Nishizawa H, Kishida K; Maeda N; Nagasawa A, Kobayashi H, Hiraoka H, Komai N, Kaibe M, Rakugi H, Ogihara T, Matsuzaw Y: Association of hypoadiponectinemia with impaired vasoreactivity. Hypertension 42: 231–234, 2003.

37. Tan KC, Xu A, Chow WS, Lam MC, Ai VH, Tam SC, Lam KS: Hypoadiponectinemia is associated with impaired endothelium-dependent vasodilation. J Clin Endocrinol Metab 89: 765–769, 2004.

38. Chen H, Montagnani M, Funahashi T, Shimomura I, Quon MJ: Adiponectin stimulates production of nitric oxide in vascular endothelial cells. J Biol Chem 278: 45021–45026, 2003.

39. Hattori Y, Suzuki M, Hattori S, Kasai K: Globular adiponectin upregulates nitric oxide production in vascular endothelial cells. Diabetologia 46: 1543–1549, 2003.

40. Hattori S, Hattori Y, Kasai K: Hypoadiponectinemia is caused by chronic blockade of nitric oxide synthesis in rats. Metabolism 54: 482–487, 2005.

41. Ouchi N, Kihara S, Arita Y, Okamoto Y, Maeda K, Kuriyama H, Hotta K, Nishida M, Takahashi M, Muraguchi M, Ohmoto Y, Nakamura T, Yamashita S, Funahashi T, Matsuzawa Y: Adiponectin, an adipocyte-derived plasma protein, inhibits endothelial NF-kappaB signaling through a cAMP-dependent pathway. Circulation 102: 1296–1301, 2000.

42. Ouchi N, Kihara S, Arita Y, Nishida M, Matsuyama A, Okamoto Y, Ishigami M, Kuriyama H, Kishida K, Nishizawa H, Hotta K, Muraguchi M, Ohmoto Y, Yamashita S, Funahashi T, Matsuzawa Y: Adipocyte-derived plasma protein, adiponectin, suppresses lipid accumulation and class A scavenger receptor expression in human monocyte-derived macrophages. Circulation 103: 1057–1063, 2001.

43. Ouchi N, Kihara S, Arita Y, Maeda K, Kuriyama H, Okamoto Y, Hotta K, Nishida M, Takahashi M, Nakamura T, Yamashita S, Funahashi T, Matsuzawa Y: Novel modulator for endothelial adhesion molecules: adipocyte-derived plasma protein adiponectin. Circulation 100: 2473–2476, 1999.

44. Engeli S, Feldpausch M, Gorzelniak K, Hartwig F, Heintze U, Janke J, Mohlig M, Pfeiffer AF, Luft FC, Sharma AM: Association between adiponectin and mediators of inflammation in obese women. Diabetes 52: 942–947, 2003.

45. Wolf AM, Wolf D, Rumpold H, Enrich B, Tilg H: Adiponectin induces the anti-inflammatory cytokines IL-10 and IL-1RA in human leukocytes. Biochem Biophys Res Commun 323: 630–635, 2004.

46. Arita Y, Kihara S, Ouchi N, Maeda K, Kuriyama H, Okamoto Y, Kumada M, Hotta K, Nishida M, Takahashi M, Nakamura T, Shimomura I, Muraguchi M, Ohmoto Y, Funahashi T, Matsuzawa Y: Adipocyte-derived plasma protein adiponectin acts as a platelet-derived growth factor-BB-binding protein and regulates growth factor-induced common postreceptor signal in vascular smooth muscle cell. Circulation 105: 2893–2898, 2002.

47. Esposito K, Pontillo A, Di Palo C, Giugliano G, Masella M, Marfella R, Giugliano D: Effect of weight loss and lifestyle changes on vascular inflammatory markers in obese women: a randomized trial, JAMA 289: 1799–1804, 2003.

48. Ouchi N, Kihara S, Funahashi T, Nakamura T, Nishida M, Kumada M, Okamoto Y, Ohashi K, Nagaretani H, Kishida K, Nishizawa H, Maeda N, Kobayashi H, Hiraoka H, Matsuzawa Y: Reciprocal association of C-reactive protein with adiponectin in blood stream and adipose tissue, Circulation 107: 671–674, 2003.

49. Shibata R, Sato K, Pimentel DR, Takemura Y, Kihara S, Ohashi K, Funahashi T, Ouchi N, Walsh K: Adiponectin protects against myocardial ischemia-reperfusion injury through AMPK- and COX-2-dependent mechanisms. Nat Med 11: 1096–1103, 2005.

50. Fujioka D, Kawabata KI, Saito Y, Kobayashi T, Nakamura T, Kodama Y, Takano H, Obata JE, Kitta Y, Umetani K, Kugiyama K: Role of adiponectin receptors in endothelin-induced cellular hypertrophy in cultured cardiomyocytes and their expression in infarcted heart. Am J Physiol Heart Circ Physiol 290:H2409–H2416, 2006.

51. Kumada M, Kihara S, Sumitsuji S, Kawamoto T, Matsumoto S, Ouchi N, Arita Y, Okamoto Y, Shimomura I, Hiraoka H, Nakamura T, Funahashi T, Matsuzawa Y: Association of hypoadiponectinemia with coronary artery disease in men. Arterioscler Thromb Vasc Biol 23: 85–89, 2003.

52. Rothenbacher D, Brenner H, März W and Koenig W: Adiponectin, risk of coronary heart disease and correlations with cardiovascular risk markers, Eur Heart J 26: 1640–1646, 2005.

53. Kojima S, Funahashi T, Sakamoto T, Miyamoto S, Soejima H, Hokamaki J, Kajiwara I, Sugiyama S, Yoshimura M, Fujimoto K, Miyao Y, Suefuji H, Kitagawa A, Ouchi N, Kihara S, Matsuzawa Y, Ogawa H: The variation of plasma concentrations of a novel, adipocyte derived protein, adiponectin, in patients with acute myocardial infarction. Heart 89: 667, 2003.

54. Schulze MB, Shai I, Rimm EB, Li T, Rifai N, Hu FB: Adiponectin and future coronary heart disease events among men with type 2 diabetes, Diabetes 54: 534–539, 2005.

55. Lindsay RS, Resnick HE, Zhu J, Tun ML, Howard BV, Zhang Y, Yeh J, Best LG: Adiponectin and coronary heart disease: the Strong Heart Study. Arterioscler Thromb Vasc Biol 25: e15–e16, 2005.

56. Maahs DM, Ogden LG, Kinney GL, Wadwa P, Snell-Bergeon JK, Dabelea D, Hokanson JE, Ehrlich J, Eckel RH, Rewers M: Low plasma adiponectin levels predict progression of coronary artery calcification. Circulation 111: 747–753, 2005.

57. Otsuka F, Sugiyama S, Kojima S, Maruyoshi H, Funahashi T, Matsui K, Sakamoto T, Yoshimura M, Kimura K, Umemura S, Ogawa H: Plasma adiponectin levels are associated with coronary lesion complexity in men with coronary artery disease. J Am Coll Cardiol 48: 1155–1162, 2006.

58. Koenig W, Khuseyinova N, Baumert J, Meisinger C, Lowel H: Serum concentrations of adiponectin and risk of type 2 diabetes mellitus and coronary heart disease in apparently healthy middle-aged men: results from the 18-year follow-up of a large cohort from southern Germany. J Am Coll Cardiol 48: 1369–1377, 2006.

59. Norhammar A, Tenerz A, Nilsson G, Hamsten A, Efendic S, Ryden L, Malmberg K: Glucose metabolism in patients with acute myocardial infarction and no previous diagnosis of diabetes mellitus: a prospective study. Lancet 359: 2140–2144, 2002.

60. Hashimoto K, Ikewaki K, Yagi H, Nagasawa H, Imamoto S, Shibata T, Mochizuki S: Glucose intolerance is common in Japanese patients with acute coronary syndrome who were not previously diagnosed with diabetes. Diabetes Care 28: 1182–1186, 2005.

61. Shioji K, Moriwaki S, Takeuchi Y, Uegaito T, Mutsuo S, Matsuda M: Relationship of serum adiponectin level to adverse cardiovascular events in patients who undergo percutaneous coronary intervention. Circ J 71: 675–680, 2007.

62. Wolk R, Berger P, Lennon RJ, Brilakis ES, Davison DE, Somers VK: Association between plasma adiponectin levels and unstable coronary syndromes. Eur Heart J 28: 292–298, 2007.

63. Pischon T, Girman CJ, Hotamisligil GS, Rifai N, Hu FB, Rimm EB: Plasma adiponectin levels and risk of myocardial infarction in men. JAMA 291: 1730–1737, 2004.

64. Cavusoglu E, Ruwende C, Chopra V, Yanamadala S, Eng C, Clark LT, Pinsky DJ, Marmur JD: Adiponectin is an independent predictor of all-cause mortality, cardiac mortality, and myocardial infarction in patients presenting with chest pain. Eur Heart J 27: 2300–2309, 2006.

65. Pilz S, Mangge H, Wellnitz B, Seelhorst U, Winkelmann BR, Tiran B, Boehm BO, Marz W: Adiponectin and mortality in patients undergoing coronary angiography. J Clin Endocrinol Metaboli 91: 4277–4286, 2006.

66. Rutter MK, Parise H, Benjamin EJ, Levy D, Larson MG, Meigs JB, Nesto RW, Wilson PW, Vasan R: Impact of glucose intolerance and insulin resistance on cardiac structure and function: sex-related differences in the Framingham Heart Study. Circulation 107: 448-454, 2003.

67. Kenchaiah S, Evans JC, Levy D, Wilson PW, Benjamin EJ, Larson MG, Kannel WB, Vasan RS: Obesity and the risk of heart failure. N Eng J Med 347: 305–313, 2002.

68. Zhou YT, Grayburn P, Karim A, Shimabukuro M, Higa M, Baetens D, Orci L, Unger RH: Lipotoxic heart disease in obese rats: implications for human obesity. Proc Natl Acad Sci 97: 1784–1789, 2000.

69. Shibata R, Ouchi N, Ito M, Kihara S, Shiojima I, Pimentel DR, Kumada M, Sato K, Schiekofer S, Ohashi K, Funahashi T, Colucci WS, Walsh K: Adiponectin-mediated modulation of hypertrophic signals in the heart. Nat Med 10: 1384–1389, 2004.

70. Kistorp C, Faber J, Galatius S, Gustafsson F, Frystyk J, Flyvbjerg A, Hildebrandt P: Plasma adiponectin, body mass index, and mortality in patients with chronic heart failure. Circulation 112: 1756–1762, 2005.

71. Nakamura T, Funayama H, Kubo N, Yasu T, Kawakami M, Saito M, Momomura S, Ishikawa SE: Association of hyperadiponectinemia with severity of ventricular dysfunction in congestive heart failure. Circulation J 70: 1557–1562, 2006.

72. George J, Patal S, Wexler D, Sharabi Y, Peleg E, Kamari Y, Grossman E, Sheps D, Keren G, Roth A: Circulating adiponectin concentrations in patients with congestive heart failure. Heart 92: 1420–1424, 2006.

73. Ohashi K, Ouchi N, Kihara S, Funahashi T, Nakamura T, Sumitsuji S, Kawamoto T, Matsumoto S, Nagaretani H, Kumada M, Okamoto Y, Nishizawa H, Kishida K, Maeda N, Hiraoka H, Iwashima Y, Ishikawa K, Ohishi M, Katsuya T, Rakugi H, Ogihara T, Matsuzawa Y: Adiponectin I164T mutation is associated with the metabolic syndrome and coronary artery disease. J Am Coll Cardiol 43: 1195–1200, 2004.

74. Jung CH, Rhee EJ, Kim SY, Shin HS, Kim BJ, Sung KC, Kim BS, Lee WY, Kang JH, Oh KW, Lee MH, Kim SW, Park JR: Associations between two single nucleotide polymorphisms of adiponectin gene and coronary artery diseases. Endocr J 53: 671–677, 2006.

75. Lacquemant C, Froguel P, Lobbens S, Izzo P, Dina C, Ruiz J: The adiponectin gene SNP+45 is associated with coronary artery disease in Type 2 (non-insulin-dependent) diabetes mellitus. Diabet Med 21: 776–781, 2004.

76. Hoefle G, Muendlein A, Saely CH, Risch L, Rein P, Koch L, Schmid F, Aczel S, Marte T, Langer P, Drexel H: The -11377 C>G promoter variant of the adiponectin gene, prevalence of coronary atherosclerosis, and incidence of vascular events in men. Thromb Haemost 97: 451–457, 2007.

77. Filippi E, Sentinelli F, Romeo S, Arca M, Berni A, Tiberti C, Verrienti A, Fanelli M, Fallarino M, Sorropago G, Baroni MG: The adiponectin gene SNP+276G>T associates with early-onset coronary artery disease and with lower levels of adiponectin in younger coronary artery disease patients (age <or=50 years). J Mol Med 83: 711–719, 2005.

78. Bacci S, Menzaghi C, Ercolino T, Ma X, Rauseo A, Salvemini L, Vigna C, Fanelli R, Di Mario U, Doria A, Trischitta V: The +276 G/T single nucleotide polymorphism of the adiponectin gene is associated with coronary artery disease in type 2 diabetic patients. Diabetes Care 27: 2015–2020, 2004.

79. Qi L, Li T, Rimm E, Zhang C, Rifai N, Hunter D, Doria A, Hu FB: The +276 polymorphism of the APM1 gene, plasma adiponectin concentration, and cardiovascular risk in diabetic men. Diabetes 54: 1607–1610, 2005.

80. Nagasawa A, Fukui K, Funahashi T, Maeda N, Shimomura I, Kihara S, Waki M, Takamatsu K, Matsuzawa Y: Effects of soy protein diet on the expression of adipose genes and plasma adiponectin. Horm Metab Res 34: 635–639, 2002.

81. Flachs P, Mohamed-Ali V, Horakova O, Rossmeisl M, Hosseinzadeh-Attar MJ, Hensler M, Ruzickova J, Kopecky J: Polyunsaturated fatty acids of marine origin induce adiponectin in mice fed a high-fat diet. Diabetologia 49: 394–397, 2006.

82. Neschen S, Morino K, Rossbacher JC, Pongratz RL, Cline GW, Sono S, Gillum M, Shulman GI: Fish oil regulates adiponectin secretion by a peroxisome proliferator-activated receptor-gamma-dependent mechanism in mice. Diabetes 55: 924–928, 2006.

83. Hotta K, Funahashi T, Arita Y, Takahashi M, Matsuda M, Okamoto Y, Iwahashi H, Kuriyama H, Ouchi N, Maeda K, Nishida M, Kihara S, Sakai N, Nakajima T, Hasegawa K, Muraguchi M, Ohmoto Y, Nakamura T, Yamashita S, Hanafusa T, Matsuzawa Y: Plasma concentrations of a novel, adipose-specific protein, adiponectin, in type 2 diabetic patients, Arterioscler Thromb Vasc Biol 20: 1595–1599, 2000.

84. Kobayashi H, Ouchi N, Kihara S, Walsh K, Kumada M, Abe Y, Funahashi T, Matsuzawa Y: Selective suppression of endothelial cell apoptosis by the high molecular weight form of adiponectin, Circ Res 94:e27–e31, 2004.

85. Yang WS, Lee WJ, Funahashi T, Tanaka S, Matsuzawa Y, Chao CL, Chen CL, Tai TY, Chuang LM: Weight reduction increases plasma levels of an adipose-derived anti-inflammatory protein, adiponectin. J Clin Endocrinol Metab 86: 3815–3819, 2001.

86. Miyazaki T, Shimada T, Mokuno H, Daida H: Adipocyte derived plasma protein, adiponectin, is associated with smoking status in patients with coronary artery disease, Heart 89: 663, 2003.

87. Imatoh T, Miyazaki M, Kadowaki K, Babazono A, Sato M, Une H Interaction of low serum adiponectin levels and smoking on coronary stenosis in Japanese men. Int J Cardiol 110: 251–255, 2006.

88. Iwashima Y, Katsuya T, Ishikawa K, Kida I, Ohishi M, Horio T, Ouchi N, Ohashi K, Kihara S, Funahashi T, Rakugi H, Ogihara T: Association of hypoadiponectinemia with smoking habit in men, Hypertension 45: 1094–1100, 2006.

89. Hallakou S, Foufelle F, Doare L, Kergoat M, Ferre P: Pioglitazone induces in vivo adipocyte differentiation in the obese Zucker fa/fa rat. Diabetes 46: 1393–1399, 1997.

90. Gurnell M, Wentworth JM, Agostini M, Adams M, Collingwood TN, Provenzano C, Browne PO, Rajanayagam O, Burris TP, Schwabe JW, Lazar MA, Chatterjee VK: A dominant-negative peroxisome proliferator-activated receptor gamma (PPARgamma) mutant is a constitutive repressor and inhibits PPARgamma-mediated adipogenesis. J Biol Chem 275: 5754–5759, 2000.

91. Tontonoz P, Hu E, Devine J, Beale EG, Spiegelman BM: PPAR gamma 2 regulates adipose expression of the phosphoenolpyruvate carboxykinase gene. Mol Cell Biol 15: 351–357, 1995.

92. Olswang Y, Cohen H, Papo O, Cassuto H, Croniger CM, Hakimi P, Tilghman SM, Hanson RW, Reshef L: A mutation in the peroxisome proliferator-activated receptor gamma-binding site in the gene for the cytosolic form of phosphoenolpyruvate carboxykinase reduces adipose tissue size and fat content in mice. Proc Natl Acad Sci USA 99: 625–630, 2002.

93. Walczak, R: Tontonoz P: PPARadigms and PPARadoxes: expanding roles for PPARgamma in the control of lipid metabolism. J Lipid Res 43: 177–186, 2002.

94. Civitarese AE, Ukropcova B, Carling S, Hulver M, DeFronzo RA, Mandarino L, Ravussin E, Smith SR: Role of adiponectin in human skeletal muscle bioenergetics. Cell Metab 4: 75–87, 2006.

95. Furuhashi M, Ura N, Higashiura K, Murakami H, Tanaka M, Moniwa N, Yoshida D, Shimamoto K: Blockade of the renin-angiotensin system increases adiponectin concentrations in patients with essential hypertension. Hypertension 42: 76–81, 2003.

96. Kon KK, Quon MJ, Han SH, Chung WJ, Lee Y, Shin EK: Anti-inflammatory and metabolic effects of candesartan in hypertensive patients. Int J Cardiol 108: 96–100, 2005.

97. Watanabe S, Okura T, Kurata M, Irita J, Manabe S, Miyoshi K, Fukuoka T, Murakami K, Higaki J: The effect of losartan and amlodipine on serum adiponectin in Japanese adults with essential hypertension. Clin Ther 28: 1677–1685, 2006.

98. Hattori Y, Akimoto K, Gross SS, Hattori S, Kasai K: Angiotensin-II-induced oxidative stress elicits hypoadiponectinaemia in rats. Diabetologia 48: 1066–1074, 2005.

99. Kurata A, Nishizawa H, Kihara S, Maeda N, Sonoda M, Okada T, Ohashi K, Hibuse T, Fujita K, Yasui A, Hiuge A, Kumada M, Kuriyama H, Shimomura I, Funahashi T: Blockade of angiotensin II type-1 receptor reduces oxidative stress in adipose tissue and ameliorates adipocytokine dysregulation. Kidney Int 70: 1717–1724, 2006.

100. Bensaid M, Gary-Bobo M, Esclangon A, Maffrand JP, Le Fur G, Oury-Donat F, Soubrie P: The cannabinoid CB1 receptor antagonist SR141716 increases Acrp30 mRNA expression in adipose tissue of obese fa/fa rats and in cultured adipocyte cells. Mol Pharmacol 63: 908–914, 2003.

101. Despres JP, Golay A, Sjostrom L: Rimonabant in Obesity-Lipids Study Group. Effects of rimonabant on metabolic risk factors in overweight patients with dyslipidemia. N Engl J Med 353: 2121–2134, 2005.

IV SEX HORMONES AND VASCULAR DISEASE

11 Testosterone and Cardiovascular Disease

Allen D. Seftel and Dr. Spencer Land

CONTENTS

SUMMARY

The effects of testosterone (T) on cardiovascular disease in both men and women are summarized in this chapter. The epidemiologic data suggest that hypogonadism is associated with a higher prevalence of hypertension, hyperlipidemia, diabetes, obesity, asthma/COPD. Physiologically, androgen binding protein is expressed in the cardiac myocyte. Testosterone also affects basal levels of intracellular calcium in the cardiac myocyte, as well as improving calcium sparks and improving myocyte contractility. In dogs, orchiectomy significantly increased the duration of QT and QTc intervals, QTc dispersion, and the dofetilide-induced lengthening of QTc, while testosterone treatment of castrated females had opposite effects. Intraventricular conduction (QRS duration) was independent of the endocrine status of the animals. Ovarectomy or estrogen treatment of castrated males failed to alter significantly these parameters except for QTc-dispersion. Clinically, the effects of testosterone on cardiovascular disease risk appear to be dependent on plasma levels of testosterone. Decreased FT and TT levels have recently been associated with ischemic stroke in men. Testosterone appears to be linearly inversely related to the intima-media thickness (IMT) of the carotid artery. Men have a higher incidence of CVD than women of similar age, and it has been suggested that testosterone may influence the development of CVD. Observational evidence suggests that serum levels of testosterone and inflammatory cytokines are interlinked, suggesting that the underlying testosterone status may modulate IL-1β production in men with CHD.

In men with CHD, both long-term physiologic testosterone therapy and short-term exposure to supraphysiologic doses of testosterone are reported to increase flow-mediated brachial artery

From: *Contemporary Endocrinology: Cardiovascular Endocrinology: Shared Pathways and Clinical Crossroads*
Edited by: V. A. Fonseca © Humana Press, New York, NY

vasodilation, which occurs as a result of increased nitric oxide release from the endothelium in response to changes in sheer stress.

In women, low SHBG and high FAI are strongly associated with CVD risk factors in racially diverse women. Androgens likely play a role in the CVD risk profile of peri-menopausal women.

Androgens and SHBG are re-emerging as potential mediators of CVD risk in women at midlife.

High androgen levels may increase cardiovascular risk in women through adverse effects on lipids, blood pressure, and glucose metabolism.

In general, the literature on this topic is scant. While no one can definitively state that treatment or no treatment with testosterone is beneficial to helping reduce the risk of CVD, it appears that hypogonadism is associated with various cardiovascular morbidities in men.

Key Words: Testosterone, Cardiovascular disease

DEFINITION AND EPIDEMIOLOGY

Testosterone is a male hormone responsible for the growth and development of the male sex organs and maintenance of secondary sex characteristics. Hypogonadism in men is a clinical syndrome that results from failure of the testes to produce physiological levels of testosterone (androgen deficiency) and the normal number of spermatozoa due to disruption of one or more levels of the hypothalamic-pituitary-gonadal axis *(1)*.

The Hypogonadism In Males (HIM) study *(2)*, a cross-sectional, epidemiologic survey, examined the prevalence of hypogonadism and its associated signs and symptoms in men aged >45 years. From a random sample of 2650 primary care practices, 130 participated in the study. All men aged 45 years and older who were seen in the offices between 8 a.m. and noon during a 2-week period were invited to participate in the survey. In addition to meeting the age requirement, each eligible patient had to provide a blood sample and answer a brief set of questions about his medical and social histories, concomitant medications, and signs and symptoms of hypogonadism. Blood was tested for total testosterone (TT), free testosterone (FT), bioavailable testosterone (BT), and sex hormone-binding globulin (SHBG). Hypogonadism was defined as TT <300 ng/dl. Patients in the HIM study were considered to be hypogonadal if they had TT <10.41 nmol/l (300 ng/dl) or if they were currently receiving treatment for hypogonadism. Of 2165 patients enrolled in the study, 836 (38.7%) had hypogonadism, with 80 (9.6%) receiving testosterone. The mean TT level was 245.6 ± 4.12 ng/dl in men with hypogonadism compared to 439.9 ± 3.52 ng/dl in eugonadal men. Concentrations of FT and BT were significantly lower ($P < 0.001$) in men with hypogonadism than in eugonadal men. Importantly, this study noted that a higher proportion of hypogonadal patients than eugonadal patients reported a history of hypertension, hyperlipidemia, diabetes, and obesity ($P<0.001$), highlighting the potential association between hypogonadism and cardiovascular disease (CVD) (Table 1).

CVD is a leading cause of death among the elderly in Western countries and is a major determinant of chronic disability, while the burden of atherosclerosis especially afflicts the increasing older segment of the population *(3)*. Two of the strongest independent risk factors for coronary heart disease are increasing age and male sex *(4)*. Despite a wide variance in coronary heart disease (CHD) mortality between countries, a consistent male:female ratio of approximately 2:1 is observed *(4)*.

In the Tromsø Study, a population-based health survey, testosterone levels were inversely associated with anthropometrical measurements, and the lowest levels of TT and FT were found in men with the most pronounced central obesity. TT was inversely associated with systolic blood pressure, and men with hypertension had lower levels of both TT and FT. Furthermore,

Table 1
Prevalence of medical disease in hypogonadal patients vs eugonadal patients in the HIM study

Condition	Hypogonadal patients $N = 836$	Eugonadal patients $(n = 1326)$	P value
Hypertension	547(65.4)	678(51.1)	< 0.001
Hyperlipidemia	506(60.5)	670(50.5)	< 0.001
Diabetes	258(30.9)	237(17.9)	< 0.001
Obesity	270(32.3)	225(17.0)	< 0.001
Prostatic disease/disorder	165(19.7)	226(17.0)	0.12
Chronic pain	155(18.5)	211(16.0)	0.13
Insomnia/sleep disturbance	129(15.4)	185(14.0)	0.34
Asthma/COPD	102(12.2)	118(8.9)	0.013
Headaches (within the last 2 weeks)	70(8.4)	125(9.4)	0.4
Rheumatoid arthritis	28(3.3)	29(2.2)	0.1
Osteoporosis	15(1.8)	15(1.1)	0.19
Not reported	0(0.0)	4(0.3)	NR

From Mulligan et al. (Ref. (2), with permission)

men with diabetes had lower testosterone levels compared to men without a history of diabetes, and an inverse association between testosterone levels and glycosylated hemoglobin was found. Thus, there are strong associations between low levels of testosterone and the different components of the metabolic syndrome. Thus, testosterone may have a protective role in the development of metabolic syndrome and subsequent diabetes mellitus and CVD in aging men (5).

Derby et al. prospectively followed 942 men in the Massachusetts Male Ageing Study with complete anthropometry and hormone data at baseline (1987–1989, ages 40–70) and 8–10 years follow-up (1995–1997). FT and TT, dehydroepiandrosterone sulphate (DHEAS), and SHBG were assessed using standardized methods. Health behaviors and medical history were obtained by structured interview. Repeated measures regression was used to describe trends in steroid hormones and SHBG in relation to obesity status, adjusting for age, smoking, alcohol, comorbidities, and physical activity. Obesity was associated with decreased levels of TT and FT, and of SHBG at follow-up relative to baseline. For any given baseline concentration of TT, FT, or SHBG, follow-up levels were lowest among men who remained obese or who became obese during follow-up. This was true for all three indices of obesity. Central adiposity was associated with lower DHEAS levels at follow-up, while elevated body mass index (BMI) was not. These authors felt that obesity may predict greater decline in testosterone and SHBG levels with age. Central adiposity may be a more important predictor of decline in DHEAS than is BMI (6).

Thus, there is ample epidemiologic evidence to link testosterone with CVD.

This chapter will provide data exploring the association between cardiovascular disease and testosterone.

PHYSIOLOGY

Testosterone is also known as a steroid hormone. Steroid hormones are derived from cholesterol, which can lead to cardiovascular disease if too much plaque build-up occurs.

Low levels of circulating sex hormone reduce feedback inhibition on gonadotropin-releasing hormone (GnRH) synthesis (the long loop), leading to elevated follicle-stimulating hormone (FSH) and luteinizing hormone (LH). The latter peptide hormones bind to gonadal tissue and stimulate P450ssc activity, resulting in sex hormone production via cAMP and PKA-mediated pathways. In males, LH binds to Leydig cells, stimulating production of the principal Leydig cell hormone, testosterone. Testosterone is secreted to the plasma and also carried to Sertoli cells by androgen-binding protein (ABP). In females, LH binds to thecal cells of the ovary, where it stimulates the synthesis of androstenedione and testosterone by the usual cAMP- and PKA-regulated pathway. An additional enzyme complex known as aromatase is responsible for the final conversion of the latter two molecules into the estrogens.

Cardiomyocytes are known to be androgen targets. Changing systemic steroid levels are thought to be linked to various cardiac ailments, including dilated cardiomyopathy (DCM). The mode of action of gonadal steroid hormones on the human heart is unknown to date. Schock et al. used high-resolution immunocytochemistry on semithin sections (1 μm thick), in situ hybridization, and mass spectrometry to investigate the expression of ABP in human myocardial biopsies taken from male patients with DCM. They observed distinct cytoplasmic ABP immunoreactivity in a fraction of the myocytes. In situ hybridization with synthetic oligonucleotide probes revealed specific hybridization signals in these cells. A portion of the ABP-positive cells contained immunostaining for androgen receptor. With SELDI TOF mass spectrometry of affinity purified tissue extracts of human myocardium, they confirmed the presence of a 50-kDa protein similar to ABP. These observations provide evidence of an intrinsic expression of ABP in human heart. ABP may be secreted from myocytes in a paracrine manner perhaps to influence the bioavailability of gonadal steroids in myocardium (7).

Detailed evaluation of chronic and acute actions of testosterone on the function of cardiac I(Ca,L) and intracellular Ca2+ handling is limited (8). Er et al. performed whole-cell and single-channel analysis of I(Ca,L), recordings of Ca2+ sparks, measurements of contractility and quantitative real-time RT-PCR in rat cardiomyocytes following testosterone pretreatment and acute testosterone application. Pretreatment with testosterone 100 nM for 24–30 h increased whole-cell I(Ca,L) from 3.8+/–0.8 pA/pF (n = 10) to 10.1+/–0.31 pA/pF (n = 9) at +10 mV ($P<0.001$). Increase of I(Ca,L) density was caused by both, increased expression levels of the alpha 1C subunit of L-type calcium channel and a pronounced increment of the single-channel activity (availability 81.8+/–3.15% versus 37.1+/–7.01%; open probability 12.8+/–3.09% versus 1.0+/–0.62%, $P<0.01$). Moreover, testosterone pretreatment significantly increased the frequency of Ca2+ sparks and improved myocytes contractility without altering SR Ca2+ load. All chronic effects could be inhibited by flutamide. In contrast acute testosterone administration significantly reduced I(Ca,L) density. Indeed, on the single-channel level acute testosterone application completely reversed the chronic testosterone-mediated effects, and antagonized the chronic testosterone effects on Ca2+ spark frequency, which was unaffected by flutamide. Thus, testosterone pretreatment activates I(Ca,L) via nuclear receptor-mediated pathways, while testosterone acutely blocks I(Ca,L) in a direct manner. These data suggest that testosterone chronically affects the basal level of intracellular Ca2+ handling, which in addition rapidly may be modulated by acute changes of hormone levels.

Other researchers examined the effects of testosterone and estrogen on the ECG parameters and expression of cardiac ion channels in male and female dogs, and to compare the dofetilide-induced lengthening of QTc interval in control, castrated, and hormone-treated animals (9). ECG records were taken from male and female anesthetized dogs (n = 10 in each group) before castration, after castration, and following inverted hormone substitution. The animals were challenged with dofetilide at each stage of the experiment. Finally, the hearts were excised and expression of ion channels was studied using Western blot technique. The heart rate was decreased and PQ interval increased by deprivation of sex hormones in both genders (orchiectomy or ovarectomy), while inverted hormonal substitution restored control values. Orchiectomy significantly increased the duration of QT and QTc intervals, QTc-dispersion, and the dofetilide-induced lengthening of QTc, while testosterone treatment of castrated females had opposite effects. Intraventricular conduction (QRS duration) was independent of the endocrine status of the animals. Ovarectomy or oestrogen treatment of castrated males failed to alter significantly these parameters except for QTc-dispersion. Expression of ion channel proteins responsible for mediation of I(K1) and I(to) currents (Kir2.1 and Kv4.3, respectively), was significantly higher in the testosterone-treated castrated females and normal males than in the oestrogen-treated castrated males and normal females. Repolarization of canine ventricular myocardium is significantly modified by testosterone, but not oestrogen, in both genders. This effect is likely due to augmentation of expression of K(+)-channel proteins, and thus may provide protection against arrhythmias via increasing the repolarization reserve. Thus, it appears that there is evidence of direct effect of T on cardiac myocytes.

In sum, the epidemiologic and cell physiology data suggest a strong correlation between testosterone and CVD.

TESTOSTERONE, CARDIOVASCULAR DISEASE, AND AGING

In aging men testosterone levels decline. Concomitantly, cognitive function, muscle and bone mass, libido, and sexual activity declines and cardiovascular diseases increase *(10)*. This decline in testosterone usually begins around age 30, which continuously persists throughout the aging process *(10)*. The effects of testosterone on cardiovascular disease risk appear to be dependent on plasma levels of testosterone *(4)*. Decreased FT and TT levels have recently been associated with ischemic stroke in men, further implicating testosterone in the pathophysiology of vascular disease *(11)*. Acute testosterone administration increases time of onset of exercise-induced myocardial ischemia in men with CAD and decreased plasma testosterone concentrations *(11)*.

CVD is the prime cause of death among the elderly in industrialized countries and it is a major determinant of chronic disability *(12)*. In men, a beneficial effect of testosterone and of DHEAS on cardiovascular risk factors has been described *(12)*. In the Van den Beld et al. study, among 403 independently living, elderly men, several associations between circulating hormone levels and ultrasonographic measures of atherosclerosis were observed *(10)*. Van den Beld et al. reported that testosterone appeared to be linearly inversely related to the intima-media thickness (IMT) of the carotid artery in 403 independently living elderly men, aged 73–94 years *(10)*. This study demonstrated a strong inverse association between serum levels of testosterone and the degree of carotid atherosclerosis *(10)*. Hak et al. reported an inverse association between levels of testosterone and aortic atherosclerosis in 504 nonsmoking men, aged 55 years and over, participating in the Rotterdam study *(10)*.

Other factors that feed into the risk of CVD include geography and ethnic differences *(12)*. The narrowing sex gap after middle age is a possible cause of the role of sex hormones in CHD *(12)*. No single study showed an association between increased testosterone level and symptoms of CAD *(13)*. The findings of these observational studies support the hypothesis that low testosterone is a component of the multidimensional metabolic syndrome *(13)*. Some observational studies have shown a consistent association between low testosterone and high cholesterol; studies of testosterone therapy have shown inconsistent results *(13)*. Overall, there is evidence to support the conclusion that the cardiovascular effects of testosterone therapy may be considered neutral to beneficial *(13)*.

Men have a higher incidence of CVD than women of similar age, and it has been suggested that testosterone may influence the development of CVD *(5)*. In two recent cross-sectional studies of elderly men, IMT of the carotid artery, an indicator of general atherosclerosis, was associated with lower testosterone levels *(6)*. In a population-based study of 482 men, TT levels were significantly related to the carotid IMT. The association was independent of age, CVD risk factors, and lifestyle factors but was not independent of BMI *(7)*. Although it is known that testosterone levels influence lipoprotein patterns, only a few studies have directly examined the relation between testosterone and markers of atherosclerotic CVD *(8)*.

Muller et al. suggested that testosterone may affect the development of CVD by modulating risk factors such as diabetes, obesity, hypertension, and hypercholesterolemia *(9)*. In this study population, serum total testosterone (T), total estradiol (E2), and free E2 were not significantly associated with age. Serum free testosterone (Tf) was significantly inversely related to age. Serum total testosterone concentrations were inversely related to BMI *(10)*. Baseline FT levels were more strongly related to atherosclerosis than the other sex hormone levels when using standardized linear regression coefficients *(3)*. In this report, FT, but not TT, was associated with progression of atherosclerosis in older men, aged 77–94 years *(3)*. In conclusion, this study found an inverse association between TT levels and atherosclerosis, measured using IMT of the carotid artery that was present *(3)*.

Increased wall thickness of the carotid artery was related to lower serum testosterone, estrone, and free IGF-I concentrations in subjects with prevalent CVD as well as in subjects free of CVD *(12)*.

CYTOKINES, TESTOSTERONE, AND ATHEROSCLEROSIS

Proinflammatory cytokines such as interlukin (IL)-1β and tumor necrosis factor (TNF)-α are key mediators of the atherosclerotic process *(10)*. Observational evidence suggests that serum levels of testosterone and inflammatory cytokines are interlinked *(10)*. Such data suggest that the underlying testosterone status may modulate IL-1β production in men with CHD *(12)*. Young hypogonadal men with delayed puberty are reported to exhibit higher serum levels of inflammatory cytokines than healthy controls. Testosterone replacement therapy was sufficient to significantly lower serum levels of TNF-α *(12)*. Similar results were observed in a larger study using the same testosterone regimen and randomized, placebo-controlled crossover protocol in 27 hypogonadal men with concomitant CVD, 20 of whom had CHD *(12)*. These data provide evidence that testosterone is important in regulation of cytokine function in men with CHD *(12)*.

TESTOSTERONE AND STROKE AND MYOCARDIAL INFARCTION RISK

Low SHBG and high free androgen index (FAI) were strongly and consistently related to elevated CVD risk factors even after controlling for BMI *(13)*. The CVD risk factors were higher insulin, glucose, hemostatic/inflammatory markers, and adverse lipids *(13)*. High testosterone levels have been found to be associated with high high-density lipoprotein (HDL) cholesterol and low triglyceride levels in several cross-sectional and one longitudinal study in agreement with our results *(14)*. Furthermore, a decrease in endogenous testosterone was associated with an increase in triglycerides *(14)*. This indicates a possible beneficial effect of chronic testosterone treatment on myocardial ischemia; however, these findings were limited by the methodology used *(4)*.

In a recent study using an experimental model, *(1)* the dose-dependent effects of testosterone on plaque development, *(2)* the expression of the androgen receptor in arteries, and *(3)* possible dose-dependent changes of androgen receptor expression induced by testosterone were evaluated *(11)*. Testosterone reduces TNF-α induced VCAM-1 expression in HUVECs of female origin, an activity blocked by estrogen receptor antagonism and aromatase inhibition in human aortic endothelial cells *(11)*. These data suggest that testosterone may exert a beneficial effect upon adhesion molecule expression *(15)*. Alternatively, this effect may represent an endogenous mechanism whereby testosterone aids the removal of damaged endothelial cell, by enhancing their programmed cell death *(12)*. Plasminogen activator inhibitor (PAI-1) is a predictor of myocardial infarction and progression of atherosclerosis in patients with stable coronary artery disease (CAD) *(12)*. Serum levels of testosterone are negatively correlated with those of PAI-1 *(12)*.

These data provide evidence that testosterone possesses a number of beneficial cardiovascular actions, and that low serum testosterone would appear to be linked to increased cardiovascular risk. These actions may combine to impair the atherosclerotic process, attenuate plaque rupture, and provide improvements in anginal symptoms *(12)*. FT and BT are generally considered to be the most accurate estimations of an individual's androgen status since, unlike the measurement of TT, they take into consideration the proportion of testosterone tightly bound to SHBG, and considered to be biologically inactive *(12)*. FT represents a small part of TT (1–2%) and is influenced by both TT and SHBG levels*(12)*. Cardiovascular risk factors include lipid fractions, blood pressure, and blood glucose *(12)*. Cardiovascular events include cardiovascular death, nonfatal myocardial infarction, angina or claudication, revascularization and stroke *(4)*. In a meta analysis, Haddad et al. *(16)* reviewed the data regarding the effect of testosterone preparations on lipid fractions in men with low-normal or normal testosterone levels. Testosterone reduced total cholesterol levels by 16mg/dl, while all other lipid fractions were not significantly affected *(16)*.

The previous stated data excludes unfavorable elevations in LDL-C levels of more than 3mg/dl and in triglyceride levels of more than 41 mg/dl and excludes unfavorable reductions in HDL-C levels of less than 7 mg/dl*(16)*. Testosterone preparations had nonsignificant effects on systolic and diastolic blood pressure that were consistent across trials[59]. Most studies that reported cardiac events had neither strict outcome definitions nor independent and blinded judicial assessors of these outcomes *(16)*. For each hormone, we used proportional hazards regression that adjusted for (1) age alone and (2) age, smoking, systolic and diastolic blood pressure, antihypertensive medication use, ratio of total and HDL cholesterol, diabetes mellitus, and BMI *(16)*.

Adiposity is a strong correlate of sex hormone levels and of SHBG. SHBG strongly influences measurements of total circulating sex hormone levels and the amount of bound hormone versus free hormone *(16)*. Serum levels of testosterone or DHEAS were not associated with CVD risk in either age-adjusted or multivariable-adjusted models *(17)*. In this study, TT and estradiol level were measured, excluding those of unbound hormones. The relationship between serum testosterone levels and CVD may vary according to genetically determined differences in androgen sensitivity, a premise not evaluated by this study *(17)*.

A study by Phillips et al. of 55 men (aged 39–89 years) found an inverse relation between serum testosterone and degree of CAD *(17)*. In summary, testosterone, estrone, and free IGF-I concentrations appear to be linearly inversely related to atherosclerosis, as measured by the IMT of the carotid artery in elderly men *(17)*. The fact that the associations were as strong in the group free of cardiovascular disease as in the group with prevalent disease suggests that testosterone, estrone, and free IGF-I levels may play a protective role in the development of atherosclerosis in aging men *(10)*.

An acute study in men with CAD demonstrated endothelium-independent increases in coronary blood flow induced by physiologic concentrations of testosterone. These data indicate a possible role for testosterone in the modulation of coronary vascular tone and suggest that testosterone may improve myocardial ischemia in men with established CAD *(10)*. In the present study of men with atherosclerotic CAD and low plasma testosterone levels, acute intravenous testosterone delayed the onset of electrocardiographic signs of myocardial ischemia by approximately 20% *(10)*. A significant increase was found of the amount of androgen receptor mRNA in testosterone segments at concentrations of 1 ng/ml and 10 ng/ml testosterone *(13)*. It was hypothesized that vascular androgen receptor might play an important role in signaling the testosterone effects on the level arterial vessel wall *(13)*. Testosterone in male rabbits had an inhibitory effect on plaque development, but in female rabbits an atheroprogressive action of testosterone was found *(15)*. In conclusion, our present data suggest the involvement of the arterial androgen receptor in mediating the beneficial vascular effects of testosterone *(15)*.

Contrary to widespread (but untested) belief, there is little evidence to suggest that exposure to testosterone underlies the higher incidence of CHD in men *(15)*. Serum levels of testosterone are actually reduced in men with CHD with approximately one in four individuals exhibiting serum levels of testosterone within the hypogonadal range *(15)*. Although no studies report a detrimental influence of physiologic testosterone replacement therapy in men with CHD, it is not yet clear whether testosterone administration would be of benefit to all men with the disease, that is, those for whom therapy is not indicated on the basis of their serum testosterone *(12)*. Currently available evidence weakly supports the inference that testosterone use in men is not associated with important cardiovascular events *(12)*.

Six randomized controlled trials reported on cardiovascular events with consistent results. There were 14 events in 161 men who received testosterone and 7 events in 147 men in the control groups *(12)*. The best available evidence suggests small and clinically negligible effects of testosterone use on lipid fractions, blood pressure, and glycemic control in men with different degrees of androgen deficiency *(16)*. In particular, among hypogonadal men who received intramuscular testosterone, we found nonsignificant effects on total cholesterol and HDL-C levels *(16)*. As patients and clinicians consider the use of testosterone in the management of symptoms consistent with hypogonadism, they should be concerned about potential adverse consequences of its long-term use *(16)*. Men in the highest quartile of estradiol had a 33% multivariable-adjusted lower risk for CVD events compared with men in the first quartile *(16)*. In supplementary analyses evaluating the estradiol–testosterone ratio, a higher ratio was associated with a lower CVD risk *(16)*. We did not detect a statistically significant relationship between hypogonadism and CVD risk *(17)*. We did not observe any association between serum testosterone level or DHEAS level and CVD incidence *(17)*. In men, estrogen is mainly synthesized by local tissue aromatization of androgenic precursors from the testes and adrenal gland, and estrogen levels do not seem to decrease with age to the same extent as testosterone *(17)*.

Low FT levels were related to IMT of the common carotid artery in elderly men independently of cardiovascular risk factors *(17)*. Subjects with baseline FT levels in the lowest tertile had a significantly more marked progression of IMT compared with subjects in the second and third tertiles *(17)*. Results suggest that FT levels and high estradiol levels were related to thickening of the IMT of the common carotid artery. These associations were independent of cardiovascular risk factors *(3)*. Our results are in agreement of other observational studies describing lower levels of TT and FT in association with atherosclerosis and CAD *(3)*. Animal studies evaluating the effect of androgens on the progression of atherosclerosis have shown beneficial effects when male animals were tested and detrimental when androgens were administered to female animals *(3)*. This study found a more consistent relation between free sex hormone levels and atherosclerosis compared with total hormone levels and atherosclerosis *(3)*. In summary, male low FT levels are associated with progression of atherosclerosis in the oldest independently of other cardiovascular risk factors *(3)*.

WOMEN, TESTOSTERONE, AND CARDIOVASCULAR DISEASE

Women are known to suffer coronary disease 10–20 years later than men. One hypothesis states endogenous ovarian hormones offer a protective effect on the development of CHD *(3)*. Low SHBG and high FAI are strongly associated with CVD risk factors in racially diverse women. Androgens likely play a role in the CVD risk profile of peri-menopausal women *(3)*. Androgens and SHBG are re-emerging as potential mediators of CVD risk in women at midlife *(14)*. High androgen levels may increase cardiovascular risk in women through adverse effects on lipids, blood pressure, and glucose metabolism *(14)*. In the total population, median level of SHBG, testosterone, FAI, estradiol, FEI, FAI/FEI, and testosterone/estradiol did not significantly differ among women with cardiovascular events and those who remained free of cardiovascular events *(14)*. Among postmenopausal women not taking hormone therapy, the study found that women with low SHBG or high FAI were at increased risk of CVD events *(18)*.

Recent randomized trial evidence demonstrated increased risk of CVD with hormone therapy, raising concern that higher estrogen levels might increase the risk also *(18)*. There were weak trends toward increased risk of CVD among women with higher androgen/estrogen (FAI/FEI) ratios *(18)*. Polycystic ovary syndrome can cause more extensive atherosclerosis on angiography than women without the condition *(18)*. Furthermore, in women, substantial evidence exists for a protective role of endogenous sex hormones and of estrogen therapy in the development of atherosclerosis *(18)*.

MEN, ESTROGEN, AND CARDIOVASCULAR DISEASE

Few studies have examined the relation between estrogens and atherosclerosis in men. In women, estrogen replacement therapy is associated with plaque regression in the carotid artery as well as a delay in the thickening of the intima layer of the carotid artery *(18)*. Although power to infer conclusions was limited, this study was able to show that the associations between IMT and testosterone, IMT and estrone, and IMT and free IGF-I in subjects free of symptomatic CVD were as powerful as those in subjects with prevalent CVD *(10)*. Genetic variation in estrogen receptor-a has been associated with prevalent CVD and androgen and estrogen receptor expression in coronary arteries has been reported to influence coronary atherosclerosis in men *(10)*. Testosterone and DHEAS levels were not associated with CVD risk. Estrogen levels were inversely related *(10)*.

In this studies' population, serum total testosterone and insulin were not significantly associated with age *(17)*. However, serum testosterone concentrations were inversely related to mean IMT of the bifurcation and combined IMT after adjustment for age *(17)*. Serum total testosterone concentrations were inversely related to BMI *(10)*. Mean serum testosterone concentrations were significantly higher in subjects who had never smoked compared with subjects who had *(10)*.

REPLACEMENT THERAPY

In men with CHD, both long-term physiologic testosterone therapy and short-term exposure to supraphysiologic doses of testosterone is reported to increase flow-mediated brachial artery vasodilation, which occurs as a result of increased nitric oxide release from the endothelium in response to changes in sheer stress *(10)*. The increased male incidence of CHD, combined with the well-documented adverse cardiovascular effects associated with high-dose anabolic steroids, has led to the supposition that testosterone provokes, or contributes to, the atherosclerotic process *(10)*. These studies vary in their definition of atherosclerosis, but are consistent in their conclusion that serum levels of testosterone are not elevated in men with CHD. Such findings would suggest that testosterone does not exacerbate coronary atherosclerosis, at least at the time when the condition becomes symptomatic *(12)*. Most of these studies actually report that serum levels of testosterone are reduced in men with CHD, which raises the possibility that testosterone deficiency may contribute to the atherosclerotic process *(12)*. This study provides strong evidence that men with significant CHD have reduced serum levels of testosterone and that testosterone replacement therapy is clinically indicated in a high proportion of these men *(12)*. In summary, the majority of these studies provide evidence for a protective role of testosterone against atherogenesis in male animal models, an action that is independent of changes in serum lipid levels *(12)*.

CONCLUSION

Prescription data tracking has shown that over the past few years, there has been a significant increase in the use of testosterone therapy in the US *(12)*. More widespread use raises concern about the undesirable cardiovascular consequences of testosterone administration *(12)*. Thus, to this day, the extent and direction of the cardiovascular consequences of testosterone remain unclear *(13)*. Treatment with oral testosterone or DHEA prevented this increase in atheroma formation, while treatment with intramuscular testosterone was associated with a significant reduction in plaque formation *(16)*. Recent research demonstrates that testosterone replacement therapy in men with CHD and low serum testosterone is effective in reducing myocardial ischemia, and also exhibits a favorable effect on serum lipids and cytokines *(16)*. The literature on this topic is scant and no one can clearly say that treatment or no treatment with testosterone is beneficial to helping reduce the risk of CVD. The correlation between testosterone and CVD is a weak correlation and needs to be further studied to determine a clear relationship.

REFERENCES

1. Bhasin S, Cunningham GR, Hayes FJ, et al. Testosterone therapy in adult men with androgen deficiency syndromes: an Endocrine Society clinical practice guideline. J Clin Endocrinol Metab. 2006;91:1995–2010.
2. Mulligan T, Frick MF, Zuraw QC, Stemhagen A, McWhirter C. Prevalence of hypogonadism in males aged at least 45 years: the HIM study. Int J Clin Pract. 2006;60:762–769.
3. Muller M, Van den Beld A, et al. Endogenous sex hormones and progression of carotid atherosclerosis in elderly men. Circulation 2004;109:2074–2079.
4. Svartberg J, Muhlen D, et al. Low testosterone levels are associated with carotid atherosclerosis in men. J Inter Med 2006;259:576–582.
5. Svartberg J: Epidemiology: testosterone and the metabolic syndrome. Int J Impotence Res 2007;19:124–128.
6. Derby CA, Zilber S, Brambilla D, Morales KH, McKinlay JB. Body mass index, waist circumference and waist to hip ratio and change in sex steroid hormones: the Massachusetts Male Ageing Study. Clin Endocrinol (Oxf) 2006;65(1):125–31.
7. Schock HW, Herbert Z, Sigusch H, Figulla HR, Jirikowski GF, Lotze U. Expression of androgen-binding protein (ABP) in human cardiac myocytes. Horm Metab Res 2006;38(4):225–9.

8. Er F, Michels G, Brandt MC, Khan I, Haase H, Eicks M, Lindner M, Hoppe UC. Impact of testosterone on cardiac L-type calcium channels and Ca2+ sparks: acute actions antagonize chronic effects. Cell Calcium 2007;41(5):467–77.

9. Fülöp L, Bányász T, Szabó G, Tóth IB, Bíró T, Lôrincz I, Balogh A, Petô K, Mikó I, Nánási PP. Effects of sex hormones on ECG parameters and expression of cardiac ion channels in dogs. Acta Physiol (Oxf) 2006 Nov–Dec;188(3–4):163–71.

10. Van den Beld A, Bots M, et al. Endogenous hormones and carotid atherosclerosis in elderly men. Am J Epidemiol 2003;157:25–31.

11. Webb C, Adamson D, et al. Effect of acute testosterone on myocardial ischemia in men with coronary artery disease. Am J Cardiol 1999; 83: 437–439.

12. Jones R, Nettleship J, et al. Testosterone and atherosclerosis in aging men. Am. J Cardiovasc Drugs 2005;5: 141–154.

13. Shabsigh R, Katz M, et al. Cardiovascular issues in hypogonadism and testosterone therapy. Am J Cardiol 2005;96:67M–72M.

14. Sutton-Tyrell K, Wildman R, et al. Sex hormone-binding globulin and the free androgen index are related to cardiovascular risk factors in multiethnic pre- and peri- menopausal women enrolled in SWAN across the nation. Circulation 2005;111:1242–1249.

15. Hanke H, Lenz C, et al. Effect of testosterone on plaque development and androgen receptor expression in the arterial vessel wall. Circulation 2001;103:1382–1385.

16. Haddad R, Kennedy C, et al. Testosterone and cardiovascular risk in men. Mayo Clinic Proc 2007;82:29–39.

17. Arnlov J, Pencina M, et al. Endogenous sex hormones and cardiovascular disease incidence in men. Ann Intern Med 2006;145(3):176–185.

18. Rexrode K, Manson J, et al. Sex hormone levels and risk of cardiovascular events in postmenopausal women. Circulation 2003;108:1688–1693.

12 Sexual Dysfunction and Cardiovascular Risk – Links and Solutions

Glenn Matfin, BSc (Hons), M.B. Ch.B., DGM, FFPM, FACE, FACP, FRCP

CONTENTS

INTRODUCTION
NORMAL PHYSIOLOGY OF ERECTION
PATHOPHYSIOLOGY OF ED
ED AS A RISK MARKER OF CVD
EVALUATION OF ED
EFFICACY OF TREATMENT FOR ED
CONCLUSION
REFERENCES

SUMMARY

Erectile dysfunction (ED) is an increasingly common problem, affecting up to 30 million men in the US and 140 million men worldwide. The prevalence and incidence of ED is closely related to an aging population and also to an increase in other associated risk factors (such as type 2 diabetes mellitus (T2DM), hypertension, atherosclerosis, smoking and polypharmacy). Several of these risk factors for ED are also components of the metabolic syndrome. The metabolic syndrome refers to a clustering of established and emerging cardiovascular (CV) risk factors within a single individual. The diagnosis of the metabolic syndrome in an individual increases the risk of subsequent cardiovascular disease (CVD) approximately twofold and T2DM fivefold.

Endothelial dysfunction is a major unifying etiology for many of the aspects of the metabolic syndrome, especially T2DM and CVD. It also plays a major role in ED. In fact, the presentation of ED should alert the physician to an underlying CV problem particularly in a patient with T2DM. This should lead to screening for CV risk factors and appropriate risk stratification for asymptomatic men with ED. Men with ED and other CV risk factors should be counseled in lifestyle modification, and treated where indicated with agents aimed at reducing CV risk (i.e., statins, aspirin, antihypertensives, etc).

Treatment of ED in general and in men with diabetes has been revolutionized with the introduction of phosphodiesterase type 5 (PDE5) inhibitors. However, men with diabetes tend to respond

From: *Contemporary Endocrinology: Cardiovascular Endocrinology: Shared Pathways and Clinical Crossroads*
Edited by: V. A. Fonseca © Humana Press, New York, NY

less well to these agents. This decreased responsiveness may relate to the severity of ED in diabetes. Alternative therapeutic strategies may be needed to overcome this problem. The safety of PDE5 inhibitors in men with ED and concomitant CVD seems to be generally accepted, especially when these agents are used according to the respective prescribing information and as per current guidelines.

Key Words: Erectile dysfunction, Diabetes, Metabolic syndrome, Cardiovascular disease, Phosphodiesterase type 5 (PDE5) inhibitors

INTRODUCTION

Erectile dysfunction (ED) has largely replaced the term "impotence". It is defined as the persistent inability to achieve and maintain an erection sufficient to permit satisfactory sexual intercourse *(1)*. ED is an increasingly common problem, affecting approximately 20–30 million men in the US *(2)*. The prevalence and incidence of ED is closely related to an aging population and also to an increase in other associated risk factors (such as type 2 diabetes mellitus (T2DM), hypertension, atherosclerosis, smoking, and polypharmacy). Several of these risk factors for ED are also components of the metabolic syndrome *(3)*. The metabolic syndrome refers to a clustering of established and emerging cardiovascular (CV) risk factors within a single individual *(4)*. Both the established risk factors, such as T2DM, dyslipidemia, hypertension, and other emerging risk factors are closely related to central obesity (especially intra-abdominal adiposity) and insulin resistance. The emerging risk factors include dysfunction of inflammation, coagulation, platelets, fibrinolysis, lipoproteins, endothelium, and miscellaneous biological processes. The diagnosis of the metabolic syndrome in an individual increases the risk of subsequent cardiovascular disease (CVD) approximately twofold and T2DM fivefold *(4)*.

Endothelial dysfunction is a major unifying etiology for many of the aspects of the metabolic syndrome, especially T2DM and CVD. It also plays a major role in ED *(3)*. In fact, the presentation of ED should alert the physician to an underlying CV problem particularly in a patient with T2DM *(3,5)*.

The purpose of this review is to highlight what is known about the relationship between ED and CVD with particular emphasis on the diabetes patient, and also to discuss the pathophysiological links between these conditions, that may have implications for treatment. Treatment of ED in general and in men with diabetes has been revolutionized with the introduction of phosphodiesterase type 5 (PDE5) inhibitors *(6,7)*.

NORMAL PHYSIOLOGY OF ERECTION

The cylindrical body or shaft of the penis is composed of three masses of erectile tissue held together by fibrous strands and covered with a thin layer of skin. The two lateral masses of tissue are called the corpora cavernosa. The third, ventral mass is called the corpus spongiosum. The corpora cavernosa and corpus spongiosum are cavernous sinuses that normally are relatively empty but become engorged with blood during penile erection *(8,9)*.

Erection is a neurovascular process which involves increased inflow of blood into the corpora cavernosa due to relaxation of the trabecular smooth muscle that surrounds the sinusoidal spaces and compression of the veins controlling outflow of blood from the venous plexus. Erection is mediated by parasympathetic impulses that pass from the sacral segments of the spinal cord through the pelvic nerves to the penis. Parasympathetic stimulation results in release of nitric oxide (NO), a nonadrenergic-noncholinergic (NANC) neurotransmitter, which causes relaxation of trabecular smooth muscle of the corpora cavernosa. This relaxation permits inflow of blood into the sinuses of the cavernosa at pressures approaching those of the arterial system and because the erectile tissues of the cavernosa are surrounded by a nonelastic fibrous covering, high pressure in the sinusoids causes ballooning of the erectile tissue to such an extent that the penis becomes hard and elongated. In the flaccid or detumescent state, locally released endothelin-1 (ET-1, a potent vasoconstrictor) and also increased sympathetic discharge through α-adrenergic receptors maintains contraction of the arteries that supply the penis and vascular sinuses of the corpora cavernosa and corpus spongiosum *(8,9)*.

Parasympathetic innervation must be intact and NO synthesis must be active for erection to occur. NO activates guanylyl cyclase, an enzyme that increases the concentration of cyclic guanosine monophosphate (cGMP), which in turn causes smooth muscle relaxation. Other smooth muscle relaxants (e.g., prostaglandin E_1 (PGE_1) analogs and α-adrenergic antagonists), if present in high enough concentrations, can independently cause sufficient cavernosal relaxation to result in erection. Many of the drugs that have been developed to treat ED act at the levels of these mediators *(6–9)*.

PATHOPHYSIOLOGY OF ED

ED is commonly classified as psychogenic, organic, or mixed psychogenic and organic *(9)*. Organic causes span a wide range of pathologies. They include neurogenic, hormonal, vascular, drug-induced, and penile-related etiologies.

ED in patients with diabetes usually has a multifactorial etiology. It can result from impairments in nearly every step responsible for the production of penile erection *(9)*. Table 1 lists some of these impairments and other indirectly acting mechanisms responsible for ED in diabetics. ED in men with diabetes is correlated with the glycosylated hemoglobin A_{1c} (A1C),

Table 1
Pathophysiology and factors complicating erectile
dysfunction (ED) in patients with diabetes

- Hyperglycemia and increasing age cause glycation of elastic fibers with failure of relaxation of the corpora cavernosa.
- Multiple drug treatments associated with ED – for example, diuretics, beta-blockers
- Dyslipidemia
- Endothelial dysfunction of the sinusoidal endothelial cells results in a decrease in NO release and impaired vasodilation.
- Peripheral vascular disease resulting in reduced arterial and arteriolar inflow
- Advanced glycation end products (AGE) increase reactive oxidizing substances and reduce NO production.
- Failed neural signal transmission to and from the spinal cord due to diabetic neuropathy and reduced production of neuronal nitric oxide synthase (nNOS) reduced levels of neuronal NO release to the cavernosal smooth muscle.
- Hypogonadism (especially hypogonadotropic)
- Obesity
- Inflammation

but it is not known whether improving glycemic control will improve ED. The presence of peripheral neuropathy also increases the risk of ED possibly due to undiagnosed autonomic neuropathy.

Patients with diabetes often suffer from other comorbid states including hypertension, obesity, and dyslipidemia. These and several other risk factors for ED are similar to those for CVD, and are key components of the metabolic syndrome. ED is often the first warning sign of underlying CV problems that are more common in persons, of either sex, affected by diabetes. The same vascular/endothelial injuries that occur in the coronary arteries likely occur in the cavernosal arteries, the primary vessels supplying penile erectile tissue.

The Metabolic Syndrome

The metabolic syndrome is a "cluster" of CV risk factors frequently, but not always, associated with obesity. Reaven first drew attention to the association of insulin resistance and T2DM, high plasma triglycerides and low plasma HDL cholesterol (HDL), and hypertension *(10)*.

Table 2
Original (as described by Reaven[10]) and expanded features of the metabolic syndrome

Metabolic Syndrome

Features defining the Metabolic Syndrome **(also known Syndrome X, Insulin Resistance Syndrome, etc.)**	
Original Features (as described by Reaven[10]):	Expanded Features include:
• Insulin resistance	• Obesity
• Hyperinsulinemia	• Abdominal (or central) obesity, especially intraabdominal (or visceral) obesity
• Hyperglycemia	• Prothrombotic tendency (e.g., high plasminogen activator inhibitor 1, PAI-1)
• Hypertriglyceridemia	• Small, dense low-density lipoprotein (sdLDL)
• Decreased HDL	• Increased apolipoprotein B
• Hypertension	• Increased leptin
	• Decreased adiponectin
	• Proinflammatory tendency (e.g., increased hsCRP)
	• Endothelial dysfunction
	• Renin-angiotensin system activation
	• Hyperuricemia
	• Polycystic ovarian syndrome (PCOS)
	• Sleep apnea syndrome
	• Microalbuminuria
	• Autonomic dysfunction
	• Non alcoholic fatty liver disease (NAFLD) / Non alcoholic steatohepatitis (NASH)
	• Hypogonadism
	• Certain cancers?
	• *Erectile dysfunction*

Since its original description there has been much experimental, clinical, and epidemiological data to support the association of this syndrome with CVD and T2DM *(4,11)*.

Additionally, other CV factors have been frequently included in the description of the syndrome (Table 2). These include inflammation, abnormal fibrinolysis, and endothelial dysfunction *(5,11–13)*. It is unclear to what extent the components of this syndrome develop independently of each other or spring from "common soil" genetic or other abnormalities (e.g., inflammation) *(14)*. Due to the frequent coexistence of these abnormalities the syndrome has become a major clinical and public health problem.

Some components of this syndrome have also been associated with ED, although it is not clear whether the risk of ED (or even CVD) is greater when all components of the syndrome are present than the risk associated with each of its components. Metabolic syndrome was linked with a significantly increased risk of advanced ED in men older than 50 years, according to data obtained from 1952 men in Vienna *(15)*. This risk appeared to be correlated with a surrogate of central obesity (i.e., intra-abdominal adiposity). ED can be considered both a component of the metabolic syndrome (Table 2), because it is a risk marker for CVD and T2DM, but also as a marker of the metabolic syndrome itself *(3,16)*. The diagnosis of ED should not only alert the clinician to screen for CVD and other CV risk factors, but also to search for other features of the metabolic syndrome as needed. Some of the various components of the metabolic syndrome related to ED will be discussed next.

Diabetes

ED is common in men with diabetes. At least 50% of men with diabetes have this complication *(2)*. After the age of 60, 55%–95% of men with diabetes are affected by ED compared with approximately 50% in an unselected population in the Massachusetts Aging Male Survey *(17)*. ED typically occurs about 5–10 years earlier in men with diabetes than age-matched controls *(18)*. ED in diabetes can result from defects in virtually all stages of achieving and maintaining an erection including endothelial dysfunction, damage to nerves (e.g., neuropathy), impaired blood flow (e.g., micro- and macrovasculopathy), and several other factors (Table 1).

ENDOTHELIAL FUNCTION AND ENDOTHELIAL DYSFUNCTION

The endothelium is important in the maintenance of vascular health. It is a critical determinant of vascular tone and patency, reactivity, inflammation, vascular remodeling, and blood fluidity. The importance of endothelial dysfunction in the pathogenesis of CVD in the metabolic syndrome and diabetes has only recently been recognized *(19–21)*.

NO is the most potent known vasodilator and is secreted by the endothelium. It is synthesized from L-arginine by the endothelial enzyme NO synthase (eNOS). The bioavailability of NO can be decreased by various mechanisms – decreased production by eNOS, enhanced NO breakdown due to increased oxidative stress, or both. eNOS deactivation is often associated with an increase in plasma levels of its endogenous inhibitor, asymmetric dimethyl-L-arginine (ADMA)*(22)*.

Endothelial dysfunction results in the increased synthesis of ET-1, a potent vasoconstrictor, decreased production of prostacyclin, increased vascular adhesion of monocytes and platelets, increased prothrombotic activity, and decreased fibrinolytic activity, changes that all contribute to the atherosclerotic process *(13)*.

It has become clear that among its many actions insulin is also a vasoactive hormone *(23,24)*. Its effect to cause endothelial-NO-dependent vasodilation is physiologic and dose-dependent

(25). Insulin has been shown to induce expression of the enzyme NOS *(26)*, and this effect is inhibited by cytokines important in the pathogenesis of insulin resistance *(27)*. Importantly, the effect of insulin on NOS is mediated through the same intracellular signaling pathway as insulin's effects on glucose metabolism *(28)*. Thus insulin resistance in glucose metabolism and in the vasculature can be explained on the basis of a single defect. Recent data suggest that insulin's metabolic and vascular actions are closely linked. Insulin-resistant states exhibit diminished insulin-mediated glucose uptake into peripheral tissues as well as impaired insulin-mediated vasodilation and impaired endothelium-dependent vasodilation to the muscarinic receptor agonist acetylcholine. Thus, insulin action in peripheral tissues is probably linked to its action on endothelium.

Endothelial dysfunction, characterized by a decrease in the bioavailability of endothelial NO, may be an initiating event in the pathogenesis of atherosclerosis and has been observed in individuals with diabetes and pre-diabetes *(29)*. Endothelial dysfunction in diabetes and pre-diabetes appears to be multifactorial in origin. Contributory factors include not only hyperglycemia and insulin resistance, but also the effect of accumulation of advanced glycation end-products (AGEs), increased polyol pathway flux, increased hexosamine pathway flux, and protein kinase C (PKC) activation *(19)*.

The link between ED and endothelial dysfunction has been suggested by many studies including the one by De Angelis and colleagues *(30)*. Thirty men with diabetes and symptomatic ED were matched for age and disease with 30 potent men with T2DM. The decrease in blood pressure and platelet aggregation in response to L-arginine (the physiological precursor of NO) was lower in patients with ED. Indices of coagulation activation (e.g., D-dimers) and reduced fibrinolysis (e.g., plasminogen activator inhibitor-1, PAI-1) were also found to be higher in the men with ED. The investigators concluded that ED in men with diabetes correlates with endothelial dysfunction.

Esposito and colleagues demonstrated that obese men with ED had evidence of abnormal endothelial function, which was indicated by reduced blood pressure and platelet aggregation responses to L-arginine and elevated serum concentrations of markers of low-grade inflammation, such as interleukin-6 (IL-6), IL-8, and high-sensitivity C-reactive protein (hsCRP) *(31)*. Erectile function score (higher score correlates with better erectile function) was positively associated with mean blood pressure responses to L-arginine and negatively associated with body mass index (BMI), waist–hip ratio (WHR, a measure of central obesity), and hsCRP *(31)*. The relationship between BMI and the International Index of Erectile Function score (IIEF score, a commonly used tool for measuring erectile function) was continuous in this population, with no evidence of a threshold effect. These associations remained statistically significant after performing a multivariate analysis in which IIEF score was the dependent variable and BMI, WHR, level of physical activity, indices of endothelial function, baseline IIEF score, and serum hsCRP concentrations were the independent variables that explained almost 68% of the variability in score changes. This association between the IIEF score and indices of endothelial dysfunction supports the presence of common vascular pathways underlying both conditions in obese men. ED and endothelial dysfunction may thus have some shared pathways through a defect in NO activity, which may be inhibited through age-, disease-, and behavioral-related pathways.

Increased levels of ADMA are associated with endothelial dysfunction and increased risk of CVD. Elevated ADMA levels have been observed in various conditions, including hypertension, dyslipidemia, hyperglycemia, hyperhomocysteinemia, and renal failure, and are believed to be one cause of endothelial dysfunction in these conditions. Increases in plasma ADMA concentrations may contribute to the endothelial dysfunction observed in insulin-resistant individuals and also to macrovascular disease in diabetes and the metabolic syndrome *(32)*.

The relationship between insulin resistance and plasma ADMA was studied by Stuhlinger et al. *(33)*. They demonstrated a correlation between insulin resistance and plasma ADMA concentrations, independent of other factors that typically are associated with insulin resistance and risk of coronary heart disease *(33)*.

Elevations in plasma and tissue ADMA levels may also be associated with ED *(34,35)*. Masuda et al. demonstrated an increase in cavernosal tissue ADMA levels, 2 weeks after cavernosal ischemia was induced by partial vessel occlusion in rabbits *(35)*.

GLUCOSE

There is a growing body of evidence that ED correlates with the level of glycemic control. In animal experiments, glycated hemoglobin significantly impairs endothelial NO-mediated corpus cavernosal relaxation in vitro. This is partly due to the generation of superoxide anions and the extracellular inactivation of NO *(36)*. ED in men with diabetes has been previously associated with poor metabolic control but very few studies have examined this relationship using modern validated methods of assessing both glycemia and ED. A retrospective analysis of a cohort of men with T2DM demonstrated that A1C was an independent predictor of erectile function score *(18)*. An inverse correlation between severity of ED assessed by the IIEF score and A1C as also been demonstrated *(37)*. However, it is not known whether improving diabetic control will improve ED or make it easier to treat with current agents. Given the association of A1C with microvascular disease, improved glycemia should, at least, slow down progression of ED.

NEUROPATHY

ED resulting from diabetic neuropathy is initially due to damage affecting the small nerve fibers innervating the corpora, but later on, the larger, myelinated nerves can also become involved. Endothelial dysfunction and NO are also linked to microvascular complications of diabetes, including neuropathy. The role of neuronal NOS (nNOS) was studied in rats with uncontrolled diabetes. These had decreased expression of nNOS in the dorsal root ganglia and diminished withdrawal responses to noxious mechanical stimuli. Cyclic GMP levels paralleled nNOS expression. Insulin treatment led to improved nerve conduction and increased nNOS expression. This suggests that decreased nNOS-cGMP system in the dorsal root ganglion may play a role in the pathogenesis of diabetic neuropathy *(38)*. It might provide a link between diabetic neuropathy and endothelial dysfunction in patients with diabetes and ED.

The ability to increase blood flow depends on an intact neurogenic vascular response. Diabetic autonomic neuropathy leads to impaired endothelium-dependent and endothelium-independent vasodilation even in the absence of clinical macrovascular disease *(38)*. The interaction between endothelial dysfunction and autonomic neuropathy results in an inability to increase blood flow under conditions of stress or increased demands.

Inflammation

Atherosclerosis is now considered a disease to which inflammation contributes substantially *(39)*, and markers of inflammation are elevated in individuals with established coronary artery disease (CAD) and in those at risk for CVD. CRP is an acute-phase protein produced in the liver that is an extremely sensitive marker of systemic inflammation and tissue damage. Its hepatic production is controlled by inflammatory cytokines, for example, IL-6, IL-1, and tumor necrosis factor-α (TNF-α). Elevations of CRP within the normal range, measured by hsCRP assay, have been observed in subjects with confirmed atherosclerosis, pre-diabetes (impaired fasting glucose (IFG), and/or impaired glucose tolerance (IGT)), insulin resistance, diabetes, and the metabolic syndrome (13). Elevations of plasma levels of hsCRP appear to be predictive of future CVD and incident diabetes. In addition to its role as a biomarker for macrovascular disease, hsCRP is also a biomarker of endothelial dysfunction (22).

Billups and colleagues examined the relation of traditional and emerging risk factors for CVD to the severity of penile vascular disease in 137 men with ED and without clinical CAD (40). Plasma hsCRP levels correlated significantly with increasing severity of penile vascular disease as measured by penile Doppler. The association between endothelial dysfunction, inflammation, and ED was further explored in a study aimed to establish a link between ED in men with diabetes and infections with *Chlamydia pneumoniae* or cytomegalovirus, or with low-grade inflammation (41). In this study of 90 men with diabetes, there was a clear association between exposure to *Chlamydia pneumoniae* and cytomegalovirus, and elevated hsCRP concentrations, in subjects with ED. This lends further support that implicates infection in the development of vascular disease.

Obesity

Cross-sectional studies have demonstrated that men with a BMI higher than 28.7 have a 30% higher risk for ED than those with a normal BMI ($\leq$25) (42). The prevalence of obesity and its associated vascular risk factors in men reporting symptoms of ED is remarkably high (43,44). In the Massachusetts Male Aging Study, Derby and colleagues found that men who were overweight at baseline were at an increased risk of developing ED regardless of whether they lost weight during follow-up (45). By contrast, men who initiated physical activity in midlife had a 70% reduced risk for ED relative to those who remained sedentary. In quantitative terms, this means that sedentary men may be able to reduce their risk of ED by adopting regular physical activity at a level of at least 200 kcal/day, which corresponds to walking briskly for 2 miles.

Results from the Health Professional Follow-up Study(31,742 men aged 50–93 with no history of prostate cancer) revealed that men who were most physically active (3 h of running per week or the equivalent), had a 30% lower risk of ED when compared with men who reported little or no physical activity (42). Conversely, watching more than 20 h per week of TV, smoking, and being overweight were associated with increased risk of ED (42).

Lipids

Total cholesterol and HDL are important predictors of ED. In a study of 3250 men (mean age 51 years) followed for a mean of 22 months, 71 developed ED during follow-up. Those subjects with total cholesterol greater than 240 mg/dl had a 1.83 times increased risk of ED. An HDL greater than 60 mg/dl meant a 0.30 times risk for ED. This suggests that a high total cholesterol and a low HDL are risks for ED (46).

Influence of Therapies Used in Diabetes and in the Metabolic Syndrome on ED

Many drugs used in the treatment of diabetes and the various components of the metabolic syndrome can impact on ED (6,9). Medication history is very important to consider in ED patients, especially in men with diabetes who are often on multiple drugs to treat hypertension, dyslipidemia, depression, glaucoma, neuropathic pain, and diabetes itself.

The major culprits which can induce ED are antihypertensives, especially nonselective beta-blockers and diuretics. The main problem in diabetes and the metabolic syndrome is that often these agents cannot be replaced – beta-blocker therapy is essential in patients with CAD or heart failure; depression and painful conditions should be adequately treated. All these problems are very real to the patient and may exacerbate ED if not adequately managed. The clinician should try and optimize therapy using agents that are least likely to cause ED. Angiotensin-converting enzyme inhibitors (ACE-I), angiotensin II receptor blockers (ARBs), statins, and thiazolidinediones (TZDs) either enhance NO levels or block production of oxygen radicals, which quench NO and prevent vasodilation.

ED AS A RISK MARKER OF CVD

ED is associated with many of the traditional CV risk factors (aging, diabetes, hypertension, hyperlipidemia, and smoking). ED has also recently been recognized to be associated with nontraditional CV risk factors (such as endothelial dysfunction). The presence of ED, therefore, can be an early warning sign of underlying vascular disease (coronary, cerebrovascular, and peripheral) which in patients with diabetes may be asymptomatic (5). It has been proposed that the smaller penile arteries (diameter 1–2 mm) suffer obstruction from plaque burden earlier than the larger coronary (3–4 mm), carotid (5–7 mm), or ileofemoral (6–8 mm) arteries, hence ED may be symptomatic before a coronary event (5).

Gazzaruso and colleagues evaluated the prevalence of ED in 133 uncomplicated diabetic men with angiographically verified silent CAD and in 127 diabetic men without myocardial ischemia at exercise electrocardiogram (ECG), 48-h ambulatory ECG, and stress echocardiography (47). Patients were screened for ED using the IIEF questionnaire. The prevalence of ED was significantly higher in patients with than in those without silent CAD (33.8% vs. 4.7%). Multiple logistic regression analysis showed that ED, apolipoprotein(a) polymorphism, smoking, microalbuminuria, HDL, and low-density lipoprotein (LDL) were significantly associated with silent CAD; among these risk factors, ED appeared to be the most efficient predictor of silent CAD (odds ratio, 14.8). Thus there may be a strong and independent association between ED and silent CAD in apparently uncomplicated T2DM patients, and ED may be a potential marker to identify diabetic patients to screen for silent CAD. Moreover, the high prevalence of ED among diabetics with silent CAD suggests the need to perform an exercise ECG before starting a treatment for ED, especially in patients with additional CV risk factors (5).

In the Detection of Ischemia in Asymptomatic Diabetics (DIAD) study, 1,123 patients with T2DM, aged 50–75 years, with no known or suspected CAD, were randomly assigned to either stress testing (assessed by adenosine technetium-99m sestamibi single-photon emission-computed tomography [SPECT] myocardial perfusion imaging) and 5-year clinical follow-up or to follow-up only (48). A total of 113 out of 522 patients (22%) had silent ischemia, including 83 with regional myocardial perfusion abnormalities and 30 with normal perfusion but other abnormalities (i.e., adenosine-induced ST-segment depression, ventricular dilation, or rest ventricular dysfunction). Moderate or large perfusion defects were present in 33 patients. The strongest predictors for abnormal tests were abnormal Valsalva (odds ratio 5.6), male sex (2.5), and diabetes duration (5.2). Other traditional cardiac risk factors or inflammatory and prothrombotic markers were not predictive. Selecting only patients who met American Diabetes Association (ADA) guidelines would have failed to identify 41% of patients with silent ischemia. Thus, silent myocardial ischemia occurs in greater than one in five asymptomatic patients with T2DM and cardiac autonomic dysfunction was a strong predictor of ischemia. These findings may have implications for guidelines for stress testing in diabetics. Further research is needed to clarify the importance of stress testing and its implications in patients with diabetes and ED who are free of cardiac symptoms.

Indeed, the severity of ED can correlate with the severity of coronary atherosclerosis *(49)*. In view of these findings, appropriate investigation and management of existing vascular disease should be undertaken by the healthcare provider, as part of the global care of the ED patient *(5, 50,51)*. The optimal cardiac management of the ED patient was part of the objectives of the second Princeton Consensus Conference (Princeton II) *(5)*. Recommendations included screening for CV risk factors and appropriate risk stratification for asymptomatic men with ED. Men with ED and other CV risk factors should be counseled in lifestyle modification, and treated where indicated with agents aimed at reducing CV risk (i.e., statins, aspirin, antihypertensives, etc).

Another consideration with respect to the presence of coexisting vascular disease in the ED patient is the safety of sexual activity itself. Sexual activity can trigger myocardial infarction, but the overall risk is low (1–3 per million). Expressed as a multiple of the metabolic equivalent (MET) of energy expenditure expanded in the resting state (MET=1), sexual intercourse is typically associated with a workload of 2–3 METs before orgasm and 3–4 METs during orgasm. This workload is similar to walking one mile in 20 minutes on the flat, or climbing up two flights of stairs. If the ED patient can manage this level of workload, he should be safe from the CV standpoint (although more rigorous sexual activity can involve 5–6 METs or greater). If there is any doubt, a thorough CV work-up should be considered *(5,50,51)*. The Princeton II consensus guidelines recommend that all men with ED should undergo a full medical assessment *(5)*. Baseline physical activity needs to be established and CV risk graded low, intermediate, or high (Table 3). Most patients with low or intermediate CV risk can have their

Table 3
Princeton II consensus guidelines – low-, intermediate-, and high-cardiovascular risk groups *(5)*

Risk from sexual activity in cardiovascular diseases		
Low-Risk Patient	**Intermediate-Risk Patient**	**High-Risk Patient**
Typically implied by the ability to perform exercise of modest intensity without symptoms	Evaluate to reclassify as high or low risk	Defer resumption of sexual activity until cardiological assessment and treatment
Asymptomatic, <3 CVD risk factors, excluding gender	Asymptomatic, ≥3 CVD risk factors, excluding gender	Hypertrophic obstructive and other cardiomyopathies
Controlled hypertension		Uncontrolled hypertension
Mild, stable angina	Moderate, stable angina	Unstable or refractory angina
Post-succesful coronary revascularization	Noncardiac atherosclerotic sequelae (PVD, history of stroke, or TIA)	High-risk arrhythmias
Uncomplicated past MI (>6–8 weeks)	Recent MI (>2 weeks but <6 weeks)	Recent MI (<2 weeks)
Mild valvular disease		Moderate/severe valvular disease
Left ventricular dysfunction (NYHA Class I)	CHF (NYHA Class II)	CHF (NYHA Class III/IV)

MI: Myocardial infarction; NYHA: New York Heart Association; CVD: Cardiovascular disease; CHF: Congestive heart failure; TIA: Transient ischemic attack; PVD: Peripheral vascular disease.

ED managed in the outpatient or primary care setting. High risk patients need more thorough CV work-up. Exercise testing can guide advice in the presence of reasonable concern (sexual workload is equivalent to 3–4 min on the standard Bruce treadmill protocol).

EVALUATION OF ED

A diagnosis of ED requires careful history (medical, sexual, and psychosocial), physical examination, and laboratory tests aimed at determining what other tests are needed to rule out organic causes of the disorder. Many medications, including prescribed, over-the-counter (OTC), and illicit drugs, can cause ED, a careful drug history is indicated. As well as potentially causing ED, many OTC agents are taken as therapies for ED and androgen replacement. For ED patients who do not respond to standard therapy, further evaluation is warranted.

EFFICACY OF TREATMENT FOR ED

ED is a distressing condition that can have a serious negative impact on not just the individuals sex life, but also his and his partner's overall quality of life. Despite this, up to 90% of sufferers are still reluctant to present to their doctor. An important aspect of ED which is sometimes underappreciated, is that this is a disorder of couples'. Any attempt at therapy should be cognizant of the needs and desires of both parties (6). ED therapies usually include first-line treatments such as lifestyle and drug therapy modification, psychosexual counseling and education, androgen replacement therapy (when deficiency is confirmed), and oral drug therapy (PDE5 inhibitors). Further therapy may include intracavernosal drug therapy, vacuum-tumescence devices, and surgical treatment (prosthesis and vascular surgery). Fortunately, the treatment options for ED have expanded in recent years, especially with the introduction of PDE5 inhibitors. However, a significant proportion of men with diabetes and ED are still frustrated by poor responses to the available treatment modalities (52,53). This often leads to noncompliance and increasing psychological distress as patients run out of therapeutic options.

The multifactorial etiology of diabetic ED increases the complexity of managing this problem, so clinicians need to be aware of the underlying pathophysiology to ensure the best possible outcomes in management. A multidisciplinary approach should be considered to deal with the different comorbidities, including psychiatric, endocrine, CV, and urologic issues. Most treatments deal with only one part of the ED equation. This leads to partial or poor responses. Ongoing research is looking at agents, or combinations thereof, that will deal with all aspects of diabetic ED. The most promising therapeutic agents available so far are the PDE5 inhibitors.

PDE5 Inhibitors

The treatment options for ED have expanded in recent years, especially with the introduction of PDE5 inhibitors. Sildenafil was the first drug in this class and has been extensively studied. Tadalafil and vardenafil are the newer generation of agents in this class and are potent and selective inhibitors of cGMP-specific PDE5. An erection occurs when penile cavernosal smooth muscle relaxes under the influence of NO which is released by cavernous nerves and vascular endothelial cells. NO activates guanylyl cyclase, an enzyme that increases the concentration of cGMP, which in turn causes smooth muscle relaxation. PDE5 inhibitors act by preventing the breakdown of cGMP, thus facilitating the corporal smooth muscle relaxation in response to sexual stimulation.

A meta-analysis of 11 randomized, double-blind, placebo-controlled trials of sildenafil in patients with diabetes reported improved erections in 59% of those with type 1 diabetes and 63% in those with T2DM *(52)*. Improvement was noted regardless of age, race, ED severity, and duration, or the presence of various comorbidities *(54)*. The response rate in men with diabetes is less than the 83% improvement in nondiabetic individuals with ED. Discontinuation rates range from 5% to 17% primarily because of insufficient clinical response *(52)*.

Vardenafil and tadalafil appear to be as effective as sildenafil. Tadalafil has the advantage of a longer duration of action (17.5 h half-life compared with approximately 4 h for sildenafil and vardenafil). For tadalafil, 76% of men with diabetes taking the 20-mg dose had improved erections with 58% of the total group having had satisfactory erections to complete intercourse. In nondiabetic men the rates were 81% and 75%, respectively *(55)*.

In one of the few studies done exclusively in 216 patients with diabetes, treatment with tadalafil significantly improved all primary efficacy variables, regardless of baseline A1C level *(56)*. Therapy with tadalafil also significantly improved a number of secondary outcome measures, including changes in other IIEF domains, individual IIEF questions, and percentage of positive responses to a global assessment question measuring erection improvement. Tadalafil was well-tolerated, with headache and dyspepsia being the most frequent adverse events with active treatment in this population. A retrospective analysis of pooled data from 12 placebo-controlled trials was conducted to characterize the efficacy and safety of tadalafil for the treatment of ED in men with diabetes compared with that in men without diabetes *(40)*. Despite more severe baseline ED in men with diabetes, tadalafil was efficacious and well-tolerated in this population. As reported for other PDE5 inhibitors, the response to tadalafil was slightly lower in men with diabetes compared to men without diabetes. Thus, tadalafil therapy significantly enhanced erectile function and was well tolerated by men with diabetes and ED.

Vardenafil led to similar results in nondiabetic men with a 71%–75% improvement in erections with 10-mg and 20-mg doses. In men with diabetes the response to the 10-mg dose was 57% and to the 20-mg dose was 72% *(57)*.

One of the side-effects of sildenafil is the visual complaint of seeing a "bluish-haze". This is due to an inhibition of PDE6, which is present in the retina. The newer PDE5 inhibitors tadalafil and vardenafil appear to have an absence of color vision changes due to a better PDE5:PDE6 selectivity ratio *(6)*. In addition, rare post-marketing reports of decreased vision have been attributed to nonarteritic anterior ischemic optic neuropathy (NAION) in temporal association with use of PDE5 inhibitors. Clinicians should advise patients to stop use of all PDE5 inhibitors and seek medical attention in the event of sudden vision loss. Other side-effects common to this class of drug include the typical vasomotor disturbances of headache, flushing, and rhinitis. All of the PDE5 inhibitors currently available are generally well-tolerated. Differences in efficacy and safety (which might be anticipated due to marked differences in potency and half-life) remain to be evaluated from further clinical trials, and post-marketing studies and surveillance. However, a recent Cochrane systematic review of PDE5 inhibitors for ED in patients with diabetes concluded that they are a valuable treatment option for these patients *(7)*. They also concluded that they were generally safe and well-tolerated. This meta-analysis was based on eight randomized controlled trials in which 976 men received PDE5 inhibitor and 741 received placebo for the treatment of ED. Overall, 80% of the participants had diabetes. Reasons for nonresponse to PDE5 inhibitors in ED patients can include failure to understand instructions, fear of adverse events, anxiety about reestablishing intimacy, and poor dose titration. The Cochrane systematic review did suggest that higher doses of PDE5 inhibitors may be needed in diabetic patients with higher glucose levels *(7)*. A recent study showed the benefit of using higher doses of sildenafil and re-education for ED patients who have previously stopped medication for lack of effect *(58)*. Significant improvements were seen in the patients, with 23.6% of men achieving normal erectile function at the end of the study.

The major concern regarding the use of PDE5 inhibitors in ED is the concomitant use of nitrate therapy (such as sublingual nitroglycerin) and PDE5 inhibitors. This combination of agents is contraindicated due to the profound hypotension (and even death) that can occur. Hemodynamically, PDE5 inhibitors have mild nitrate-like activity (sildenafil was originally intended as an antianginal agent). In healthy volunteers, a single dose of sildenafil 100 mg transiently lowered blood pressure by an average of 10/7 mmHg with a return to baseline at 6 h post-dose. Short-acting nitrates for angina should not be taken within 24 h of the short-acting PDE5 inhibitors (i.e., sildenafil and vardenafil) and vice versa *(5)*. As tadalafil is a long-acting PDE5 inhibitor, at least 48 h should elapse between the last tadalafil dose and readministration of a nitrate *(5)*. In contrast, long-acting nitrates should not be taken within a week of PDE5 inhibitors. Concerns regarding the CV safety of the PDE5 inhibitors has largely been dispelled in consensus statements, when these agents are used according to the specific prescribing information and in-line with published guidelines *(5,50,51,59)*.

Recent studies show that both acute and chronic sildenafil therapy improves brachial artery flow-mediated dilation, an effect of intrinsic, endothelial NO release (Fig. 1) *(60)*. This enhanced dilation suggests that sildenafil directly improves endothelial function. Similar findings were noted in other studies *(19,61)*. In addition, sildenafil dilates epicardial coronary arteries and inhibits platelet activation in patients with CAD *(62)*. Other studies are underway to test the hypothesis that chronic sildenafil use improves biochemical markers of endothelial dysfunction.

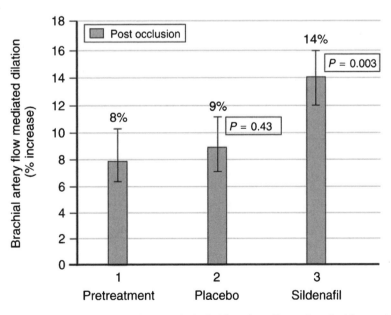

Fig. 1. Effect of sildenafil taken for 2 weeks on endothelial function. (Reproduced with permission from Ref. *(60)*).

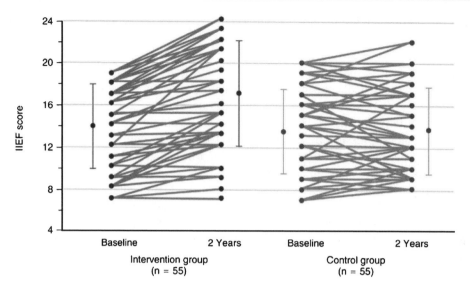

Fig. 2. Effect of lifestyle changes on erectile dysfunction in obese men. IIEF, International index of erectile function. (Reproduced with permission from Ref. *(34)*).

Can Treating the Metabolic Syndrome Improve ED?

There is currently no approved pharmacological therapy for the metabolic syndrome, and lifestyle change consisting of dietary changes and exercise leading to weight loss are the cornerstone of therapy. Lifestyle change has been shown to not only prevent diabetes *(63)* but also improve endothelial function and decrease markers of inflammation *(64,65)*.

Ameliorating certain modifiable risk factors, such as sedentary lifestyle or obesity, might prevent the subsequent occurrence of ED or improve existing ED *(66)*. Esposito and colleagues tested this hypothesis in a randomized controlled trial involving 110 men with obesity who had ED but no significant comorbid conditions (such as other features of the metabolic syndrome – hypertension, diabetes, and CVD). Men were assigned to either an intensive weight loss group or usual general weight loss guidance *(31)*. After 2 years, almost one-third of the obese men in the intensive group had reversed their ED after exercising more and losing weight (Fig. 2). Various measures of nontraditional CV risk factors were also measured. Changes in hsCRP was independently associated with improvements in ED. Serum concentrations of hsCRP decreased more in the intervention group (from 3.3 mg/l to 1.9 mg/l (mean decrease –1.4)) than in the control group (from 3.4 mg/l to 3.4 mg/l (Mean decrease 0)) ($P = 0.02$) *(31)*.

Given the correlation of hyperlipidemia and ED, a recent small study showed improvement of ED by cholesterol lowering using daily atorvastatin for 4 months *(67)*. It is unclear whether this is a direct effect of lipid lowering or an indirect effect from improved endothelial dysfunction *(67)*.

CONCLUSION

ED is an increasingly common problem. Several of the risk factors for ED are also components of the metabolic syndrome. Endothelial dysfunction is a major unifying etiology for many of the aspects of the metabolic syndrome, especially T2DM and CVD. It also plays a major role in ED. ED can be considered a risk marker for the presence of CVD, and the metabolic syndrome and its associated conditions. Appropriate screening and management of CVD and CV risk factors should be performed in the ED patient.

The etiology of ED in patients with diabetes is multifactorial. Diabetes is a complex chronic disorder associated with various factors which could exacerbate ED (including other components of the metabolic syndrome): including obesity, poor glycemic control, dyslipidemia, micro- and macrovascular disease, autonomic neuropathy, inflammation, and drug therapies for comorbid states – all interact to some degree and exacerbate erectile failure. Every effort should be made to correct or improve all causes of ED, whether organic, psychogenic, iatrogenic, or mixed. A multidisciplinary approach is recommended to deal with the comorbidities so as to ensure the best possible outcomes for patients with ED and diabetes. Treatment of ED in general and in men with diabetes has been revolutionized with the introduction of PDE5 inhibitors.

REFERENCES

1. NIH Consensus Conference. Impotence. NIH Consensus Development Panel on Impotence. *JAMA* 1993; 270: 83–90.
2. Selvin E, Burnett AL, Platz EA: Prevalence and risk factors for erectile dysfunction in the US. *Am J Med* 2007; 120: 151–157.
3. Matfin G, Jawa A, Fonseca VA: Erectile dysfunction: interrelationship with the metabolic syndrome. *Curr Diab Rep* 2005; 5: 64–69.
4. Matfin G: Diabetes mellitus and the metabolic syndrome. In: Porth CM, ed. Essentials of Pathophysiology, 2nd ed. Philadelphia, PA: Lippincott Williams & Wilkins, 2005:987–1015.
5. Rosen RC, Jackson G, Kostis JB: Erectile dysfunction and cardiac disease: recommendations of the Second Princeton Conference. *Curr Urol Rep* 2006; 7: 490–496.
6. Matfin G: New treatments for erectile dysfunction. *Fertil Steril* 2003; 80 Suppl 4: 40–45.
7. Vardi M, Nini A: Phosphodiesterase inhibitors for erectile dysfunction in patients with diabetes mellitus. *Cochrane Database of Systematic Reviews* 2007, Issue 1. Art. No.: CD002187. DOI: 10.1002/14651858.CD002187.pub3.
8. Matfin G: Disorders of the male genitourinary system. In: Porth CM, ed. Essentials of Pathophysiology, 2nd ed. Philadelphia, PA: Lippincott Williams & Wilkins, 2005:901–923.
9. Lue TF: Erectile dysfunction. *N Eng J Med* 2000; 342: 1802–1813.
10. Reaven GM: Banting lecture 1988. Role of insulin resistance in human disease. *Diabetes* 1988; 37:1595–1607.
11. Grundy SM, Cleeman JI, Daniels SR, et al.: Diagnosis and management of the metabolic syndrome: An American Heart Association/National Heart, Lung, and Blood Institute Scientific Statement. *Circulation* 2005; 112: 2735–2752.
12. Fonseca VA: Risk factors for coronary heart disease in diabetes. *Ann Intern Med* 2000;133:154–156.
13. Fonseca V, Desouza C, Asnani S, Jialal I: Nontraditional risk factors for cardiovascular disease in diabetes. Endocr Rev 2004; 25:153–175.
14. Stern MP: Diabetes and cardiovascular disease. The "common soil" hypothesis. *Diabetes* 1995; 44:369–374.
15. Heidler S, Temml C, Broessner C: Is the metabolic syndrome an independent risk factor for erectile dysfunction? *J Urol* 2007; 177: 651–654.
16. Kupellian V, Shabsigh R, Arujo AB, et al.: Erectile dysfunction as a predictor of the metabolic syndrome in aging men: results from the Massachusetts Male Aging Study. *J Urol* 2006; 176: 222–226.
17. Feldman HA, Goldstein I, Hatzichristou DG, et al.: Impotence and its medical and psychosocial correlates: results of the Massachusetts Male Aging Study. *J Urol* 1994; 151: 54–61.
18. Romeo JH, Seftel AD, Madhun ZT, Aron DC: Sexual function in men with diabetes type 2: association with glycemic control. *J Urol* 2000; 163: 788–791.
19. Gkaliagkousi E, Shah A, Ferro A: Pharmacological and non-pharmacological treatment of endothelial dysfunction: relevance to diabetes. *Br J Diabetes Vasc Dis* 2007; 7:5–10.
20. Matfin G, Jawa A, Fonseca VA: Erectile dysfunction in diabetes: an endothelial disorder. In: Fonseca V, ed. Clinical Diabetes: Translating Research into Practice. Philadelphia, PA: Saunders, 2006:165–178.
21. Pegge NC, Twomey AM, Vaughton K, et al.: The role of endothelial dysfunction in the pathophysiology of erectile dysfunction in diabetes and in determining response to treatment. Diabet Med 2006; 23:873–878.

22. Theuma P, Fonseca VA: Novel cardiovascular risk factors and macrovascular and microvascular complications of diabetes. *Curr Drug Targets* 2003; 4: 477–486.

23. Baron AD: Insulin resistance and vascular function. *J Diabetes Complicat* 2002; 16: 92–102.

24. Baron AD: Insulin and the vasculature – old actors, new roles. *J Invest Med* 1996; 44:406–412.

25. Grover A, Padginton C, Wilson MF, et al. Insulin attenuates norepinephrine-induced venoconstriction. An ultrasonographic study. *Hypertension* 1995; 25:779–784.

26. Aljada A, Dandona P: Effect of insulin on human aortic endothelial nitric oxide synthase. *Metabolism* 2000; 49:147–150.

27. Aljada A, Ghanim H, Assian E, Dandona P: Tumor necrosis factor-alpha inhibits insulin-induced increase in endothelial nitric oxide synthase and reduces insulin receptor content and phosphorylation in human aortic endothelial cells. *Metabolism* 2002; 51:487–491.

28. Zeng G, Quon MJ.: Insulin-stimulated production of nitric oxide is inhibited by wortmannin. Direct measurement in vascular endothelial cells. *J Clin Invest* 1996; 98:894–898.

29. Caballero AE, Arora S, Saouaf R, et al.: Microvascular and macrovascular reactivity is reduced in subjects at risk for type 2 diabetes. *Diabetes* 1999; 48:1856–1862.

30. De Angelis L, Marfella MA, Siniscalchi M, et al.: Erectile and endothelial dysfunction in Type II diabetes: a possible link. *Diabetologia* 2001; 44:1155–1160.

31. Esposito K, Giugliano F, Di Palo C, et al.: Effect of lifestyle changes on erectile dysfunction in obese men: a randomized controlled trial. *JAMA* 2004; 291:2978–2984.

32. Chan NN, Chan JC.: Asymmetric dimethylarginine (ADMA): a potential link between endothelial dysfunction and cardiovascular diseases in insulin resistance syndrome? *Diabetologia* 2002, 45: 1609–1616.

33. Stuhlinger MC, Abbasi F, Chu JW, Lamendola C, et al.: Relationship between insulin resistance and an endogenous nitric oxide synthase inhibitor. *JAMA* 2002; 287: 1420–1426.

34. Mass R, Schwedhelm E, Albsmeier J, Boger RH: The pathophysiology of erectile dysfunction related to endothelial dysfunction and mediators of vascular function. *Vasc Med* 2002; 7: 213–225.

35. Masuda H, Tsujii T, Okuno T, et al.: Accumulated endogenous NOS inhibitors, decreased NOS activity, and impaired cavernosal relaxation with ischemia. *Am J Physiol Regul Integr Comp Physiol* 2002; 282: R1730–R1738.

36. Cartledge JJ, Eardley I, Morrison JF: Impairment of corpus cavernosal smooth muscle relaxation by glycosylated human haemoglobin. *BJU Int* 2000, 85: 735–741.

37. Fonseca V, Seftel A, Denne J, Fredlund P: Impact of diabetes mellitus on the severity of erectile dysfunction and response to treatment: analysis of data from tadalafil clinical trials. *Diabetologia* 2004; 47:1914–1923.

38. Veves A, Akbari CM, Primavera J, et al.: Endothelial dysfunction and the expression of endothelial nitric oxide synthetase in diabetic neuropathy, vascular disease, and foot ulceration. *Diabetes* 1998; 47: 457–463.

39. Ross R: Atherosclerosis – an inflammatory disease. *N Eng J Med* 1999; 340:115–126.

40. Billups KL, Kaiser DR, Kelly AS et al.: Relation of C-reactive protein and other cardiovascular risk factors to penile vascular disease in men with erectile dysfunction. *Int J Impot Res* 2003; 15:231–236.

41. Blans MCA, Visseran FLJ, Banga JD et al.: Infection induced inflammation is associated with erectile dysfunction in men with diabetes. *Eur J Clin Invest* 2006; 36: 497–502.

42. Bacon CG, Mittleman MA, Kawachi I, et al.: Sexual function in men older than 50 years of age: results from the health professionals follow-up study. *Ann Intern Med* 2003; 139:161–168.

43. Walczak MK, Lokhandwala N, Hodge MB, Guay AT.: Prevalence of cardiovascular risk factors in erectile dysfunction. *J Gend Specif Med* 2002; 5:19–24.

44. Chung WS, Sohn JH, Park YY.: Is obesity an underlying factor in erectile dysfunction? *Eur Urol* 1999; 36: 68–70.

45. Derby CA, Mohr BA, Goldstein I, et al.: Modifiable risk factors and erectile dysfunction: can lifestyle changes modify risk? *Urology* 2000; 56(2):302–306.

46. Wei M, Macera CA, Davis DR, et al.: Total cholesterol and high density lipoprotein cholesterol as important predictors of erectile dysfunction. *Am J Epidemiol* 1994, 140: 930–937.

47. Gazzaruso C, Giordanetti S, De Amici E, et al.: Relationship between erectile dysfunction and silent myocardial ischemia in apparently uncomplicated type 2 diabetic patients. *Circulation* 2004; 110: 22–26.

48. Wackers FJ, Young LH, Inzucchi SE, et al.: Detection of silent myocardial ischemia in asymptomatic diabetic subjects: The DIAD study. *Diabetes Care* 2004; 27:1954–1961.

49. Greenstein A, Chen J, Miller H, Matzkin H, Villa Y, Braf Z: Does severity of ischemic coronary disease correlate with erectile function? *Int J Impot Res* 1997, 9: 123–126.

50. Russell ST, Khandheria BK, Nehra A: Erectile dysfunction and cardiovascular disease. *Mayo Clin Proc* 2004, 79: 782–794.

51. Jackson G: Treatment of erectile dysfunction in patients with cardiovascular disease : guide to drug selection. *Drugs* 2004, 64: 1533–1545.
52. Fink HA, Mac DR, Rutks IR, et al.: Sildenafil for male erectile dysfunction: a systematic review and meta-analysis. *Arch Intern Med* 2002, 162: 1349–1360.
53. Guay AT, Perez JB, Velasquez E, et al.: Clinical experience with intraurethral alprostadil (MUSE) in the treatment of men with erectile dysfunction. A retrospective study. Medicated urethral system for erection. *Eur Urol* 2000; 38: 671–676.
54. Carson CC, Burnett AL, Levine LA, Nehra A: The efficacy of sildenafil citrate (Viagra) in clinical populations: an update. *Urology* 2002; 60: 12–27.
55. Brock GB, McMahon CG, Chen KK, et al.: Efficacy and safety of tadalafil for the treatment of erectile dysfunction: results of integrated analyses. *J Urol* 2002; 168: 1332–1336.
56. Saenz dT, Anglin G, Knight JR, Emmick JT.: Effects of tadalafil on erectile dysfunction in men with diabetes. *Diabetes Care* 2002; 25:2159–2164.
57. Porst H, Rosen R, Padma-Nathan H, et al.: The efficacy and tolerability of vardenafil, a new, oral, selective phosphodiesterase type 5 inhibitor, in patients with erectile dysfunction: the first at-home clinical trial. *Int J Impot Res* 2001; 13: 192–199.
58. Gruenwald I, Shenfield O, Chen J, et al.: Positive effects of counseling and dose adjustment in patients with erectile dysfunction who had failed treatment with sildenafil. *Eur Urol* 2006; 50: 134–140.
59. Cheitlin MD, Hutter AM, Jr., Brindis RG, et al.: Use of sildenafil (Viagra) in patients with cardiovascular disease. Technology and Practice Executive Committee. *Circulation* 1999; 99: 168–177.
60. DeSouza C, Parulkar A, Lumpkin D, Akers D, Fonseca VA: Acute and prolonged effects of sildenafil on brachial artery flow-mediated dilatation in type 2 diabetes. *Diabetes Care* 2002; 25: 1336–1339.
61. Katz SD, Balidemaj K, Homma S, et al.: Acute type 5 phosphodiesterase inhibition with sildenafil enhances flow-mediated vasodilation in patients with chronic heart failure. *J Am Coll Cardiol* 2000; 36: 845–851.
62. Halcox JP, Nour KR, Zalos G, et al.: The effect of sildenafil on human vascular function, platelet activation, and myocardial ischemia. *J Am Coll Cardiol* 2002; 40: 1232–1240.
63. Knowler WC, Barrett-Connor E, Fowler SE, et al.: Reduction in the incidence of type 2 diabetes with lifestyle intervention or metformin. *N Eng J Med* 2002; 346:393–403.
64. Esposito K, Di Palo C, Marfella R, Giugliano D: The effect of weight loss on endothelial functions in obesity: response to Sciacqua et al. *Diabetes Care* 2003; 26:2968–2969.
65. Esposito K, Pontillo A, Di Palo C, et al.: Effect of weight loss and lifestyle changes on vascular inflammatory markers in obese women: a randomized trial. *JAMA* 2003; 289:1799–1804.
66. Saigal CS.: Obesity and erectile dysfunction: common problems, common solution? *JAMA* 2004; 291:3011–3012.
67. Saltzman EA, Guay AT, Jacobson J: Improvement in erectile function in men with organic erectile dysfunction by correction of elevated cholesterol levels: a clinical observation. *J Urol* 2004; 172: 255–258.

V OF INTEREST

13 Natriuretic Peptides and Cardiovascular Regulation

Kailash N. Pandey, PhD

CONTENTS

SUMMARY

Atrial natriuretic factor/peptide (ANF/ANP) is the first described member in the natriuretic peptides (NPs) hormone family, which elicits natriuretic, diuretic, vasorelaxant, and antimitogenic effects, all of which are largely directed to the reduction of blood volume and blood pressure. Two other members, brain natriuretic peptide (BNP) and C-type natriuretic peptide (CNP) also exhibit biochemical and structural characteristics similar to ANP, but each derived from a separate gene. However, ANP, BNP, and CNP have highly homologous structure, bind to specific cell-surface receptors, and elicit some discrete biological functions. Till date, three subtypes of NPs receptors, namely, NP receptor-A, -B, and -C (NPRA, NPRB, and NPRC, respectively) are known. Interestingly, both ANP and BNP activate NPRA, which contains intracellular guanylyl cyclase (GC) catalytic domain and produces second messenger cGMP in response to hormone binding; however, CNP binds NPRB, which also contains GC catalytic domain and produces cGMP, but all three NPs indiscriminately bind to NPRC, which lacks intracellular GC catalytic domain. The biochemical,

From: *Contemporary Endocrinology: Cardiovascular Endocrinology: Shared Pathways and Clinical Crossroads*
Edited by: V. A. Fonseca © Humana Press, New York, NY

molecular, and pharmacological aspects of NPs and their prototype receptors have revealed hallmark functions of physiological and pathophysiological importance, including renal, cardiovascular, neuronal, and immunological aspects in health and disease.

Key Words: Natriuretic peptide receptors, hypertension, blood pressure, signaling mechanisms

INTRODUCTION

The pioneer discovery by de Bold et al. *(1)* demonstrated that atrial extracts contained natriuretic activity which led them to isolate "atrial natriuretic factor/peptide (ANF/ANP)" and to establish the field of natriuretic peptides (NPs). The NPs are a group of peptide hormones that play important roles in the control of renal, cardiovascular, endocrine, and skeletal homeostasis *(2–5)*. ANP is the first described member in the NP hormone family that elicits natriuretic, diuretic, vasorelaxant, and antimitogenic effects, all of which are directed to the reduction of body fluid and blood pressure homeostasis *(4,6)*. Later, two other members, B-type or brain NP (BNP) and C-type NP (CNP), were identified *(7,8)*. ANP and BNP are primarily stored in the granules of heart, circulate in the plasma, and display the most variability in primary structure, whereas CNP is largely present in the endothelial cells and is highly conserved among the species. Three subtypes of NP receptors have been identified, namely NP receptor-A (NPRA), NP receptor-B (NPRB), and NP receptor-C (NPRC). Both NPRA and NPRB contain an extracellular ligand-binding domain, a single transmembrane spanning region, and an intracellular protein kinase-like homology domain (KHD) and guanylyl cyclase (GC) catalytic domain *(9,10)*. Interestingly, both ANP and BNP activate NPRA, which produces second messenger cGMP in response to hormone binding; however, CNP activates NPRB, which also produces cGMP, but all three NPs indiscriminately bind to NPRC, which lacks the KHD and GC catalytic domain *(11)*. The discovery of structurally related NPs indicated that the physiological control of blood pressure and body fluid homeostasis is complex. This complexity is further enhanced by the prevalence of at least three subtypes of NP-specific receptors. A combination of biochemical, molecular, and pharmacological aspects of NPs and their prototype receptors have revealed hallmark functions of physiological and pathophysiological importance, including renal, cardiovascular, neuronal, and immunological aspects in health and disease *(5,12,13)*.

PROPERTIES OF NPs

ANP is primarily synthesized in the heart atrium; BNP, initially isolated from the brain but predominantly present in the heart, displays most variability in the primary structure; and CNP, isolated from porcine brain, is highly conserved among the species *(14)*. All three NPs contain highly conserved residues with a 17-member disulfide ring but deviate from each other in flanking sequences. The primary structure deduced from cDNAs suggested that ANP is synthesized first as the 152-amino-acid prepro-ANP that contained sequences of active peptides in its carboxyl-terminal region, and major form of circulatory ANP is a 28-residue molecule *(15)*. The ring conformation of ANP molecule with a disulfide-bonded loop is essential for its activities *(2)*. Furthermore, the carboxyl-terminal sequence extending from the ring structure to Asn-Phe-Arg-Tyr is also required for biological activity of ANP.

The amino acid sequence of ANP is almost identical across the mammalian species, except for position 10 which is isoleucine in rat, mouse, and rabbit; however, in human, dog, and bovine, ANPs have methionine in this position. The biologically active ANP is produced by proteolytic cleavage of pro-ANP molecule into predominantly 28-amino-acid ANP (residues

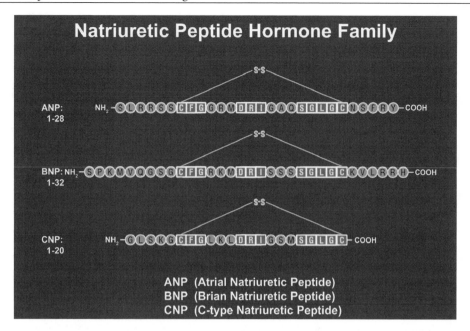

Fig. 1. The amino acid sequence comparison and structure of the mature human ANP, BNP, and CNP with conserved residues represented by shaded square boxes. The lines between the two cysteine residues (ANP, BNP, and CNP) indicate a 17-residue disulfide bridge, essential for biological activity. ANP: atrial natriuretic peptide; BNP: brain natriuretic peptide; and CNP: C-type natriuretic peptide.

99–126) and the N-terminal pro-ANP (NT-Pro ANP) molecule (residues 1–98). The active form of ANP has disulfide-bonded loop between cysteine 105 and cysteine 121, essential for the biological activity *(2)*. All ANP analogs with natriuretic or diuretic activity share this common central ring structure *(16)*. Subsequently, BNP *(17)* and CNP *(18)* were both isolated from porcine brain extracts on the basis of their potent relaxant effects. Soon, it was established that BNP is predominantly synthesized and secreted from the heart ventricles *(19)*. Similarly, CNP is predominantly localized in the central nervous system and endothelial cells and is considered a noncirculatory NP hormone *(20)*. Like ANP, both BNP and CNP are synthesized from large precursor molecules and the mature bioactive peptides contain 17-residue loop bridged by an intramolecular disulfide bond. In essence, 11 of these amino acids are identical in biologically active ANP, BNP, and CNP; however, the amino- and carboxyl-terminus vary in length and composition (Fig. 1). Among the species, BNP exhibits most variability in primary structure, and both ANP and CNP are highly conserved across the species. The mechanisms of action of NPs in relation to their structure and their physiology are still not well understood.

NPs SYNTHESIS AND SECRETION

The three NPs ANP, BNP, and CNP have highly homologous structure, but they have distinct sites of synthesis. Both ANP and BNP are predominantly synthesized in the heart, and ANP concentrations range from 50–100-fold higher than BNP. It is generally believed that following the processing of preprohormone to prohormone molecule, the cleavage and secretion of biologically active mature 28-residue ANP molecule occurs predominantly in response to atrial distension *(4)*. The atrium is the primary site of synthesis for both hormones within the heart; however, ventricle also produces both ANP and BNP but at the level 100–1000-fold less than the atrium, respectively. It has been observed that the difference in the NP concentrations also correlate with mRNA levels *(4,21)*. Interestingly, the expression of both ANP and BNP increases dramatically in both the atrium and ventricle in cardiac hypertrophy *(22,23)*; nevertheless, the ventricle becomes the primary site of synthesis and release for BNP. In patients with severe congestive heart failure (CHF), the concentrations of both ANP and BNP increase higher than control values; however, the BNP concentrations increase 10–50-fold higher than a comparative increase in ANP concentrations*(22)*. These findings indicated that ANP and BNP elicit distinct physiological and pathophysiological effects. In essence, ANP and BNP show similar hemodynamic responses; however, BNP exerts a longer duration of action and causes enhanced rather than blunted natriuretic responses as compared with ANP *(24–26)*. Cardiac atrium expresses almost 50–100-fold ANP or even higher ANP mRNA levels as compared with extracardiac tissues *(27)*. Interestingly, higher ventricular ANP is present in the developing embryo and fetus; nevertheless, both mRNA and peptide levels of ANP decline rapidly during the prenatal period *(28)*. However, ANP gene expression in ventricle is reinducible postnatally in response to phenylephrine administration, after-load stress, and myocardium infarction *(29)*. Indeed, the mRNA levels of BNP are markedly lower than ANP in heart; however, the BNP concentrations are higher in the ventricle as compared with both neonatal and adult rat hearts, but the reduction in the ventricular expression of BNP is far less than ANP in the adult hearts *(30,31)*. Although, the circulating BNP levels are far less than that of ANP levels in normal subjects, the increase in BNP concentrations in plasma can surpass the level of ANP in patients with CHF *(22,26,31–33)*.

On the contrary, CNP does not seem to behave as a cardiac hormone and its levels are extremely low in the circulation *(34)*. CNP is largely present in the central nervous system *(35)* and in the vascular endothelial cells *(36–39)*. D-type NP (DNP) represents an additional member in the NP hormone family *(40,41)*. DNP is present in the venom of the green mamba (*Dendroaspis angusticeps*) as a 38-amino-acid peptide molecule. In addition, a 32-amino-acid peptide termed urodilatin (URO) is identical to C-terminal sequence of pro-ANP and appears to be present only in urine *(42,43)*. It was initially purified from human urine and is presumed to be only synthesized in the kidney *(44)*. URO is not present in the circulation and appears to be a unique intrarenal NP with unexplored physiological significance *(44,45)*. The studies with immunohistological staining indicated that URO is largely present in the cortical tubules around the collecting ducts of the kidney *(46–48)*.

NPs RECEPTORS

The cross-linking and photoaffinity labeling studies showed the existence of ANP receptors with a wide range of molecular weights (M_r) of the 60–140 kDa *(49)*. Based on the biological activity of different ANP analogs, ANP receptors were classified as biologically active and clearance or silent receptors *(2)*. Subsequently, different subtypes of ANP receptors were identified by photoaffinity and cross-linking, which appeared to be specific to different cell types. Intriguing was the finding that using photoaffinity labeling three distinct types of NP receptors (NPRs) were classified in different cell types *(49)*. Biochemical, immunohistochemical, and molecular biological data indicated that specific NP binds and activates specific receptor, which are quite widespread in their tissue distributions *(2,49–52)*. Some additional members of the plasma membrane GCs have also been discovered; however, their specific ligands have yet to be discovered (Table 1).

Molecular cloning and expression of cDNA led to identify and characterize the primary structure of three distinct subtypes of NPRs, which are currently designated as NPRA *(9,53)*,

Table 1
Tissue distribution of various types of particulate guanylyl cyclases and soluble guanylyl
cyclase with their respective ligands and/or activators

Ligand	Guanylyl Cyclases	Tissue-Specific Distribution
ANP	GC-A/NPRA	Kidney, adrenal glands, heart, lung, vascular bed, ovary, testis, brain, and other tissues
BNP	GC-A/NPRA	Kidney, adrenal glands, heart, lung, vascular bed, ovary, testis, brain, and other tissues
CNP	GC-B/NPRB	Vascular bed, fibroblast, heart, lung, adrenal gland, brain, ovary, and other tissues
Enterotoxin/Guanylyn/ Uroguanylin	GC-C	Colon, intestine, and kidney
NO	Soluble Cyclase	Smooth muscle, platelet, kidney, lung, and other tissues
CO	Soluble Cyclase	Vasculature, kidney, lung, platelet, and other tissues

ANP: atrial natriuretic peptide; BNP: brain natriuretic peptide; CNP: C-type natriuretic peptide; NO: Nitric oxide; CO: Carbon monoxide.

NPRB *(10)*, and NPRC *(54)*. The three receptor subtypes (NPRA, NPRB, and NPRC) constitute NPR family (Fig. 2). The general topological structure of NPRA and NPRB is consistent with at least four distinct domains. As such, the entire coding region of both NPRA and NPRB is separated by a single transmembrane-spanning region into extracellular ligand-binding domain and intracellular protein kinase-like homology domain, also referred to as kinase homology domain (KHD) and GC catalytic domain *(9,10)*. NPRA and NPRB are also referred to as GC-A and GC-B, respectively, *(55)*. The transmembrane GC receptors contain a single cyclase catalytic active site per polypeptide molecule; however, based on the structure modeling data *(56,57)* two polypeptide chains seem to be required to activate the function of NPRA *(57–59)*. The dimerization region of the receptor has been suggested to be located between the KHD and GC catalytic domain that have been predicted to form an amphipathic alpha-helix structure *(27)*. The NPRB has the overall domain structure similar to that of NPRA with binding selectivity to CNP, and also generates the second messenger cGMP *(7,27,60,61)*. NPRA is the dominant form of the NPRs found in peripheral organs and mediates most of the known actions of ANP and BNP. Whereas NPRB is localized mainly in the brain and vascular tissues, it is thought to mediate the actions of CNP in the central nervous systems and also in vascular bed (Table 1).

The third member of the NPR family, NPRC, constitutes a large extracellular domain of 496 amino acids, a single transmembrane domain, and a very short 37-amino-acid cytoplasmic tail that bears no homology domain of any other known receptor proteins. The extracellular region of NPRC is approximately 30% identical to NPRA and NPRB. Ligand receptor binding studies have shown that NPRC has much less stringent specificity for structural variants of ANP than does NPRA or NPRB *(62)*. The extracellular domain of NPRC possesses two pairs of cysteine residues along with one isolated cysteine near the transmembrane domain, three potential signals for N-glycosylation, and several serines and threonines for O-linked glycosylation sites *(54)*. Earlier, it was proposed that NPRC may function as a clearance receptor to remove NPs from the circulation *(63)*; however, a number of studies provide the evidence that NPRC plays roles in biological action of NPs *(64–67)* and clearance name carries only by a default nomenclature to NPRC.

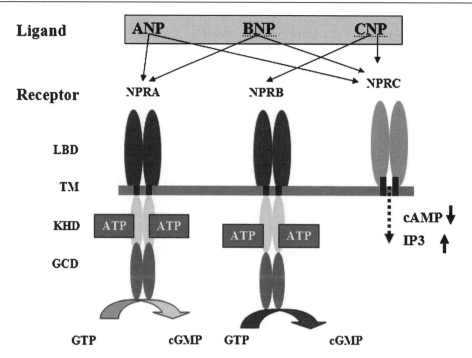

Fig. 2. A schematic representation of the natriuretic peptides (ANP, BNP, and CNP) and their specificity to activate the natriuretic peptide receptors NPRA, NPRB, and NPRC. The solid lines connect the NP receptors with their preferred ligands as indicated. The ligand-binding domains, transmembrane region, and intracellular domains have been indicated. The NPRA and NPRB are shown to generate the second messenger cGMP, and NPRC is shown to decrease cAMP and to increase inositol trisphosphate (IP_3) levels. NPRA: natriuretic peptide receptor-A; NPRB: natriuretic peptide receptor-B; NPRC: natriuretic peptide receptor-C.

INTERNALIZATION AND DOWNREGULATION OF NPRs

The downregulation of NPRA has also been observed and reported in Leydig tumor (MA-10) cells and PC-12 cells containing endogenous receptors *(68,69)* and in COS-7 and HEK-293 cells containing recombinant receptors *(5,70,71)*. Thus, downregulation of NP receptors by ligand-dependent internalization plays important role in NP receptor signaling and function. The carboxyl-terminal deletion studies of NPRA have suggested that specific sites in the GC catalytic domain and KHD seem to play critical role in the endocytosis and sequestration of GC-coupled receptor proteins *(72–75)*. It should be mentioned that a number of studies have also shown that after prolonged treatment of cultured cells with ANP, both receptor density and GC activity are decreased with simultaneous decrease in mRNA levels *(74,76–78)*. In addition, transforming growth factor-β1 (TGF-β1), ANG II, and endothelin have also been shown to reduce NPRA mRNA levels in cultured cells *(79)*. Some of these studies have established that a decrease in mRNA levels of NPRA correlated well with repressed transcriptional activity of NPRA.

It has been suggested that NPRA exists in the phosphorylated state and the addition of ANP causes a decrease in the phosphate contents as well as reduction in the ANP-dependent GC catalytic activity *(80–85)*. The apparent mechanism of desensitization of NPRA is in contrast to many other cell-surface receptors which appear to be desensitized by phosphorylation *(86–90)*. The previous findings also suggested that ANP seems to stimulate phosphorylation of its GC-coupled receptor protein *(91)*. It has been indicated that cGMP-dependent protein kinase (PKG), a serine/threonine kinase, is capable of phosphorylating NPRA in vitro *(92–98)*. These authors suggested that PKG is recruited to the plasma membrane after ANP treatment and increases the GC catalytic activity of NPRA.

The downregulation of NPRC has been shown in cultured vascular smooth muscle cells, which predominantly contain this receptor protein *(92–94,99–103)*. The kinetic studies of metabolic processing of ANP involving NPRC which does not contain GC catalytic activity has been reported by several investigators utilizing vascular smooth muscle cells *(93,104)*. The downregulation of NPRC seems to be associated with increased internalization of the ligand–receptors complexes involving receptor-mediated endocytotic mechanisms *(93)*. It has been suggested that a portion of the receptor population recycles back to the plasma membrane and newly synthesized receptors reconstitute the receptor population *(105–108)*.

NPs AND RENAL FUNCTIONS

Renal sites of ANP action include inner medullary collecting duct, glomerulus, and mesangial cells *(2,109–114)*. ANP action is perceived to facilitate the excretion of salt and water with an increase in glomerular filtration rate *(2,65)*. The intracellular actions of ANP in renal cells include the stimulation of GC activity and reduction in adenylyl cyclase and phospholipase C activities, sodium influx, and reduced calcium concentrations *(108)*. The increased production of cGMP at ANP concentrations affecting renal functions correlates with the effects of dibutyryl-cGMP, which prevents mesangial cell contraction in response to ANG II *(115,116)*. The most compelling evidence supporting a role for cGMP in mediating the renal effects of ANP was obtained with selective NPRA antagonists, A71915 and HS-121-1, to eliminate the renal effect of infused ANP, including the elevation of urinary cGMP *(109,110,117,118)*. These studies established that ANP effect in kidney is largely mediated by cGMP through the activation of NPRA. ANP markedly lowers renin secretion from kidney and also affects plasma renin concentrations *(109)*. Ample experimental data have established that ANP plays an important role in regulation of renal function by its vasodilatory and natriuretic responses and its ability to counteract the renin-angiotensin-aldosterone system (RAAS) in a tissue-specific manner *(119)*. Attempts have been made to define physiological responses in kidney by infusing the exogenous ANP *(120)*. Cardiac appendectomy has been used to prevent ANP release; however, the problem in this setting is that the missing normal cardiac function results in a lack of physiological reflexes that are normally elicited by atrial components *(121–123)*. Another approach has used monoclonal antibodies against circulating ANP; however, problems are related to nonspecific effect of the antibody or antigen complexes. One of the classical approaches has been taken to specifically inhibit the signaling pathway of NPRA to block cGMP production. Although two compounds, A71917 and HS-140-1, have been shown to diminish the effect of ANP by antagonizing NPRA, these compounds do not completely inhibit NPRA activity *(124)*. Activation of NPs (ANP, BNP), enhances the pressure–natriuresis relationship and reduces atrial pressures. It has also been suggested that chloride-mediated feedback control of NPRA occurs in the kidney and plays a role in ANP-mediated natriuresis *(110,118,125–127)*. Initial as well as recent studies have shown that ANP/NPRA system suppresses renin and decreases blood pressures *(118)*. ANP antagonizes most of the actions of angiotensin II, and thereby maintains normal cardiovascular homeostatic balance (Table 2).

The studies with *Npr1* (coding for NPRA) gene-disrupted mice demonstrated that at birth, the absence of NPRA allows greater renin and ANG II levels and increased renin mRNA expression compared with the wild-type mice *(119,128)*. However, at 3–16 weeks of age, both

Table 2
Antagonistic actions of ANP and angiotensin II on various
physiological functions involved in the regulation of blood
pressure and cardiovascular homeostasis

Physiological Function	ANP	ANG II
Aldosterone release	Inhibition	Stimulation
Renin Release	Inhibition	Inhibition
Vasopression Release	Inhibition	Stimulation
Water drinking	Inhibition	Stimulation
Central nervous system-mediated hypertension	Inhibition	Stimulation
Neurotransmission	Inhibition	Stimulation
Blood vessels tone	Relaxation	Contraction

Stimulatory and inhibitory actions of ANP or ANG II on cellular and physiological responses in target tissues and cells.

circulating and kidney renin and ANG II levels were decreased dramatically in *Npr1* homozygous null mutant mice as compared with wild-type control mice. This decrease in renin activity in adult null mutant mice is implicated due to progressive elevation in arterial pressure leading to inhibition of renin synthesis and release from the kidney juxtaglomerular cells. It has been suggested that increased levels of ANP released into the plasma in response to blood volume expansion is attributed to be mainly responsible for the natriuretic and diuretic responses *(125)*. Recent studies have examined the quantitative contributions and possible mechanisms mediating the responses of varying numbers of *Npr1* gene copies by determining the renal plasma flow (RPF), glomerular filtration rate (GFR), urine flow and sodium excretion patterns following blood volume expansion in *Npr1* homozygous null mutant (0-copy), wild-type (2-copy), and gene-duplicated (4-copy) mice in a *Npr1* gene-dose-dependent manner *(2,129,130)*. These findings demonstrated that the ANP/NPRA axis is primarily responsible for mediating the renal hemodynamic and sodium excretory responses to intravascular blood volume expansion and established that NPRA is a hallmark receptor, which plays a critical role in mediating the natriuresis, diuresis, and renal hemodynamic responses to acute blood volume expansion. Interestingly, ANP/NPRA system inhibits aldosterone synthesis and release from adrenal glomerulosa cells *(2,65,73)* suggesting that this ANP action could be physiologically important, which probably accounts for renal natriuretic and diuretic effects.

NPs AND VASCULAR FUNCTION

The findings on the effect of ANP either in intact aortic rings or in cultured vascular smooth muscle cells have always reported an elevation in the intracellular levels of cGMP. The correlative evidence between ANP-induced cGMP accumulation and vasodilation has suggested the role of cGMP as the second messenger of dilator responses to ANP *(131,132)*. ANP as well as cGMP analogs have been found to reduce the agonist-induced increases in cytosolic Ca^{2+} concentrations in vascular smooth muscle cells *(133,134)*. It has been reported that cGMP activates sarcolemmal Ca^{2+}-ATPase, and this mechanism may be important in the ANP-induced decreases in cytosolic Ca^{2+} in vascular smooth muscle cells *(135,136)*. Nevertheless, it is anticipated that the ultimate effect of ANP in vascular smooth muscle cells could be due to production of cGMP and the activation of cGMP-dependent protein kinases *(137–139)*. However, more studies are needed to define the biochemical and molecular basis of NP actions in vascular smooth muscle cells.

ANTIMITOGENIC EFFECTS OF NPs

NPs have been shown to act as a growth suppressor in a variety of cell types, including kidney *(140)*, heart *(141,142)*, neurons *(143)*, thymus *(37,137,142,144–147)*, vasculature *(148)*, and fibroblasts *(70,136,146)*. Interestingly, cGMP analogs mimic the antiproliferative action of NPs; thus, it is considered that they exert the antimitogenic effects largely through the second messenger cGMP *(149)*. ANP has been shown to inhibit collagen synthesis in cardiac fibroblasts *(150–152)* and also it inhibits hypertrophy in primary cultures of cardiac myocytes *(153)*. Similarly, PKG has been shown to suppress extracellular matrix production in vascular smooth muscle cells *(151,154)*. The expression of ANP and BNP genes are greatly augmented in hypertrophied hearts, which supports the notion that autocrine and/or paracrine effects of ANP/BNP signal plays an important role against pathological cardiac hypertrophy in disease states *(70,146,155,156)*. The mechanisms of signaling pathways which elicit antimitogenic effect of ANP/NPRA are not yet well characterized. However, both GC-linked NP receptors, NPRA and NPRB, as well as GC-unlinked NP receptor, NPRC, have been suggested to play a role in ANP-dependent antimitogenic responses *(70,155,156)*. Previous studies have demonstrated that ANP inhibits ANG II- and platelet-derived growth factor (PDGF) -dependent MAPK activity in different tissues and cell types *(148)*. CNP, which acts through NPRB, has also been shown to inhibit MAPK activity in fibroblast cells in a cGMP-dependent manner *(157,158)*. Clearly more experimentation is needed to delineate the underlying mechanisms of the antiproliferative effect of NPs in target cells.

In addition to its antimitogenic effect, ANP has been shown to induce apoptosis in cultured vascular smooth muscle cells and in neonatal rat cardiac myocytes *(158)*. ANP-induced apoptotic effect was mimicked by 8-bromo-cGMP, a membrane-permeable analog of cGMP, and by nitroprusside, an activator of soluble GC. Furthermore, ANP effect was potentiated by a cGMP-specific phosphodiesterase inhibitor zaprinast. It was indicated that norepinephrine, a myocyte growth effector, inhibited ANP-induced apoptosis via activation of β-adrenergic receptor and elevation of cAMP *(158,159)*. The existence of a complementary ANP-mediated mechanism to inhibit cell growth is not surprising. The inhibition of cell proliferation is often accompanied by an increased probability of apoptosis, whereas, growth-promoting agents tend to promote cell growth and proliferation. For instance, ANG II inhibits apoptosis; in contrast, ANP and nitric oxide, both potently inhibit cell growth and proliferation and induce apoptosis *(160,161)*. It has been suggested that the antiapoptotic Bcl-2 homologue Mcl-1 might serve as an important target in ANP-induced apoptosis of cardiac myocytes. The Bcl-2 homologue Mcl-1 was initially identified as a protein which was upregulated during the differentiation of monocytoid cell line ML-1 cells *(158,162)*. Interestingly, Mcl-1 is expressed at high levels in the heart *(163–165)*.

NPs AND PATHOPHYSIOLOGY OF CARDIOVASCULAR DISEASES

High levels of endogenous ANP are thought to compensate the condition of patients with heart failure by reducing preload and afterload. Evidence suggests that a high plasma ANP/BNP level is a prognostic predictor in humans with heart failure *(166)*. Studies with ANP-deficient genetic strains of mice demonstrated that a defect in the ANP synthesis can cause hypertension *(126,166,167)*. The blood pressures of homozygous null mutant animals were elevated by 8–12 mmHg when they were fed with standard or intermediate salt diets. Heterozygous animals showed normal blood pressures and normal amount of circulatory ANP; however, they became hypertensive and blood pressure was elevated by 20–27 mmHg if these animals were fed with high-salt diets *(168)*. Those previous findings clearly demonstrated that genetically reduced production of ANP can lead to salt-sensitive hypertension. On the other hand, the disruption of *Npr1* gene indicated that the blood pressure of homozygous mutant mice remained elevated and unchanged in response to either minimal- or high-salt diets *(169)*. These investigators suggested that NPRA may exert its major effect at the level of vasculature and probably does so independently of salt. In contrast, Oliver et al., *(118,125,126,167–174)* reported that disruption of *Npr1* gene resulted in chronic elevation of blood pressure in mice fed with high-salt diets. Indeed, more studies are needed to clarify the relationship between salt-sensitivity and blood pressures in *Npr1* gene-targeted mice.

Genetic mouse models with disruption of both ANP and NPRA genes have provided strong support for the role of this hormone-receptor system in the regulation of arterial pressure and other physiological functions *(125,167,171,173,175,176)*. Therefore, the genetic defects that reduce the activity of ANP and its receptor system can be considered as candidate contributors to essential hypertension and CHF *(118,125,170)*. Interestingly, complete absence of NPRA causes hypertension in mice and leads to altered renin and ANG II levels, cardiac hypertrophy, and lethal vascular events similar to those seen in untreated human hypertensive patients *(125, 169,172)*. In contrast, increased expression of NPRA reduces the blood pressures and increases the second messenger cGMP, corresponding to the increasing number of *Npr1* gene copies *(113,126,177)*. Transgenic mice overexpressing ANP developed sustained hypotension with arterial pressure that was 25–30 mmHg lower than their nontransgenic siblings *(178)*. A recent study demonstrated that somatic delivery of ANP gene in spontaneously hypertensive rat (SHR) induced a sustained reduction of systemic blood pressure, raising the possibility of using ANP as a therapeutic agent for treatment of human hypertension *(118)*.

Genetic defects that reduce the activity or influence the ANP/NPRA system greatly contribute to the development of hypertension. The mechanistic role of ANP/NPRA system in counteracting the pathophysiology of hypertension is not well understood. Although, the expression of ANP and BNP is markedly increased in patients with hypertrophied or failing heart, it is unclear if the NP system is activated to play a protective role by reducing the detrimental effects of high blood pressure caused by sodium retention and fluid volume, inhibiting the RAAS, or it is simply a consequence of the hypertrophic changes occurring in heart. Recent studies indicated that intrarenal renin in newborn *Npr1* homozygous null mutant pups (2 days after birth) was 2.5-fold higher than in two-copy wild-type counterparts *(118)*. However, adult (16 weeks) hypertensive *Npr1* null mutant mice showed 50–70% reduction in plasma renin concentrations and renal renin contents as compared with wild-type control animals. In contrast, the adrenal renin contents and mRNA expression levels were elevated approximately 1.5- to 2.0-fold in adult homozygous null mutant mice than wild-type mice. However, the factors that modulate renin gene expression in the adrenal gland have not been clearly identified. Together, the studies in both SHR and *Npr1* gene-knockout hypertensive mouse models suggest that in hypertension, both kidney and circulatory renin concentrations are decreased; however, as a compensatory event, the adrenal renin is increased *(129)*. Thus in light of those previous findings, it can be suggested that ANP/NPRA system may play a key regulatory role in the synthesis and maintenance of both systemic and tissue levels of RAAS components in both physiological and pathological conditions *(31)*.

NPs AS A BIOLOGICAL INDICATOR OF CARDIOVASCULAR DISORDERS

Interestingly, the half-life of BNP is greater than ANP; thus, the evaluation of the diagnostic importance of the NPs has largely favored BNP (26,31,179,180). The inactive N-terminal fragment of BNP (NT-proBNP) has even a greater half-life than the BNP. The plasma levels of both BNP and NT-proBNP are markedly elevated under the pathophysiological condition of cardiac dysfunction, including diastolic dysfunction, CHF, and pulmonary embolism (179). The basal plasma levels of BNP vary from 10 pg/ml to 50 pg/ml and NT-proBNP levels ranges from 75 pg/ml to 160 pg/ml; however, an abnormal range is considered as 100 pg/ml for BNP and 125 pg/ml for NT-proBNP (181). Nevertheless, the secretion of both ANP and BNP from ventricular myocytes increases proportionally in relation to the magnitude of cardiac dysfunction or cardiovascular disease states (182). It has been reported that BNP can be considered as an important prognostic indicator in CHF patients, however, NT-proBNP is considered to be a stronger risk bio-indicator for cardiovascular disorders (183). Nevertheless, both BNP and NT-proBNP can provide an ideal tool to be utilized as blood test markers to diagnose cardiovascular events in high-risk CHF patients. BNP and NT-proBNP have also been used as biological markers in patients with chronic kidney disease with left ventricular hypertrophy and coronary artery disease (184,185). Similarly, the levels of both BNP and NT-proBNP are also greatly increased in patients with renal insufficiency. The BNP level is increased to almost 200 pg/ml and NT-proBNP levels reaches to approximately 1200 pg/ml in patients with reduced creatinine clearance (31,164,165).

It is widely believed that ANP and BNP concentrations are markedly increased both in cardiac tissues and in plasma of CHF patients (163). Studies in patients with chronic CHF have suggested that their plasma NPs levels decreased, whereas plasma cGMP levels increased significantly from femoral artery to the femoral vein; however, in patients with mild CHF, the plasma cGMP levels correlated with ANP levels (151,152,176). Furthermore, those previous studies suggested that among patients with severe CHF, plasma cGMP levels reached a plateau despite high levels of plasma ANP, and the molar ratio of cGMP production to ANP in peripheral circulation was significantly lower than those in patients with mildCHF. The findings of those previous studies further indicated that downregulation of NPRA may also occur in the peripheral vascular bed of patients with chronic severeCHF. In hypertrophied heart, ANP and BNP genes are overexpressed, suggesting that autocrine and/or paracrine effects of NPs predominate and might serve as an endogenous protective mechanism against maladaptive pathological cardiac hypertrophy (170). Inactivation of either ANP or *Npr1* gene in mice increases the cardiac mass to a great extent (154,179). A significant inverse relationship has been found between myocardial ANP and BNP mRNAs expression or peptide levels and increases in left ventricular cardiac mass (186). Those previous findings suggested that ANP expression plays a protective role in hypertrophied heart. Furthermore, it has been shown that functional alterations of ANP promoter are linked to cardiac hypertrophy in progenies of crosses between Wistar Kyoto (WKY) and Wistar Kyoto-derived hypertensive (WKYH) rats. These authors suggested that a single-nucleotide polymorphism altered the transcriptional activity of ANP gene promoter, and implicated that ANP may protect cardiomyocytes against hypertrophy as a strong candidate gene for the determination of left ventricular mass.

CONCLUSIONS

Thus far, three related NPs and three distinct receptors have been identified which have advanced our knowledge toward understanding control of high blood pressure, hypertension, and cardiovascular disorders to a great extent. Biochemical and molecular studies have been advanced to examine receptor function and signaling mechanisms and the role of second messenger cGMP in physiology and pathophysiology of hypertension, renal hemodynamics, and cardiovascular functions. Tools have been developed to examine receptor internalization, downregulation, and/or desensitization of both GC-coupled and GC-uncoupled NP receptors in different cell systems. The development of gene-knockout and gene-duplication mouse models along with transgenic mice have provided a framework for understanding both the physiological and pathophysiological importance of NPs and their receptors and the signaling pathways involved in their mechanisms of action in hypertension and cardiovascular disease states. Although, a considerable progress has been made, the transmembrane signal transduction mechanisms of NPs and their receptors remain unresolved. Future challenges should include the identification and characterization of cellular targets of NPs and second messenger cGMP including cytosolic and nuclear proteins, role in gene transcription, cell growth and proliferation, apoptosis, and differentiation. More vigorous studies of the crosstalk with other signaling mechanisms needs to be pursued systematically. Now, NPs are considered as circulating markers of CHF; however, their therapeutic potential for the treatment of cardiovascular diseases such as hypertension, renal insufficiency, cardiac hypertrophy, CHF, and stroke is still lacking. Indeed, the alternative avenues of investigations need to be undertaken, as we are at the initial stage of the molecular therapeutic and pharmacogenomic implications.

ACKNOWLEDGMENTS

I thank my wife Kamala Pandey for her assistance during the preparation of this review. My special thanks go to Dr. Susan L. Hamilton, Department of Molecular Physiology and Biophysics at Baylor College of Medicine, and Dr. Bharat B. Aggarwal, Department of Experimental Therapeutics and Cytokine Research Laboratory at MD Anderson Cancer Center, for providing their facilities during our displacement due to Hurricane Katrina. The research in the author's laboratory is supported by the grants from the National Institutes of Health (HL 57531 and HL 62147) and Louisiana Health Excellence Fund.

REFERENCES

1. de Bold AJ, Borenstein HB, Veress AT, Sonnenberg H. A rapid and potent natriuretic response to intravenous injection of atrial myocardial extract in rats. Life Sci. 1981;28:89–94.
2. Brenner BM, Ballermann BJ, Gunning ME, Zeidel ML. Diverse biological actions of atrial natriuretic peptide. Physiol Rev 1990;70(3):665–99.
3. Drewett JG, Garbers DL. The family of guanylyl cyclase receptors and their ligands. Endocr Rev 1994;15: 135–162.
4. McGrath MF, de Bold ML, de Bold AJ. The endocrine function of the heart. Trends Endocrinol Metab 2005;16(10):469–77.
5. Pandey KN. Biology of natriuretic peptides and their receptors. Peptides 2005;26(6):901–932.
6. de Bold AJ. Atrial natriuretic factor: a hormone produced by the heart. Science 1985;230(4727):767–770.
7. Schulz S. C-type natriuretic peptide and guanylyl cyclase B receptor. Peptides 2005;26(6):1024–1034.
8. LaPointe MC. Molecular regulation of the brain natriuretic peptide gene. Peptides 2005;26:944–956.
9. Pandey KN, Singh S. Molecular cloning and expression of murine guanylate cyclase/atrial natriuretic factor receptor cDNA. J Biol Chem 1990;265(21):12342–12348.
10. Schulz S, Singh S, Bellet RA, Singh G, Tubb DJ, Chin H, et al. The primary structure of a plasma membrane guanylate cyclase demonstrates diversity within this new receptor family. Cell 1989;58:1155–1162.
11. Koller KJ, Goddel DV. Molecular biology of the natriuretic peptides and their receptors. Circulation 1992;86:1081–1088.
12. Kuhn M. Cardiac and intestinal natriuretic peptides: insights from genetically modified mice. Peptides 2005;26:1078–1085.
13. Vollmer AM. The role of atrial natriuretic peptide in the immune system. Peptides 2005;26:1087–1094.

14. Rosenzweig A, Seidman CE. Atrial natriuretic factor and related peptide hormones. Annu Rev Biochem 1991;60:229–255.
15. Maki M, Takayanagi R, Misono K, Pandey KN, Tibbetts C, Inagami T. Structure of rat atrial natriuretic factor precursor deduced from cDNA sequence. Nature 1984;309:722–724.
16. Misono KS, Fukumi H, Grammer RT, Inagami T. Rat atrial natriuretic factor: complete amino acid sequence and disulfide linkage essential for biological activity. Biochem Biophys Res Commun 1984;119: 524–529.
17. Sudoh T, Minamino N, Kangawa K, Matsuo H. Brain natriuretic peptide-32: N-terminal six amino acid extended form of brain natriuretic peptide identified in porcine brain. Biochem Biophys Res Commun 1988;155(2): 726–732.
18. Sudoh T, Minamino N, Kangawa K, Matsuo H. C-type natriuretic peptide (CNP): a new member of natriuretic peptide family identified in porcine brain. Biochem Biophys Res Commun 1990;168(2): 863–870.
19. Philips RA, Ardeljan M, Shimabukuro S, Goldman ME, Garbowit DL, Eison HB, et al. Normalisation of left ventricular mass and associated changes in neurohormones and atrial natriuretic peptide after 1 year of sustained nifedipine therapy for severe hypertension. J Am Card 1991;17:1595–1602.
20. Suga S, Nakao K, Hosoda K, Mukoyama M, Ogawa Y, Shirakami G, et al. Phenotype-related alteration in expression of natriuretic peptide receptors in aortic smooth muscle cells. Circ. Res. 1992;71:34–39.
21. Kojima M, Minamino N, Kangawa K, Matsuo H. Cloning and sequence analysis of cDNA encoding a precursor for rat brain natriuretic peptide. Biochem Biophys Res Commun 1989;159:1420–1426.
22. Mukoyama M, Nakao K, Hosoda K, Suga S, Saito Y, Ogawa Y, et al. Brain natriuretic peptide as a novel cardiac hormone in humans. Evidence for an exquisite dual natriuretic peptide system, atrial natriuretic peptide and brain natriuretic peptide. J Clin Invest 1991;87(4):1402–1412.
23. Vellaichamy E, Khurana ML, Fink J, Pandey KN. Involvement of the NF-kappa B/matrix metalloproteinase pathway in cardiac fibrosis of mice lacking guanylyl cyclase/natriuretic peptide receptor A. J Biol Chem 2005;280(19):19230–19242.
24. Yoshimura M, Yasue H, Morita E, Sakaino N, Jougasaki M, Kurose M, et al. Hemodynamic renal and hormonal responses to brain natriuretic peptide infusion in patients with congestive heart failure. Circulation 1991;84:1581–1588.
25. Omland T, Aakvaag A, Banarjee V, Caidahl K, Lie R, Nilsen D, et al. Plasma brain natriuretic peptide as an indicator of left ventricular systolic function and long-term survival after acute myocardial infarction: Comparison with plasma atrial natriuretic peptide and N-terminal proatrial natriuretic peptide. Circulation 1996;93:1963–1969.
26. Jaffe AS, Babuin L, Apple FS. Biomarkers in acute cardiac disease: the present and the future. J Am Coll Cardiol 2006;48:1–11.
27. Garbers DL, Lowe DG. Guanylyl cyclase receptors. J Biol Chem 1994;269:30714–30744.
28. Cameron V, Aitken G, Ellmers L, Kennedy M, Espiner E. The sites of gene expression of atrial, brain, and C-type natriuretic peptides in mouse fetal development: temporal changes in embryos and placenta. Endocrinology 1996;137:817–824.
29. Larsen TH, Saetersdal T. Regional appearance of atrial natriuretic peptide in the ventricles of infarcted rat hearts. Virchows. Arch B. Cell Pathol Inc Mol Pathol 1993;64:309–314.
30. Glembotski CC. Cellular and molecular biology of B-type natriuretic peptide. In: Samson WK, Levin ER, editors. In: Contemp Endocrinol Natriuretic peptides in Health and Disease. Totowa, NJ: Humana Press; 1997. p. 95–106.
31. Reinhart K, Meisner M, Brunkhorst FM. Markers for sepsis diagnosis: what is useful? Crit Care Clin 2006;22:503–519.
32. Hanford DS, Glembotski CC. Stabilization of the B-type natriuretic peptide mRNA in cardiac myocytes by alpha-adrenergic receptor activation: potential roles for protein kinase C and mitogen-activated protein kinase. Mol Endocrinol 1996;10:1719–1727.
33. Hanford DS, Thuerauf DJ, Murray SF, Glembotski CC. Brain natriuretic peptide is induced by α1-adrenergic agonists as a primary response gene in cultured rat cardiac myocytes. J Biol Chem 1994;269:26227–26233.
34. Igaki T, Itoh H, Suga S, Hama N, Ogawa Y, Komatsu Y, et al. C-type natriuretic peptide in chronic renal failure and its action in humans. Kidney Int 1996;49: S144–S147.
35. Ogawa Y, Nakao K, Nakagawa O, Komatsu Y, Hosoda K, Suga S, et al. Human C-type natriuretic peptide characterization of the gene and peptide. Hypertension 1992;19:809–813.
36. Suga S, Itoh H, Komatsu Y, Ogawa Y, Hama N, Yoshimasa T, et al. Cytokine-induced C-type natriuretic peptide (CNP) secretion from vascular endothelial cells – evidence for CNP as a novel autocrine/paracrine regulator from endothelial cells. Endocrinology 1993;133:3038–3041.

37. Suga S, Nakao K, Itoh H, Komatsu Y, Ogawa Y, Hama N, et al. Endothelial production of C-type natriuretic peptide and its marked augmentation by transforming growth factor-beta: possible existence of vascular natriuretic peptide system. J Clin Invest 1992; 90:1145–1149.

38. Tamura N, Ogawa Y, Yasoda A, Itoh H, Saito Y, Nakao K. Two cardiac natriuretic peptide genes (atrial natriuretic peptide and brain natriuretic peptide) are organized in tandem in the mouse and human genomes. J Mol Cell Cardiol 1996;28(8):1811–1815.

39. Chen HH, Burnett JC, Jr. C-type natriuretic peptide: the endothelial component of the natriuretic peptide system. J Cardiovas Pharmacol 1998;32:S22–S28.

40. Schweitz H, Vigne P, Moinier D, Frelin CH, Lazdunski M. A new member of the natriuretic peptide family is present in the venom of the green mamba (*Dendroaspis angusticeps*). J Biol Chem 1992;267:13928–13932.

41. Lisy O, Jougasaki M, Heublein DM, Schirger JA, Chen HH, Wennberg PW, et al. Renal actions of synthetic *Dendroaspis* natriuretic peptide. Kidney Int 1999;56:502–508.

42. Schulz-Knappe P, Forssmann K, Herbst F, Hock D, Pipkorn R, Forssmann WD. Isolation and structural analysis of urodilatin, a new peptide of the cardiodilatin (ANP)-family extracted from human urine. Klin. Wochenschr. 1988;66:752–759.

43. Feller SM, Mägert HJ, Schulz-Knappe P, Forssmann WG. Urodilatin (hANF 95–126) – characteristics of a new atrial natriuretic factor peptide. In: Struthers AD, editor. Atrial Natriuretic Factor. Oxford: UK Blackwell; 1990. pp. 209–226.

44. Goetz KL. Renal natriuretic peptide (urodilatin?) and atriopeptin: evolving concepts. Am J Physiol 1991;261(6 Pt 2):F921–F932.

45. Saxenhofer H, Roselli A, Weidmann P, Forssmann WG, Bub A, Ferrari P, et al. Urodilatin, a natriuretic factor from kidneys can modify renal and cardiovascular function in men. Am J Physiol 1990; 259:F832-F838.

46. Bub A, Marxen P, Forssmann WG. Urodilatin (Uro) binding sites in rat kidney. Anat Rec 1993;41:14.

47. Forssmann WG, Meyer M, Schulz-Knappe P. Urodilatin from cardiac hormones to clinical trials. Exp Nephrol 1994;2:318–323.

48. Meyer M, Richter R, Brunkhorst R, Wrenger E, Schulz-Knappe P, Kist A, et al. Urodilatin is involved in sodium homeostasis and exerts sodium-state dependent natriuretic and diuretic effects. Am J Physiol 1996;271: 489–497.

49. Pandey KN, Pavlou SN, Inagami T. Identification and characterization of three distinct atrial natriuretic factor receptors. Evidence for tissue-specific heterogeneity of receptor subtypes in vascular smooth muscle, kidney tubular epithelium, and Leydig tumor cells by ligand binding, photoaffinity labeling, and tryptic proteolysis. J Biol Chem 1988;263(26):13406–13413.

50. Levin ER, Gardner DG, Samson WK. Natriuretic peptides. N Eng J Med. 1998;339:321–328.

51. Pandey K. Vascular action natriuretic peptide receptor: Totawa, NJ: Humana Press Inc.,pp. 255–267; 1996.

52. Pandey KN. Physiology of the natriuretic peptides gonadal function. In: Samson WK, Levin ER, editors. Contemporary Endocrinology: Natriuretic Peptides in Health and Disease. Totawa NJ: Humana Press; 1997. pp. 171–191.

53. Lowe DG, Chang M-S, Hellmis R, Chen E, Singh S, Garbers DL, et al. Human atrial natriuretic peptide receptor defines a new paradigm for second messenger signal transduction. EMBO J. 1989;8:1377–1384.

54. Fuller F, Porter JG, Arfsten AE, Miller J, Schilling JW, Scarborough RM, et al. Atrial natriuretic peptide clearance receptor. Complete sequence and functional expression of cDNA clones. J Biol Chem 1988;263: 9395–9401.

55. Garbers DL. Guanylyl cyclase receptors and their endocrine, paracrine, and autocrine ligands. Cell 1992;71(1):1–4.

56. van den Akker F, Zhang X, Miyagi M, Huo X, Misono KS, Yee VC. Structure of the dimerized hormone-binding domain of a guanylyl-cyclase-coupled receptor. Nature 2000;406(6791):101–104.

57. Misono KS, Ogawa H, Qiu Y, Ogata CM. Structural studies of the natriuretic peptide receptor: a novel hormone-induced rotation mechanism for transmembrane signal transduction. Peptides 2005;26(6):957–968.

58. Wilson EM, Chinkers M. Identification of sequences mediating guanylyl cyclase dimerization. Biochemistry 1995;34:4696–4701.

59. Labrecque J, McNicoll N, Marquis M, De Lean A. A disulfide-bridged mutant of natriuretic peptide receptor-A displays constitutive activity. Role of receptor dimerization in signal transduction. J Biol Chem 1999;274: 9752–9759.

60. Koller KJ, Lowe DG, Bennett GL, Minamino N, Kangawa K, Matsuo H, et al. Selective activation of the B natriuretic peptide receptor by C-type natriuretic peptide (CNP). Science 1991;252:120–123.

61. Lucas KA, Pitari GM, Kazerousnian S, Ruiz-Stewart I, Park J, Schulz S, et al. Guanylyl cyclases and signaling by cGMP. Pharmacol Rev 2000;52:375–413.

62. Bovy PR. Structure activity in the atrial natriuretic peptide (ANP) family. Med Res Rev 1990;10:115–142.

63. Maack T, Suzuki M, Almeida FA, Nussenzveig D, Scarborough RM, McEnroe GA, et al. Physiological role of silent receptors of atrial natriuretic factor. Science 1987;238:675–678.

64. Anand-Srivastava MB. Natriuretic peptide receptor-C signaling and regulation. Peptides 2005;26(6):1044–1059.

65. Anand-Srivastava MB, Trachte GJ. Atrial natriuretic factor receptors and signal transduction mechanisms. Pharmacol Rev 1993;45(4):455–497.

66. He XL, Dukkipati A, Wang X, Garcia KC. A new paradigm for hormone recognition and allosteric receptor activation revealed from structural studies of NPR-C. Peptides 2005;26:1035–1043.

67. Zhou H, Murthy KS. Identification of the G-protein activation sequence of the single-transmembrane natriuretic peptide receptor C (NPR-C). Am J Cell Physiol 2003;284:C1255–C1261.

68. Rathinavelu A, Isom GE. Differential internalization and processing of atrial natriuretic factor B and C receptors in PC-12 cells. Biochem J 1991;276:493–497.

69. Pandey KN. Stoichiometric analysis of internalization, recycling, and redistribution of photoaffinity-labeled guanylate cyclase/atrial natriuretic factor receptors in cultured murine Leydig tumor cells. J Biol Chem 1993;268(6):4382–4390.

70. Pandey KN, Nguyen HT, Li M, Boyle JW. Natriuretic peptide receptor-A negatively regulates mitogen-activated protein kinase and proliferation of mesangial cells: role of cGMP-dependent protein kinase. Biochem Biophys Res Commun 2000;271(2):374–379.

71. Pandey KN. Internalization and trafficking of guanylyl cyclase/natriuretic peptide receptor-A. Peptides 2005;26(6):985–1000.

72. Cao L, Chen SC, Humphreys MH, Gardner DG. Ligand-dependent regulation of NPR-A gene expression in inner medullary collecting duct cells. Am J Physiol 1998(275):F119–F125.

73. Cao L, Wu J, Gardner DG. Atrial natriuretic peptide suppresses the transcription of its guanylyl cyclase-linked receptor. J Biol Chem 1995;270(42):24891–24897.

74. Fujio N, Gossard F, Bayard F, Tremblay J. Regulation of natriuretic peptide receptor A and B expression by transforming growth factor-beta 1 in cultured aortic smooth muscle cells. Hypertension 1994;23(6 Pt 2):908–913.

75. Hum D, Besnard S, Sanchez R, Devost D, Gossard F, Hamet P, et al. Characterization of a cGMP-response element in the guanylyl cyclase/natriuretic peptide receptor A gene promoter. Hypertension 2004;43(6):1270–1278.

76. Garg R, Pandey KN. Angiotensin II-mediated negative regulation of Npr1 promoter activity and gene transcription. Hypertension 2003;41(3 Pt 2):730–736.

77. Chen YO, Gardner DG. Endothelin inhibits NPR-A and stimulates eNOS gene expression in rat IMCD cells. Hypertension 2003;41:675–681.

78. Arise KK, Pandey KN. Inhibition and down-regulation of gene transcription and guanylyl cyclase activity of NPRA by angiotensin II involving protein kinase C. Biochem Biophys Res Commun 2006;349(1):131–135.

79. Potter LR, Garbers DL. Dephosphorylation of the guanylyl cyclase-A receptor causes desensitization. J Biol Chem 1992;267(21):14531–14534.

80. Sibley DR, Benovic JL, Caron MG, Lefkowitz RJ. Regulation of transmembrane signaling by receptor phosphorylation. Cell 1987; 48:913–933.

81. Hugnir RI, Greengard P. Regulation of neurotransmitter receptor desensitization by protein phosphorylation. Neuron 1990;5:555–567.

82. Goodman OBJ, Krupnick JG, Santini F, Gurevich VV, Penn RB, Gagnon AW, et al. β-arrestin acts as a clathrin adaptor in endocytosis of the β2-adrenergic receptor. Nature 1996;383:447–450.

83. Zhang G, Liu Y, Arnold ER, Hurley JH. Structure of the adenylyl cyclase catalytic core. Nature 1997;386:247–253.

84. Lefkowitz RJ, Pitcher J, Krueger K, Daaka Y. Mechanisms of β-adrenergic receptor desensitization and resensitization. Adv Pharmacol 1998;42:416–420.

85. Sorkin A, von Zastrow M. Signal transduction and endocytosis close encounters of many kinds. Nat Rev Mol Cell Biol 2002;3:600–614.

86. Ballerman BJ, Marala RB, Sharma RK. Characterization and regulation by protein kinase C of renal glomerular atrial natriuretic peptide receptor-coupled guanylate cyclase. Biochem Biophys Res Commun 1988;157:755–761.

87. Duda T, Sharma RK. Regulation of guanylate cyclase activity by atrial natriuretic factor and protein kinase C. Mol Cell Biochem 1990; 93:179–184.

88. Pandey KN. Stimulation of protein phosphorylation by atrial natriuretic factor in plasma membranes of bovine adrenal cortical cells. Biochem Biophys Res Commun 1989;163(2):988–994.

89. Potter LR, Hunter T. Phosphorylation of the kinase homology domain is essential for activation of the A-type natriuretic peptide receptor. Mol Cell Biol 1998;18:2164–2172.

90. Larose L, Rondeau JJ, Ong H, De Lean A. Phosphorylation of atrial natriuretic factor R1 receptor by serine/threonine protein kinases: evidences for receptor regulation. Mol Cell Biochem 1992;115(2):203–211.

91. Airhart N, Yang YF, Roberts CT, Jr., Silberbach M. Atrial natriuretic peptide induces natriuretic peptide receptor-cGMP-dependent protein kinase interaction. J Biol Chem 2003;278(40):38693–38698.

92. Cahill PA, Redmond EM, Keenan AK. Vascular atrial natriuretic factor receptor subtypes are not independently regulated by atrial peptides. J Biol Chem 1990;265:21896–21906.

93. Pandey KN. Kinetic analysis of internalization, recycling and redistribution of atrial natriuretic factor-receptor complex in cultured vascular smooth-muscle cells. Ligand-dependent receptor down-regulation. Biochem J 1992;288(Pt 1):55–61.

94. Anand-Srivastava MB. Down-regulation of atrial natriuretic peptide ANP-C receptor is associated with alteration in G-protein expression in A10 smooth muscle cells. Biochemistry 2000;39:6503–6513.

95. Neuser D, Bellermann P. Receptor binding, cGMP stimulation and receptor desensitization by atrial natriuretic peptides in cultured A10 vascular smooth muscle cells. FEBS Lett 1986;209: 347–351.

96. Hirata Y, Hirose S, Takada S, Takagi Y, Matsubara H. Down-regulation of atrial natriuretic peptide receptor and cyclic GMP response in cultured rat vascular smooth muscle cells. Eur J Pharmacol 1987;135:439–442.

97. Roubert P, Lonchampt MO, Chabrier PE, Plas P, Goulin J, Braquet P. Down-regulation of atrial natriuretic factor receptors and correlation with cGMP stimulation in rat cultured vascular smooth muscle cells. Biochem Biophys Res Commun 1987;148:61–67.

98. Hughes RJ, Struthers RS, Fong AM, Insel PA. Regulation of the atrial natriuretic peptide receptor on a smooth muscle cell. Am J Physiol 1987; 253:C809-C816.

99. Hirata Y, Takata S, Tomita M, Takaichi S. Binding, internalization, and degradation of atrial natriuretic peptide in cultured vascular smooth muscle cells of rat. Biochem Biophys Res Commun 1985;132:976–984.

100. Napier M, Arcuri K, Vandlen R. Binding and internalization of atrial natriuretic factor by high-affinity receptors in A10 smooth muscle cells. Arch Biochem Biophys 1986;248:516–522.

101. Murthy KK, Thibault G, Cantin M. Binding and intracellular degradation of atrial natriuretic factor by cultured vascular smooth muscle cells. Mol Cell Endocrinol 1989;67:195–206.

102. Nussenzveig DR, Lewicki JA, Maack T. Cellular mechanisms of the clearance function of type-C receptors of atrial natriuretic factor. J Biol Chem 1990;265:20952–20958.

103. Cohen D, Koh GY, Nikonova LN, Porter JG, Maack T. Molecular determinants of the clearance function of type-C receptor of natriuretic peptides. J Biol Chem 1996;271:9863–9869.

104. Hirata Y, Takata S, Takagi Y, Matsbara H, Omae T. Regulation of atrial natriuretic peptide receptors in cultured vascular smooth muscle cells of rat. Biochem Biophys Res Commun 1986;138:405–412.

105. Nonguchi H, Knepper MA, Mangiello VC. Effects of atrial natriuretic factor on cyclic guanosine monophosphate and cyclic adenosine monophosphate accumulation in microdissected nephron segments from rats. J Clin Invest 1987;79:500–507.

106. Kremer S, Troyer D, Kreisberg J, Skorecki K. Interaction of atrial natriuretic peptide-stimulated guanylyl cyclase and vasopressin-stimulated calcium signaling pathways in the glomerular mesangial cells. Arch Biochem Biophys 1988;260:763–767.

107. Light DB, Schwiebert EM, Karlson KH, Stanton BA. Atrial natriuretic peptide inhibits a cation channel in renal inner medullary collecting duct cells. Science 1989;243:383–385.

108. Appel RG. Mechanism of atrial natriuretic factor-induced inhibition of rat mesangial cell mitogenesis. Am. J. Physiol. 1990;259:E312–E318.

109. Meyer M, Forsmann WG. Renal actions of atrial natriuretic peptide. In: Samson WK, Levin ER, editors. Contemporary Endocrinology: Natriuretic Peptides in Health and Disease. Totawa, NJ: Humana Press; 1997. pp. 147–170.

110. Burnett JCJ, Granger JP, Opgenorth TJ. Effects of synthetic atrial natriuretic factor on renal function and renin release. Am J Physiol 1984;247:F863–F866.

111. Camarago MJ, Kleinert HD, Atlas SA, Sealey JE, Laragh JH, Maack T. Ca2+-dependent hemodynamic and natriuretic effects of atrial extract in isolated rat kidney. Am J Physiol 1984;246:F447–F456.

112. Freeman RH, Davis JO, Vari RC. Renal response to atrial natriuretic factor in conscious dogs with caval constriction. Am J Physiol 1985;248:R495–R500.

113. Melo LG, Steinhelper ME, Pang SC, Tse Y, Ackermann U. ANP in regulation of arterial pressure and fluid-electrolyte balance: lessons from genetic mouse models. Physiol Genomics 2000;3:45–58.

114. Villrreal D, Freeman RH. Natriuretic peptides and salt sensitivity. In: Samson WK, Levin ER, editors. Contemporary Endocrinology: Natriuretic Peptides in Health and Disease. Totowa, NJ: Humana Press Inc; 1997. pp. 239–258.

115. von Geldern TW, Budzik GP, Dillon TP, Holleman WH, Holst MA, Ksio Y, et al. Atrial natriuretic peptide antagonists: biological evaluation and structural correlations. Mol Pharmacol 1990;38:771–778.

116. Sano T, Morishita Y, Matsuda Y, Yamada K. Pharmacological profile of HS-142–1, a novel nonpeptide atrial natriuretic peptide antagonist of microbial origin I. Selective inhibition of the actions of natriuretic peptides in anesthetized rats. J Pharmacol Exp Thr 1992;260:825–831.

117. Obana K, Naruse M, Naruse K, Sakurai H, Demura H, Inagami T, et al. Synthetic rat atrial natriuretic factor inhibits in vitro and in vivo renin secretion in rats. Endocrinology 1985;117(3):1282–1284.

118. Shi SJ, Nguyen HT, Sharma GD, Navar LG, Pandey KN. Genetic disruption of atrial natriuretic peptide receptor-A alters renin and angiotensin II levels. Am J Physiol 2001;281(4):F665–F673.

119. Paul RV, Ferguson T, Navar LG. ANF secretion and renal responses to volume expansion with equilibrated blood. Am J Physiol 1988;255:F936–F943.

120. Schwab TR, Edwards BS, Heublein DM, Burnett JCJ. Role of atrial natriuretic peptide in volume-expansion natriuresis. Am J Physiol 1986;251:R310–R313.

121. Ohyama Y, Miyamoto R, Morishita Y, Matsuda Y, Saito Y, Minamino N, et al. Stable expression of natriuretic peptide receptors effects of HS-142–1, a non-peptide ANP antagonist. Biochem Biophys Res Commun 1992;189:336–342.

122. Delporte C, Poloczek P, Tastenoy M, Winard J, Christopher J. Atrial natriuretic peptide binds to ANP-R 1 receptors in neuroblastoma cells or is degraded extracellularly at the Ser-Phe bond. Eur J Pharmacol 1992;227:247–256.

123. Kumar R, Cartledge WA, Lincoln TM, Pandey KN. Expression of guanylyl cyclase-A/atrial natriuretic peptide receptor blocks the activation of protein kinase C in vascular smooth muscle cells. Role of cGMP and cGMP-dependent protein kinase. Hypertension 1997;29(1 Pt 2):414–421.

124. Misono KS. Atrial natriuretic factor binding to its receptor is dependent on chloride concentration: a possible feedback control mechanism in renal salt regulation. Circ. Res. 2000;86:1135–1139.

125. Shi SJ, Vellaichamy E, Chin SY, Smithies O, Navar LG, Pandey KN. Natriuretic peptide receptor A mediates renal sodium excretory responses to blood volume expansion. Am J Physiol. 2003;285(4):F694–F702.

126. Melo LG, Veress AT, Ackermann U, Steinhelper ME, Pang SC, Tse Y, et al. Chronic regulation of arterial blood pressure in ANP transgenic and knockout mice: role of cardiovascular sympathetic tone. Cardiovasc Res 1999;43(2):437–444.

127. Obana K, Naruse N, Inagami T, Brown AB, Naruse K, Kurimoto F, et al. Atrial natriuretic factor inhibits vasopressin secretion from rat posterior pituitary. Biochem Biophys Res Commun 1985;132:1088–1094.

128. Antunes-Rodrigues J, Machado BH, Andrade HA, Mauad H, Ramalho MJ, Reis LC, et al. Carotid aortic and renal baroreceptors mediate the atrial natriuretic peptide release induced by blood volume expansion. Proc Natl Acad Sci USA 1992;89:6829–6831.

129. Zhao D, Vellaichamy E, Somanna NK, Pandey KN. Guanylyl cyclase/natriuretic peptide receptor-A gene disruption causes increased adrenal angiotensin II and aldosterone levels. Am J Physiol Renal Physiol 2007;293(1):F121–F127.

130. Atarashi K, Mulrow PJ, Franco-Saenz R, Snajdar R, Rapp J. Inhibition of aldosterone production by an atrial extract. Science 1984;224(4652):992–994.

131. Hassid A. Atriopeptin II decreases cytosolic free Ca^{2+} in cultured vascular smooth muscle cells. Am J Physiol 1986;251:C681–C686.

132. Lincoln TM, Komalavilas P, Cornwell TL. Pleiotropic regulation of vascular smooth muscle tone by cyclic GMP-dependent protein kinase. Hypertension 1994;243:383–385.

133. Rashatwar SS, Cornwell TL, Lincoln TM. Effect of 8-bromo cGMP on Ca^{2+}-ATPase by cGMP dependent protein kinase. Proc Natl Acad Sci U.S.A 1987; 84:5685–5689.

134. Cornwell TL, Lincoln TM. Regulation of intracellular Ca^{2+} levels in cultured vascular smooth muscle cells. Reduction of Ca^{2+} by atriopeptin and 8-bromo-cyclic GMP is mediated by cyclic GMP-dependent protein kinase. J Biol Chem 1989;264:1146–1155.

135. Kumar R, von Geldern TW, Calle RA, Pandey KN. Stimulation of atrial natriuretic peptide receptor/guanylyl cyclase-A signaling pathway antagonizes the activation of protein kinase C-alpha in murine Leydig cells. Biochimica et Biophysica Acta 1997;1356(2):221–228.

136. Lincoln TM, Komalavilas P, Cornwell TL. Pleiotropic regulation of vascular smooth muscle tone by cyclic GMP-dependent protein kinase. Hypertension 1994;23:383–385.

137. Appel RG. Growth-regulatory properties of atrial natriuretic factor. Am J Physiol 1992;262:F911–F918.

138. Sugimoto T, Kikkawa R, Haneda M, Shigeta Y. Atrial natriuretic peptide inhibits endothelin-1 induced activation of mitogen-activated protein kinase in cultured rat mesangial cells. Biochem Biophys Res Commun 1993;195:72–78.

139. Isono M, Haneda M, Maeda S, Omatsu-Kanbe M, Kikkawa R. Atrial natriuretic peptide inhibits endothelin-1-induced activation of JNK in glomerular mesangial cells. Kidney International 1998;53(5):1133–1142.

140. Cao L, Gardner DG. Natriuretic peptides inhibit DNA synthesis in cardiac fibroblast. Hypertension 1995;25:227–234.

141. Hu RM, Levin ER. Astrocyte growth is regulated by neuropeptides through Tis 8 and basic fibroblast growth factor. J Clin Invest 1994;93:1820–1827.

142. Biesiada E, Razandi M, Levin ER. Egr-1 activates basic fibroblast growth factor transcription. J Biol Chem 1996;271:18576–18581.

143. Vollmer AM, Schmidt KN, Schulz R. Natriuretic peptide receptors on rat thymocytes: inhibition of proliferation by atrial natriuretic peptide. Endocrinology 1996;137:1706–1713.

144. Itoh H, Pratt RE, Dzau V. Atrial natriuretic polypeptide inhibits hypertrophy of vascular smooth muscle cells. J Clin Invest 1990;86:1690–1697.

145. Morishita R, Gibbons GH, Pratt RE, Tomita N, Kaneda Y, Ogihara T, et al. Autocrine and paracrine effects of atrial natriuretic peptide gene transfer on vascular smooth muscle and endothelial cellular growth. J Clin Invest 1994;94:824–829.

146. Hutchinson HG, Trinadade PT, Cunanan DB, Wu CF, Pratt RE. Mechanisms of natriuretic-peptide-induced growth inhibition of vascular smooth muscle cells. Cardiovas Res 1997;35:158–167.

147. Suhasini M, Li H, Lohmann SM, Boss GR, Pilz RB. Cyclic-GMP-dependent protein kinase inhibits the Ras/mitogen-activated protein kinase pathway. Mole Cell Biol 1998;18:6983–6994.

148. Chrisman TD, Garbers DL. Reciprocal antagonism coordinates C-type natriuretic peptide and mitogen-signaling pathways in fibroblasts. J Biol Chem 1999;274:4293–4299.

149. Redondo J, Bishop JE, Wilkins MR. Effect of atrial natriuretic peptide and cyclic GMP phosphodiesterase inhibition on collagen synthesis by adult cardiac fibroblasts. Br J Pharm 1998;124:1455–1462.

150. Calderone A, Thaik CM, Takahashi N, Chang DLF, Colucci WS. Nitric oxide, atrial natriuretic peptide, and cyclic GMP inhibit the growth-promoting effects of norepinephrine in cardiac myocytes and fibroblasts. J Clin Invest 1998;101: 812–818.

151. Silberbach M, Gorenc T, Hershberger RE, Stork PJS, Steyger PS, Roberts CTJ. Extracellular signal-regulated protein kinase activation is required for the anti-hypertrophic effect of atrial natriuretic factor in neonatal rat ventricular myocytes. J Biol Chem 1999;274: 24858–24864.

152. Horio T, Nishikimi T, Yoshihara F, Matsuo H, Takishita S, Kangawa K. Inhibitory regulation of hypertrophy by endogenous atrial natriuretic peptide in cultured cardiac myocytes. Hypertension 2000;35:19–24.

153. Dey NB, Boerth NJ, Murphy-Ullrich JE, Chang PL, Prince CW, Lincoln TM. Cyclic GMP-dependent protein kinase inhibits osteopontin and thrombospondin production in rat aortic smooth muscle cells. Circ Res 1998;82:139–146.

154. Masciotra S, Picard S, Deschepper CF. Cosegregation analysis in genetic crosses suggests a protective role for atrial natriuretic factor against ventricular hypertrophy. Circ Res 1999;84:1453–1458.

155. Prins BA, Weber MJ, Hu R-M, Pedram A, Daniels M, Levin ER. Atrial natriuretic peptide inhibits mitogen-activated protein kinase through the clearance receptor: potential role in the inhibition of astrocyte proliferation. J Biol Chem 1996;271:14156–14162.

156. Sharma GD, Nguyen HT, Antonov AS, Gerrity RG, von Geldern T, Pandey KN. Expression of atrial natriuretic peptide receptor-A antagonizes the mitogen-activated protein kinases (Erk2 and P38MAPK) in cultured human vascular smooth muscle cells. Mol Cell Biochem 2002;233(1–2):165–173.

157. Trindade P, Hutchinson HG, Pollman MJ, Gibbons GH, Pratt RE. Atrial natriuretic peptide (ANP) and C-type natriuretic peptide (CNP) induce apoptosis in vascular smooth muscle cells (VMSC). Circulation 1995; 92: I-696.

158. Wu CF, Bishopric NH, Pratt RE. Atrial natriuretic peptide induces apoptosis in neonatal rat cardiac myocytes. J Biol Chem 1997;272:14860–14866.

159. Pollman MJ, Yamada T, Horiuchi M, Gibbons GH. Vasoactive substances regulate vascular smooth muscle cell apoptosis. Circ Res 1996;79:748–756.

160. Kozopas KM, Yang T, Buchan HL, Zhou P, Craig RW. MCLI, a gene expressed in programmed myeloid cell differentiation, has sequence similarity to BCL2. Proc. Natl. Acad. Sci. U.S.A 1993;90:3516–3520.

161. Kiefer MC, Brauer MJ, Powers VC, Wu JJ, Umansky SR, Tomel LD, et al. Modulation of apoptosis by the widely distributed Bcl-2 homologue Bak. Nature 1995;374:736–739.

162. Krajewski S, Bodrug S, Krajewski M, Shabaik A, Gascoyne R, Berean K, et al. Immunohistochemical analysis of Mcl-1 protein in human tissues. Am J Pathol 1995;146:1309–1319.

163. Tsutamoto T, Kanamori T, Morigami N, Sugimoto Y, Yamaoka O, Kinoshita M. Possibility of downregulation of atrial natriuretic peptide receptor coupled to guanylate cyclase in peripheral vascular beds of patients with chronic severe heart failure. Circulation 1993;87(1):70–75.

164. Wei C-M, Heublein DM, Perrella MA, Lerman A, Rodeheffer RJ, McGregor CGA, et al. Natriuretic peptide system in human heart failure. Circulation 1993;88:1004–1009.

165. Chen HH, Burnett JC, Jr. The natriuretic peptides in heart failure. Proc Assoc Am Physicians 1999;111: 406–416.

166. Melo LG, Veress AT, Chong CK, Pang SC, Flynn TG, Sonnenberg H. Salt-sensitive hypertension in ANP knockout mice: potential role of abnormal plasma renin activity. Am J Physiol 1998;274:R255–R261.

167. John SW, Krege JH, Oliver PM, Hagaman JR, Hodgin JB, Pang SC, et al. Genetic decreases in atrial natriuretic peptide and salt-sensitive hypertension. Science 1995;267(5198):679–681.

168. Lopez MJ, Wong SK, Kishimoto I, Dubois S, Mach V, Friesen J, et al. Salt-resistant hypertension in mice lacking the guanylyl cyclase-A receptor for atrial natriuretic peptide. Nature 1995;378(6552):65–68.

169. Oliver PM, John SW, Purdy KE, Kim R, Maeda N, Goy MF, et al. Natriuretic peptide receptor 1 expression influences blood pressures of mice in a dose-dependent manner. Proc Natl Acad Sci U.S.A. 1998; 95:2547–2551.

170. Oliver PM, Fox JE, Kim R, Rockman HA, Kim HS, Reddick RL, et al. Hypertension, cardiac hypertrophy, and sudden death in mice lacking natriuretic peptide receptor A. Proc Natl Acad Sci U.S.A. 1997;94(26):14730–14735.

171. Kishimoto I, Dubois SK, Garbers DL. The heart communicates with the kidney exclusively through the guanylyl cyclase-A receptor: acute handling of sodium and water in response to volume expansion. Proc Natl Acad Sci U.S.A 1996;93(12):6215–6219.

172. Pandey KN, Oliver PM, Maeda N, Smithies O. Hypertension associated with decreased testosterone levels in natriuretic peptide receptor-A gene-knockout and gene-duplicated mutant mouse models. Endocrinology 1999;140(11):5112–5119.

173. Holtwick R, Baba HA, Ehler E, Risse-Vob MD, Gehrmann J, Pierkes M, et al. Left but not right cardiac hypertrophy in atrial natriuretic peptide receptor-deficient mice is prevented by angiotensin type 1 receptor antagonist losartan. J Cardiovasc Pharmacol 2002;40:725–734.

174. Holtwick R, Gotthardt M, Skryabin B, Steinmetz M, Potthast R, Zetsche B, et al. Smooth muscle-selective deletion of guanylyl cyclase-A prevents the acute but not chronic effects of ANP on blood pressure. Proc Natl Acad Sci U.S.A 2002;99(10):7142–7147. Epub 2002 May 7.

175. Zhao L, Long L, Morrell NW. NPRA-deficient mice show increased susceptibility to hypoxia-induced pulmonary hypertension. Circulation 1999;99:605–607.

176. Knowles JW, Esposito G, Mao L, Hagaman JR, Fox JE, Smithies O, et al. Pressure-independent enhancement of cardiac hypertrophy in natriuretic peptide receptor A-deficient mice. J Clin Invest 2001;107(8):975–984.

177. Steinhelper ME, Cochran KL, Field LJ. Hypotension in transgenic mice expressing atrial natriuretic factor fusion genes. Hypertension 1990;16:301–307.

178. Lin X, Hanze J, Heese F, Sodmann R, Lang RE. Gene expression of natriuretic peptide receptors in myocardial cells. Circ. Res. 1995;77:750–758.

179. Felker GM, Petersen JW, Mark DW. Natriuretic peptides in the diagnosis and management of heart failure. CMAJ 2006;175:611–617.

180. See R, de Lemos JA. Current status of risk stratification methods in acute coronary syndromes. Curr Cardiol Rep 2006;8:282–288.

181. Yoshimura M, Yasue H, Okumura K, Ogawa H, Jougasaki M, Mukoyama M, et al. Different secretion patterns of atrial natriuretic peptide and brain natriuretic peptide in patients with congestive heart failure. Circulation 1993;87:464–469.

182. Doust JA, Pietrzak E, Dobson A, Glasziou P. How well does B-type natriuretic peptide predict death and cardiac events in patients with heart failure: systematic review. BWJ 2005:330–625.

183. Khan IA, Fink J, Nass C, Chen H, Christenson R, deFilippi CR. N-terminal pro-B-type natriuretic peptide and B-type natriuretic peptide for identifying coronary artery disease and left ventricular hypertrophy in ambulatory chronic kidney disease patients. Am J Cardiol 2006;97:1530–1534.

184. Anwaruddin S, Lloyd-Jones DM, Baggish A, Chen A, Krauser D, Tung R, et al. Renal function, congestive heart failure, and amino-terminal pro-brain natriuretic petpide measurement: results from the proBNP investigation of dyspnea in the Emergency Department (PRIDE) study. J Am Coll Cardiol 2006;47:91–97.

185. McCullough PA, Duc P, Omland T, McCord J, Nowak RM, Hollander JE, et al. B-type natriuretic peptide and renal function in the diagnosis of heart failure: an analysis from the breathing not properly multinational study. Am J Kidney Dis 2003;41:571–579.

186. Deschepper CF, Masciotra S, Zahabi A, Boutin-Ganache I, Picard S, Reudelhuber TL. Function alterations of the Nppa promoter are linked to cardiac ventricular hypertrophy in WKY/WKHA rat crosses. Circ Res 2001;88:223–228.

14 Insulin-Like Growth Factors, Cardiovascular Risk Factors, and Cardiovascular Disease

Islam Bolad MBBS MD MRCP FESC and Patrice Delafontaine MD FACC FACP FAHA FESC

CONTENTS

INTRODUCTION
CARDIOVASCULAR DISEASE
CARDIOVASCULAR RISK FACTORS
CONCLUSIONS
REFERENCES

SUMMARY

Insulin-like growth factor-1 (IGF-1) is a peptide that is mostly produced in the liver. It was previously thought that IGF-1 could contribute to the development of atherosclerotic and hypertensive vascular disease. However, recent evidence suggests that this is likely not the case, and that IGF-1 may confer a protective role against atherosclerosis. Furthermore, altered IGF-1 levels and/or signaling may play a role in the pathogenesis of heart failure. We hereby review the available clinical data on the role of IGF-1 in cardiovascular disease and its relation to the cardiovascular risk factors.

Key Words: Insulin-like Growth Factor-1, Atherosclerosis, Hypertension, Metabolic syndrome, Insulin-like growth factor binding protein, Diabetes, Cardiovascular disease

INTRODUCTION

Insulin-like growth factor-1 (IGF-1) is a peptide that is mostly produced in the liver in response to growth hormone (GH) secretion, and it mediates many of the anabolic actions of GH through IGF-1 receptors (IGF-1R) *(1)*. The activity of IGF-1 is influenced by specific IGF-binding proteins (IGFBP-1 to IGFBP-6), and the activity of these in turn is regulated by phosphorylation, proteolysis, polymerization, and cell or matrix association. Circulating IGF-1 is primarily complexed to the high-molecular-weight IGFBP-3 and an acid-labile subunit which are incapable of transendothelial transport. IGF-1 can leave the circulating reservoir only in its

From: *Contemporary Endocrinology: Cardiovascular Endocrinology: Shared Pathways and Clinical Crossroads*
Edited by: V. A. Fonseca © Humana Press, New York, NY

free active form or bound to the low-molecular-weight IGFBP-1 and -2. It is technically difficult to measure the free fraction of IGF-1, and thus the total concentration of IGF-1 is commonly determined after elimination of interfering IGFBPs. It is thus important to measure IGFBP-3 and take it into account when total IGF-1 is determined and related to a biological outcome.

IGF-1 levels and the molar ratio between IGF-1 and IGFBP-3 decrease with increasing age throughout adulthood and as atherosclerosis is more prevalent with increasing age, theoretically, decreasing IGF-1 levels could be involved in the development of atherosclerosis *(2)*. Patients with GH deficiency, and thus low IGF-1 are characterized by increased mortality attributable to cardiovascular disease *(3)* which supports the hypothesis of IGF-1 being involved in the pathogenesis of ischemic heart disease (IHD) *(4)*.

During the last decade there has been accumulating evidence on the role of IGF-1 in multiple cardiovascular pathologies, including atherosclerosis, hypertension, restenosis, angiogenesis, and diabetic vascular disease *(1)*. In this review, we will discuss the available clinical data on the relation of IGF-1 to cardiovascular disease and to cardiovascular risk factors.

CARDIOVASCULAR DISEASE

We have previously shown that IGF-1 and IGF-1R expression are reduced in early and advanced atherosclerotic lesions from patients undergoing aortic, carotid, or femoral arterial surgery *(5)*. Since IGF-1 is a potent survival factor for vascular smooth muscle cells (VSMCs), poor expression of IGF-1 and IGF-1R in intimal regions with macrophage infiltration could contribute to triggering VSMC apoptosis potentially leading to plaque weakening, plaque rupture, and acute coronary events. This hypothesis is supported by the observation that atherosclerotic-plaque derived VSMCs in culture exhibit reduced IGF-1-mediated survival signaling *(6)*. Juul et al. *(7)* in the DAN-MONICA study showed that individuals without IHD but with low circulating IGF-1 levels and high IGFBP-3 levels have significantly increased risk of developing IHD during a 15-year follow-up period. They measured IGF-1 and IGFBP-3, in serum, from 231 individuals who had a diagnosis of IHD 7.6 years after blood sampling and among 374 control subjects matched for age, sex, and calendar time. At baseline when all individuals were free of known disease, subjects in the low-IGF-1 quartile had significantly higher risk of IHD during the follow-up period compared with the high-IGF-1 quartile group, when IGFBP-3, body mass index (BMI), smoking, menopause, diabetes, and use of antihypertensives were controlled for. Individuals in the high-IGFBP-3 quartile group had an increased risk of having IHD. Identification of a high-risk population with low-IGF-1 and high-IGFBP-3 levels resulted in markedly higher risk of IHD (RR 4.07; 95% CI, 1.48–11.22) compared with the index group.

In the Rancho Bernardo Study, Laughlin et al. *(8)* evaluated the prospective association of serum IGF-1 and IGFBP-1 with IHD mortality in 633 men and 552 nonestrogen-using postmenopausal women, aged 51–98 years (mean 74 years) during the period 1988–1992 and who were followed through July 2001. During the 9–13-year follow-up, there were 105 deaths caused by IHD. IGF-1 and IGFBP-1 were independently and jointly related to the risk of IHD mortality. In a proportional hazards model including both IGF-1 and IGFBP-1 and adjusting for cardiovascular disease risk factors, the relative risk of IHD mortality was 38% higher for every 40 ng/ml (1 SD) decrease in IGF-1 and three times greater for those in the lowest quintile of IGFBP-1 compared with those with higher IGFBP-1 levels. In an observational study involving 174 healthy subjects, Colao et al. *(9)* studied peak serum IGF-1 and IGFBP-3 after a GH-releasing hormone and arginine test; they found an inverse correlation between IGF-1 and IGFBP-3 levels and mean intima-media thickness of common carotid arteries.

However, not all researchers agree with this relationship between IGF-1 and its binding proteins and the development of atherosclerosis. Indirect evidence has suggested that IGF-1 could have a direct atherogenic effect on the vascular wall. Bayes-Genis et al. *(10)* showed that IGF-1 had a potent motility effect on coronary VSMC and that this effect was partially inhibited by alphaIR-3, a specific IGF-R inhibitor. As VSMC migration plays a crucial role in atherosclerosis and restenosis after angioplasty, it was concluded that IGF-1 blockade could have the potential to limit atherogenesis. Grant et al. *(11,12)* showed IGF-1 receptor expression to be increased in de novo atherosclerotic and restenotic lesions both in humans and animal models. Clemmons and collaborators have shown that inhibition of the $\alpha V\beta 3$ integrin reduces IGF-1 signaling and atherosclerotic lesion size in hypercholesterolemic pigs *(13)*.

The relationship between IGF-1 and heart failure has also been assessed. In a community-based prospective study, Vacant et al. *(14)* studied 717 elderly individuals from Framingham (mean age of 78 years) who did not have myocardial infarction or congestive heart failure at baseline and followed them for a mean of 5 years. Fifty-six participants developed congestive heart failure and it was found that there was a 27% decrease in risk for heart failure for every 1 SD increment in log IGF-1 and that individuals with serum IGF-1 levels at or above the median value had half the risk for heart failure of those with serum IGF-1 levels below the median. These comparisons were maintained in analyses adjusting for the occurrence of myocardial infarction on follow-up. Bleumink et al. *(15)* studied 4963 participants of the population-based Rotterdam Study and found that a genetically determined chronic exposure to low IGF-1 levels is associated with an increased risk for heart failure in elderly patients. Anwar has reported that in an elderly population, hospitalized for congestive heart failure, there is a reduction in total IGF-1 and IGFBP-3 and an increase in circulating, free IGF-1 *(16)*. In cachectic heart failure patients, there is an increase in circulating GH levels suggesting some degree of GH resistance *(17)*. Hambrecht et al. *(18)* found that in patients with chronic heart failure, exercise training improves local skeletal muscle IGF-1 expression without significant changes of systemic parameters of the GH/IGF-1 axis. Animal studies have suggested that a reduction in skeletal muscle IGF-1 signaling in response to high angiotensin II levels may play an important role in the skeletal muscle wasting that is characteristic of advanced heart failure *(19,20)*.

On balance, it seems that IGF-1 levels are inversely related to the development of atherosclerotic disease and heart failure. However, the potential use of IGF-1 to treat cardiovascular disease has not been explored. Side effects associated with IGF-1 treatment of the GH insensitivity syndrome (Laron syndrome) have been mostly attributed to the water-retentive effects of IGF-1 *(21)*. The equimolar combination of IGF-1 with IGFBP-3 could possibly reduce side effects *(21)*.

CARDIOVASCULAR RISK FACTORS

Metabolic Syndrome

Metabolic syndrome, also known as Syndrome X, insulin resistance syndrome, and dysmetabolic syndrome is the clustering of abdominal obesity, dyslipidemia, hyperglycemia, and hypertension that increase the chance of developing heart disease and stroke. The World Health Organization *(22)* defines it as BMI >30 kg/m^2, blood pressure of $>140/90$ mmHg, increased albumin excretion in the urine, triglycerides > 150 mg/dl and/or HDL cholesterol <35 mg/dl in men or <40 mg/dl in women.

In a cross-sectional study of 218 healthy individuals aged 55–80 years, Janssen et al. *(4)* measured fasting serum IGF-1 and IGFBP-1 levels, lipid profile, insulin, and glucose, in addition to blood pressure, BMI, and waist–hip ratio. Mean free IGF-1 levels in subjects without signs or symptoms of cardiovascular diseases were significantly higher than in those with at least one cardiovascular symptom or sign. Free IGF-1 levels were also higher in subjects who had no atherosclerotic plaques in the carotid arteries and were inversely related to serum triglycerides. IGFBP-1 showed an inverse relation with insulin, BMI, and waist–hip ratio, and a positive relation with HDL cholesterol. In a population-based study of 839 apparently healthy individuals in Cambridgeshire (UK), Kaushal et al. *(23)* found that 154 persons fulfilled criteria for the metabolic syndrome and these had lower IGFBP-1 levels compared to those without. Logistic regression analysis demonstrated a 14-fold increased risk for the metabolic syndrome in individuals with IGFBP-1 levels below the median.

In summary, evidence suggests that the IGF-1/IGFBP system is related to cardiovascular risk factors and the metabolic syndrome.

Diabetes Mellitus

It has been postulated that IGF-1 may be associated with the pathophysiology of vascular complications in diabetes. In an in vitro study, Shigematsu et al. *(24)* examined the effects of high glucose and/or IGF-1 on cell migration and angiogenesis by using human endothelial cells (ECs). They found that chronic treatment with a high concentration of D-glucose strongly stimulated cell migration, which was mimicked by a protein kinase C agonist and inhibited by protein kinase C antagonism. The cell migration was also induced by IGF-1 and this was not blocked by a phosphatidylinositol 3-kinase inhibitor. Tubular formation was induced only when the cells were exposed to a combination of high glucose and IGF-1 and was blocked by a phosphatidylinositol 3-kinase inhibitor but not by a protein kinase C inhibitor. Their results indicated that a combination of hyperglycemia and IGF-1 stimulated EC migration and angiogenesis. Recently, Clemmons et al. have suggested that activation of the $\alpha V\beta 3$ integrin in response to hyperglycemia plays a critical role in the response of VSMCs to IGF-1, leading to increased mitogenic responses *(25)*.

The association between cardiovascular risk factors and IGF-1, IGF-2, and IGFBP-1 were studied by Gibson et al. *(26)* in 74 non-insulin-dependent diabetic patients. IGF-1 was not significantly associated with cardiovascular risk factors. In the whole group, reduced IGFBP-1 levels were significantly associated with low HDL cholesterol, elevated blood pressure, BMI, insulin, and proinsulin. In the treatment groups, IGFBP-1 was lower in patients on diet alone and sulphonylurea with or without insulin relative to insulin treatment alone. These findings indicate that in non-insulin-dependent diabetic patients low IGFBP-1 levels are associated with multiple factors predisposing to atherogenesis.

It is important to note however that IGF-1 has also been shown to improve metabolic control and insulin resistance in patients with type 1 or type 2 diabetes *(27–29)*. Although there is a lack of long-term outcome data in adults receiving IGF-1, there has not been a clear association between IGF-1 therapy and diabetic retinopathy *(30)* and this issue remains to be resolved *(31)*.

Hypertension

About 35% of patients with acromegaly suffer from hypertension and a reduction of GH levels after successful therapy leads to a lowering of the blood pressure *(32)*. This suggests a relationship between GH and IGF-1 excess and the development of hypertension. Kajantie et al. *(33)* in a population-based study measured fasting serum IGF-1 and IGFBP-1 concentrations in 394 men and women (mean age 69 years) from a cohort of 7086 Finnish individuals whose weight and height were recorded at birth and from 7 years to 15 years of age. They found that serum IGF-1 was positively correlated with systolic and diastolic blood pressure and that IGFBP-1 was inversely correlated with blood pressure.

However, not all authors agree on these relationships. In an observational study, Colangelo et al. *(34)* analyzed data collected at the year 2, year 7, and year 10 examinations and assessed the association between IGF-1 and IGFBP-3 and cardiovascular disease risk factors in 544 black and 747 white male participants in the CARDIA Male Hormone Study who were aged 20–34 years at year 2. There was no consistent, independent association between IGF-1 or IGFBP-3 levels and blood pressure.

Further studies are needed to evaluate potential associations between the IGF system and blood pressure.

Lipids

We have demonstrated that oxidized low-density lipoprotein (LDL) markedly downregulates IGF-1 and IGF-1 receptor in rat and human aortic smooth muscle cells *(35,36)*. Furthermore, oxidized LDL is associated with apoptosis of VSMCs in atherosclerotic plaques *(37)*. Because IGF-1 can rescue VSMCs from oxidized LDL-induced cell death *(38)*, the ability of oxidized LDL to reduce IGF-1 survival effects in atherosclerotic plaques could contribute to plaque destabilization and acute coronary events. There is a paucity of clinical literature on the potential relationship between IGF-1 and lipid profiles. In an observational study, Colao et al. *(9)* investigated the relationships between the GH/IGF-1 axis and lipid profiles in 172 healthy individuals aged 18–80 years after a GH-releasing hormone and arginine test. They found an inverse relationship between IGF-1 and the total/HDL-cholesterol ratio suggesting a role of the IGF in the pathogenesis of atherosclerosis. Further studies are needed to evaluate the relationship between lipid levels and IGF-1.

CONCLUSIONS

Recent epidemiological evidence suggests that IGF-1 may have a protective effect in IHD contrary to the previous belief that IGF-1 is a mediator of vascular disease. It is also possible that IGF-1 may have a protective effect in congestive heart failure. The role of IGFBPs is less clear, although evidence, so far, suggests that increased levels of IGFBP-3 are associated with coronary disease.

The relation between IGF-1 and IGFBPs and specific cardiovascular risk factors is less obvious and requires further evaluation, as the results so far have not been consistent.

Measurement of circulating IGF-1 may add valuable information to cardiovascular risk assessment. Individuals with more risk factors but elevated IGF-1 may be relatively protected against cardiovascular disease. On the contrary, individuals with fewer risk factors but reduced IGF-1 level may be at increased risk from coronary disease and warrant more aggressive management.

Whether treatment with IGF-1 could reduce coronary artery disease risk remains to be evaluated.

REFERENCES

1. Delafontaine P, Song YH, Li Y. Expression, regulation, and function of IGF-1, IGF-1R, and IGF-1 binding proteins in blood vessels. Arterioscler Thromb Vasc Biol 2004;24(3):435–44.
2. Juul A, Main K, Blum WF, Lindholm J, Ranke MB, Skakkebaek NE. The ratio between serum levels of insulin-like growth factor (IGF)-I and the IGF binding proteins (IGFBP-1, 2 and 3) decreases with age in healthy adults and is increased in acromegalic patients. Clin Endocrinol (Oxf) 1994;41(1):85–93.
3. Colao A, di Somma C, Pivonello R, et al. The cardiovascular risk of adult GH deficiency (GHD) improved after GH replacement and worsened in untreated GHD: a 12-month prospective study. J Clin Endocrinol Metab 2002;87(3):1088–93.
4. Janssen JA, Stolk RP, Pols HA, Grobbee DE, Lamberts SW. Serum total IGF-I, free IGF-I, and IGFB-1 levels in an elderly population: relation to cardiovascular risk factors and disease. Arterioscler Thromb Vasc Biol 1998;18(2):277–82.
5. Okura Y, Brink M, Zahid AA, Anwar A, Delafontaine P. Decreased expression of insulin-like growth factor-1 and apoptosis of vascular smooth muscle cells in human atherosclerotic plaque. J Mol Cell Cardiol 2001;33(10):1777–89.
6. Patel VA, Zhang QJ, Siddle K, et al. Defect in insulin-like growth factor-1 survival mechanism in atherosclerotic plaque-derived vascular smooth muscle cells is mediated by reduced surface binding and signaling. Circ Res 2001;88(9):895–902.
7. Juul A, Scheike T, Davidsen M, Gyllenborg J, Jorgensen T. Low serum insulin-like growth factor I is associated with increased risk of ischemic heart disease: a population-based case–control study. Circulation 2002;106(8):939–44.
8. Laughlin GA, Barrett-Connor E, Criqui MH, Kritz-Silverstein D. The prospective association of serum insulin-like growth factor I (IGF-I) and IGF-binding protein-1 levels with all cause and cardiovascular disease mortality in older adults: the Rancho Bernardo Study. J Clin Endocrinol Metab 2004;89(1):114–20.
9. Colao A, Spiezia S, Di Somma C, et al. Circulating insulin-like growth factor-I levels are correlated with the atherosclerotic profile in healthy subjects independently of age. J Endocrinol Invest 2005;28(5):440–8.
10. Bayes-Genis A, Schwartz RS, Bale LK, Conover CA. Effects of insulin-like growth factor-I on cultured human coronary artery smooth muscle cells. Growth Horm IGF Res 2003;13(5):246–53.
11. Grant MB, Wargovich TJ, Ellis EA, et al. Expression of IGF-I, IGF-I receptor and IGF binding proteins-1, -2, -3, -4 and -5 in human atherectomy specimens. Regul Pept 1996;67(3):137–44.
12. Grant MB, Wargovich TJ, Bush DM, et al. Expression of IGF-1, IGF-1 receptor and TGF-beta following balloon angioplasty in atherosclerotic and normal rabbit iliac arteries: an immunocytochemical study. Regul Pept 1999;79(1):47–53.
13. Nichols TC, du Laney T, Zheng B, et al. Reduction in atherosclerotic lesion size in pigs by alphaVbeta3 inhibitors is associated with inhibition of insulin-like growth factor-I-mediated signaling. Circ Res 1999;85(11):1040–5.
14. Vasan RS, Sullivan LM, D'Agostino RB, et al. Serum insulin-like growth factor I and risk for heart failure in elderly individuals without a previous myocardial infarction: the Framingham Heart Study. Ann Intern Med 2003;139(8):642–8.
15. Bleumink GS, Rietveld I, Janssen JA, et al. Insulin-like growth factor-I gene polymorphism and risk of heart failure (the Rotterdam Study). Am J Cardiol 2004;94(3):384–6.
16. Anwar A, Gaspoz JM, Pampallona S, et al. Effect of congestive heart failure on the insulin-like growth factor-1 system. Am J Cardiol 2002;90(12):1402–5.
17. Anker SD, Chua TP, Ponikowski P, et al. Hormonal changes and catabolic/anabolic imbalance in chronic heart failure and their importance for cardiac cachexia. Circulation 1997;96(2):526–34.
18. Hambrecht R, Schulze PC, Gielen S, et al. Effects of exercise training on insulin-like growth factor-I expression in the skeletal muscle of non-cachectic patients with chronic heart failure. Eur J Cardiovasc Prev Rehabil 2005;12(4):401–6.
19. Brink M, Wellen J, Delafontaine P. Angiotensin II causes weight loss and decreases circulating insulin-like growth factor I in rats through a pressor-independent mechanism. J Clin Invest 1996;97(11):2509–16.
20. Song YH, Li Y, Du J, Mitch WE, Rosenthal N, Delafontaine P. Muscle-specific expression of IGF-1 blocks angiotensin II-induced skeletal muscle wasting. J Clin Invest 2005;115(2):451–8.
21. Ranke MB. Insulin-like growth factor-I treatment of growth disorders, diabetes mellitus and insulin resistance. Trends Endocrinol Metab 2005;16(4):190–7.
22. Alberti KG, Zimmet PZ. Definition, diagnosis and classification of diabetes mellitus and its complications. Part 1: diagnosis and classification of diabetes mellitus provisional report of a WHO consultation. Diabet Med 1998;15(7):539–53.

23. Kaushal K, Heald AH, Siddals KW, et al. The impact of abnormalities in IGF and inflammatory systems on the metabolic syndrome. Diabetes Care 2004;27(11):2682–8.

24. Shigematsu S, Yamauchi K, Nakajima K, Iijima S, Aizawa T, Hashizume K. IGF-1 regulates migration and angiogenesis of human endothelial cells. Endocr J 1999;46 Suppl:S59–S62.

25. Clemmons DR, Maile LA, Ling Y, Yarber J, Busby WH. Role of the integrin alphaVbeta3 in mediating increased smooth muscle cell responsiveness to IGF-I in response to hyperglycemic stress. Growth Horm IGF Res 2007 Aug; 17(4):265–70. Epub 2007 Apr 6.

26. Gibson JM, Westwood M, Young RJ, White A. Reduced insulin-like growth factor binding protein-1 (IGFBP-1) levels correlate with increased cardiovascular risk in non-insulin dependent diabetes mellitus (NIDDM). J Clin Endocrinol Metab 1996;81(2):860–3.

27. Clemmons DR, Moses AC, McKay MJ, Sommer A, Rosen DM, Ruckle J. The combination of insulin-like growth factor I and insulin-like growth factor-binding protein-3 reduces insulin requirements in insulin-dependent type 1 diabetes: evidence for in vivo biological activity. J Clin Endocrinol Metab 2000;85(4):1518–24.

28. Saukkonen T, Amin R, Williams RM, et al. Dose-dependent effects of recombinant human insulin-like growth factor (IGF)-I/IGF binding protein-3 complex on overnight growth hormone secretion and insulin sensitivity in type 1 diabetes. J Clin Endocrinol Metab 2004;89(9):4634–41.

29. Acerini CL, Patton CM, Savage MO, Kernell A, Westphal O, Dunger DB. Randomised placebo-controlled trial of human recombinant insulin-like growth factor I plus intensive insulin therapy in adolescents with insulin-dependent diabetes mellitus. Lancet 1997;350(9086):1199–204.

30. Genovese S, Riccardi G. The role of modulation of GH/IGF-I axis in the development of diabetic proliferative retinopathy. J Endocrinol Invest 2003;26(8 Suppl):114–6.

31. Wilkinson-Berka JL, Wraight C, Werther G. The role of growth hormone, insulin-like growth factor and somatostatin in diabetic retinopathy. Curr Med Chem 2006;13(27):3307–17.

32. Bondanelli M, Ambrosio MR, degli Uberti EC. Pathogenesis and prevalence of hypertension in acromegaly. Pituitary 2001;4(4):239–49.

33. Kajantie E, Fall CH, Seppala M, et al. Serum insulin-like growth factor (IGF)-I and IGF-binding protein-1 in elderly people: relationships with cardiovascular risk factors, body composition, size at birth, and childhood growth. J Clin Endocrinol Metab 2003;88(3):1059–65.

34. Colangelo LA, Liu K, Gapstur SM. Insulin-like growth factor-1, insulin-like growth factor binding protein-3, and cardiovascular disease risk factors in young black men and white men: the CARDIA Male Hormone Study. Am J Epidemiol 2004;160(8):750–7.

35. Higashi Y, Peng T, Du J, et al. A redox-sensitive pathway mediates oxidized LDL-induced downregulation of insulin-like growth factor-1 receptor. J Lipid Res 2005;46(6):1266–77.

36. Scheidegger KJ, James RW, Delafontaine P. Differential effects of low density lipoproteins on insulin-like growth factor-1 (IGF-1) and IGF-1 receptor expression in vascular smooth muscle cells. J Biol Chem 2000;275(35):26864–9.

37. Okura Y, Brink M, Itabe H, Scheidegger KJ, Kalangos A, Delafontaine P. Oxidized low-density lipoprotein is associated with apoptosis of vascular smooth muscle cells in human atherosclerotic plaques. Circulation 2000;102(22):2680–6.

38. Li Y, Higashi Y, Itabe H, Song YH, Du J, Delafontaine P. Insulin-like growth factor-1 receptor activation inhibits oxidized LDL-induced cytochrome C release and apoptosis via the phosphatidylinositol 3 kinase/Akt signaling pathway. Arterioscler Thromb Vasc Biol 2003;23(12):2178–84.

INDEX

Note: The letter *t* and *f* in the index refers to *tables* and *figures* respectively For example 125*t* refers to *table* in page 125 and 122*f* refers to *figure* in page 122